Identification and Characterization of Genetic Components in Autism Spectrum Disorders 2019

Identification and Characterization of Genetic Components in Autism Spectrum Disorders 2019

Editor

Merlin G. Butler

MDPI • Basel • Beijing • Wuhan • Barcelona • Belgrade • Manchester • Tokyo • Cluj • Tianjin

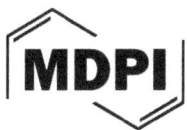

Editor
Merlin G. Butler
University of Kansas Medical
Center
USA

Editorial Office
MDPI
St. Alban-Anlage 66
4052 Basel, Switzerland

This is a reprint of articles from the Special Issue published online in the open access journal *International Journal of Molecular Sciences* (ISSN 1422-0067) (available at: https://www.mdpi.com/journal/ijms/special_issues/ASD_2019).

For citation purposes, cite each article independently as indicated on the article page online and as indicated below:

LastName, A.A.; LastName, B.B.; LastName, C.C. Article Title. *Journal Name* **Year**, *Volume Number*, Page Range.

ISBN 978-3-0365-3609-5 (Hbk)
ISBN 978-3-0365-3610-1 (PDF)

© 2022 by the authors. Articles in this book are Open Access and distributed under the Creative Commons Attribution (CC BY) license, which allows users to download, copy and build upon published articles, as long as the author and publisher are properly credited, which ensures maximum dissemination and a wider impact of our publications.

The book as a whole is distributed by MDPI under the terms and conditions of the Creative Commons license CC BY-NC-ND.

Contents

About the Editor vii

Preface to "Identification and Characterization of Genetic Components in Autism Spectrum Disorders 2019" ix

Alexander P. Gabrielli, Ann M. Manzardo and Merlin G. Butler
GeneAnalytics Pathways and Profiling of Shared Autism and Cancer Genes
Reprinted from: *Int. J. Mol. Sci.* **2019**, *20*, 1166, doi:10.3390/ijms20051166 1

Kyle W. Davis, Moises Serrano, Sara Loddo, Catherine Robinson, Viola Alesi, Bruno Dallapiccola, Antonio Novelli and Merlin G. Butler
Parent-of-Origin Effects in 15q11.2 BP1-BP2 Microdeletion (Burnside-Butler) Syndrome
Reprinted from: *Int. J. Mol. Sci.* **2019**, *20*, 1459, doi:10.3390/ijms20061459 15

Ann Katrin Sauer, Juergen Bockmann, Konrad Steinestel, Tobias M. Boeckers and Andreas M. Grabrucker
Altered Intestinal Morphology and Microbiota Composition in the Autism Spectrum Disorders Associated SHANK3 Mouse Model
Reprinted from: *Int. J. Mol. Sci.* **2019**, *20*, 2134, doi:10.3390/ijms20092134 29

Ritsuko Ohtani-Kaneko
Crmp4-KO Mice as an Animal Model for Investigating Certain Phenotypes of Autism Spectrum Disorders
Reprinted from: *Int. J. Mol. Sci.* **2019**, *20*, 2485, doi:10.3390/ijms20102485 45

Merlin G. Butler
Magnesium Supplement and the 15q11.2 BP1–BP2 Microdeletion (Burnside–Butler) Syndrome: A Potential Treatment?
Reprinted from: *Int. J. Mol. Sci.* **2019**, *20*, 2914, doi:10.3390/ijms20122914 61

Nina S. Levy, George K. E. Umanah, Eli J. Rogers, Reem Jada, Orit Lache and Andrew P. Levy
IQSEC2-Associated Intellectual Disability and Autism
Reprinted from: *Int. J. Mol. Sci.* **2019**, *20*, 3038, doi:10.3390/ijms20123038 69

Syed K. Rafi, Alberto Fernández-Jaén, Sara Álvarez, Owen W. Nadeau and Merlin G. Butler
High Functioning Autism with Missense Mutations in Synaptotagmin-Like Protein 4 (SYTL4) and Transmembrane Protein 187 (TMEM187) Genes: SYTL4- Protein Modeling, Protein-Protein Interaction, Expression Profiling and MicroRNA Studies
Reprinted from: *Int. J. Mol. Sci.* **2019**, *20*, 3358, doi:10.3390/ijms20133358 79

Noemi Di Nanni, Matteo Bersanelli, Francesca Anna Cupaioli, Luciano Milanesi, Alessandra Mezzelani and Ettore Mosca
Network-Based Integrative Analysis of Genomics, Epigenomics and Transcriptomics in Autism Spectrum Disorders
Reprinted from: *Int. J. Mol. Sci.* **2019**, *20*, 3363, doi:10.3390/ijms20133363 111

Khushmol K. Dhaliwal, Camila E. Orsso, Caroline Richard, Andrea M. Haqq and Lonnie Zwaigenbaum
Risk Factors for Unhealthy Weight Gain and Obesity among Children with Autism Spectrum Disorder
Reprinted from: *Int. J. Mol. Sci.* **2019**, *20*, 3285, doi:10.3390/ijms20133285 127

Valerie W. Hu, Christine A. Devlin and Jessica J. Debski
ASD Phenotype—Genotype Associations in Concordant and Discordant Monozygotic and Dizygotic Twins Stratified by Severity of Autistic Traits
Reprinted from: *Int. J. Mol. Sci.* **2019**, *20*, 3804, doi:10.3390/ijms20153804 157

Michael Field, Tracy Dudding-Byth, Marta Arpone, Emma K. Baker, Solange M. Aliaga, Carolyn Rogers, Chriselle Hickerton, David Francis, Dean G. Phelan, Elizabeth E. Palmer, David J. Amor, Howard Slater, Lesley Bretherton, Ling Ling and David E. Godler
Significantly Elevated *FMR1* mRNA and Mosaicism for Methylated Premutation and Full Mutation Alleles in Two Brothers with Autism Features Referred for Fragile X Testing
Reprinted from: *Int. J. Mol. Sci.* **2019**, *20*, 3907, doi:10.3390/ijms20163907 183

Harumi Jyonouchi and Lee Geng
Associations between Monocyte and T Cell Cytokine Profiles in Autism Spectrum Disorders: Effects of Dysregulated Innate Immune Responses on Adaptive Responses to Recall Antigens in a Subset of ASD Children
Reprinted from: *Int. J. Mol. Sci.* **2019**, *20*, 4731, doi:10.3390/ijms20194731 199

Liza Weinstein-Fudim, Zivanit Ergaz, Gadi Turgeman, Joseph Yanai, Moshe Szyf and Asher Ornoy
Gender Related Changes in Gene Expression Induced by Valproic Acid in A Mouse Model of Autism and the Correction by S-adenosyl Methionine. Does It Explain the Gender Differences in Autistic Like Behavior?
Reprinted from: *Int. J. Mol. Sci.* **2019**, *20*, 5278, doi:10.3390/ijms20215278 221

About the Editor

Merlin G. Butler (MD, Ph.D.) is Professor of Psychiatry & Behavioral Sciences and Pediatrics at the University of Kansas Medical Center, Kansas City, Director of the Division of Research and Genetics and Director of the University of Kansas Health System Genetics Clinic. He received his MD degree from the University of Nebraska College of Medicine in Omaha and his Ph.D. in Medical Genetics from Indiana University School of Medicine in Indianapolis where he also trained and completed post-graduate training in medical genetics accredited by the American Board of Medical Genetics (ABMG). He received ABMG board certification in both Clinical Genetics and Clinical Cytogenetics in 1984. He is also a Founding Fellow of the American College of Medical Genetics and Genomics. He previously held faculty and academic positions at Indiana University, University of Notre Dame, Vanderbilt University and University of Missouri—Kansas City prior to his arrival at the University of Kansas Medical Center in 2008.

Dr. Butler is an appointed member of local academic and state programs for genetic screening services as well as national committees engaged in the care and treatment of those with rare genetic disorders. He is also a member of federal and parent-based organizations or foundations participating in grant review study sections. He serves as a member of several editorial boards for peer-reviewed journals and Associate Editor of *Frontiers in Genetics* and *Frontiers in Pediatrics*. He is a recipient of local academic and national honors for recognition of his research and clinical service in genetic disorders. He is a member of advisory board organizations for rare disorders including Mowat-Wilson syndrome and Chairperson of the Scientific Advisory Board of the Prader-Willi Syndrome Association (USA). His research interests include the genetics of developmental disorders, congenital anomalies, connective tissue disorders, autism and mechanisms of genomic imprinting with impact on Prader-Willi, Angelman, Burnside-Butler and fragile X syndromes. He has focused his research on genotype-phenotype correlations and delineation with natural history of rare disorders as well as the use of advanced genetic technology including high-resolution microarrays, next-generation sequencing and pharmacogenetics testing in clinical practice. He has published over 500 peer-reviewed articles, over 50 book chapters and authored or edited 20 books on the principles of medical genetics and clinical description, management and care of patients with common and rare genetic disorders, specifically Prader-Willi, fragile X and Burnside-Butler syndromes, the genetics of autism and syndromic obesity, congenital anomalies, intellectual disabilities and clinical application of advanced genetic testing.

Preface to "Identification and Characterization of Genetic Components in Autism Spectrum Disorders 2019"

This textbook, *The Identification of the Genetic Components of Autism Spectrum Disorders 2019*, includes themes associated with autism spectrum disorders (ASD) and related conditions divided into three sections (clinical, genetics, other) covering the topics from 2019. These sections include information on clinical description and phenotypic subtyping, causes, diagnosis, treatment and characterization of ASD and biomarker development related to neurodevelopmental disorders; the overview of genetic, epigenetic, and environmental factors involved in ASD; characterization of findings in autism based on genomics advanced laboratory testing and genetics with bioinformatics and translational research with characterization of an emerging 15q11.2 BP1-BP2 deletion (Burnside–Butler) syndrome as a cause of autism and neurodevelopmental defects; and other factors contributing to our understanding of causation of ASD including proteomics and metabolomics with approaches towards functional insights into autism.

This textbook includes 13 chapters written by experts in the field of genetics, medical care and treatment approaches and diagnosis, autism research and discovery with characterization and analysis of genetic and environmental factors. Of these, four chapters are dedicated to clinical description and phenotype-genotype and associations with autistic traits, immune responses to antigens in children with ASD, risk factors for children with autism and of-parental-origin effects in the 15q11.2 BP1-BP2 deletion (Burnside–Butler) syndrome as a genetic cause of autism; six chapters are dedicated to basic laboratory or translational research with genetic data analysis of single genes with expression patterns, pathways, and profiling related to intellectual disabilities, fragile X syndrome and autism, as well as reviews regarding their contribution to ASD, as 90% of individuals with autism may have a genetic component contributing to their clinical findings; and 3 chapters describe altered intestinal morphology and microbiota composition in autism, animal modeling, and the possible role of magnesium in Burnside–Butler syndrome.

This textbook should be a useful resource for basic scientists and clinical researchers, medical geneticists, physicians and clinicians caring for and managing patients with the goal to translate this information directly to the clinical setting for diagnosis, care and treatment of patients with ASD. Health care providers and paraprofessionals should be interested, particularly those engaged in teaching, research, care and treatment including students at all levels of training and families regarding this important neurodevelopmental disorder which is on the rise in our society and worldwide.

Ultimately, the team of healthcare professionals required to diagnose, treat and care for the growing list of problems recognized or understudied in ASD may include psychiatrists, psychologists, clinical and laboratory geneticists, clinical geneticists and genetic counselors, neurologists, special educators and paraprofessionals, child life experts, developmental specialists and pediatricians, social workers, nurses and nurse practitioners, occupational and physical therapists, speech therapists and pathologists and public health experts with community activists should find this resource helpful in recognizing features seen in autism and understanding and identifying causes. Lastly, this book would serve as a resource for parents and other family members for better awareness about risks, features and causes of autism as well as agencies providing care, information, resource and services for those families with autism and/or related neurodevelopmental disorders.

Merlin G. Butler
Editor

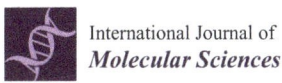

Article

GeneAnalytics Pathways and Profiling of Shared Autism and Cancer Genes

Alexander P. Gabrielli, Ann M. Manzardo and Merlin G. Butler *

Departments of Psychiatry, Behavioral Sciences & Pediatrics, University of Kansas Medical Center, Kansas City, KS 66160, USA; a228g039@kumc.edu (A.P.G.); amanzardo@kumc.edu (A.M.M.)
* Correspondence: mbutler4@kumc.edu; Tel.: +1-913-588-1800

Received: 16 January 2019; Accepted: 1 March 2019; Published: 7 March 2019

Abstract: Recent research revealed that autism spectrum disorders (ASD) and cancer may share common genetic architecture, with evidence first reported with the *PTEN* gene. There are approximately 800 autism genes and 3500 genes associated with cancer. The VarElect phenotype program was chosen to identify genes jointly associated with both conditions based on genomic information stored in GeneCards. In total, 138 overlapping genes were then profiled with GeneAnalytics, an analysis pathway enrichment tool utilizing existing gene datasets to identify shared pathways, mechanisms, and phenotypes. Profiling the shared gene data identified seven significantly associated diseases of 2310 matched disease entities with factors implicated in shared pathology of ASD and cancer. These included 371 super-pathways of 455 matched entities reflecting major cell-signaling pathways and metabolic disturbances (e.g., CREB, AKT, GPCR); 153 gene ontology (GO) biological processes of 226 matched processes; 41 GO molecular functions of 78 matched functions; and 145 phenotypes of 232 matched phenotypes. The entries were scored and ranked using a matching algorithm that takes into consideration genomic expression, sequencing, and microarray datasets with cell or tissue specificity. Shared mechanisms may lead to the identification of a common pathology and a better understanding of causation with potential treatment options to lessen the severity of ASD-related symptoms in those affected.

Keywords: autism spectrum disorders (ASD); cancer; overlapping genes and gene profiling; super-pathways; phenotypes and diseases; molecular functions and processes

---

1. Introduction

Autism spectrum disorders (ASD) include an array of conditions arising from neurodevelopmental defects during a crucial stage of brain formation characterized by deficits in communication ability, a paucity of social skills, repetitive behaviors, and narrow interests [1]. Environmental factors and perinatal care may play a role in both ASD onset and severity, but often arises from a substantial genetic burden. Colvert et al. [2] found heritability estimates of 56% to 95% among monozygotic twins, with additive genetic factors comprising a significant share of the burden.

Morphologically, the brains of individuals diagnosed with ASD contain abnormal neuronal growth patterns, including an overabundance of neurons and unusual dendritic spine profiles [3,4]. Butler and others in 2005 [5] suggested that common causal factors could contribute to both abnormal neuronal development, autism, and risk for malignancy in patients with autism, with macrocephaly and *PTEN* gene mutations seen in about one-fifth of affected individuals. *PTEN* is an important tumor-suppressor gene reported to play a role in tumor growth, hamartoma disorders (e.g., Cowden, Proteus, Bannayan–Riley–Ruvalcaba syndrome), overgrowth, and cancer [6–8]. Several of these overgrowth-related disorders are also at risk of developing malignancy, particularly colorectal cancer.

The genetic architecture of ASD was extensively surveyed through genome-wide association studies (GWAS) and candidate gene approaches [9–11]. Several pathways and mechanisms were proposed as mediating factors in the pathogenesis of disorders, although the causative agents of the vast majority of cases remain elusive. However, cross-talk between the canonical Wnt pathway, the Notch signaling cascade [12], and other disturbed genes and pathways [13,14] are believed to play a potential role and helpful in explaining an association with malignancy [15,16]. Furthermore, MAPK and calcium signaling pathways, particularly overlapping calcium-PKC–Ras–Raf–MAPK/ERK processes are strongly associated with ASD. These pathways play a central role in a large range of biological processes and, when abnormal, may compromise biological output and contribute to neuropsychiatric disorders, cell growth, and malignancy [17–20].

The *PTEN* gene product behaves as an inhibitor of the phosphoinositol 3-kinase/AKT pathway [21]. Disturbances contribute to dysregulation in the pathway leading to excessive uncontrolled cell growth and malignancy. Butler et al. [5] and Varga et al. [21] previously reported elevated frequencies of heterozygous germline *PTEN* gene mutations in the ASD population, suggesting that mutations serve as a critical component of the shared cancer and ASD etiology requiring further research. Investigation into the connection of other genetic factors contributing to ASD and cancer could be of clinical utility. Individuals diagnosed with autism should be screened more frequently for cancers for which they may have a genetic susceptibility.

In the investigation herein, we utilized GeneAnalytics, which incorporates a computer-based bioinformatics pipeline developed by GeneCards, to identify and interrogate shared genes and their architecture between cancer and ASD. We explored influential shared pathways in overlapping genes which could represent potential therapeutic targets. We reviewed reports on the overlap between approximately 800 autism and over 3500 cancer-related genes utilizing this bioinformatics/pathway analysis program. GeneCards was used as an integrated, human genomic database to leverage information from 125 scholarly databases including genetic, transcriptomic, proteomic, functional, and clinical information to interrogate genomic-related data for our study [22,23]. This novel study may supply information helpful to stimulate or address a potential medical or genetic conundrum and may provide a research-based foundation of common pathology in ASD and cancer.

2. Results

Using the VarElect program, autism and cancer genes were screened for overlapping units, according to phenotype category. VarElect identified 138 genes in common between the 792 reported known, susceptible, or clinically relevant genes for autism or ASD (17.4%), and 3.9% of approximately 3500 genes implicated in cancer. The 138 genes and their underlying biological functions were profiled by the commercially available GeneAnalytics program, previously validated in studies of random genes to test the interpretation power or relationship to the gene set under investigation [22].

The GeneAnalytics output furnished a list of diseases highly associated with the combined cancer and autism gene set. The resulting high score matches ($p < 0.05$) are presented, ranked by score, and categorized by disease type in Table 1. The number of matched genes between the indicated disease and the autism and cancer gene set is included for context. Seven diseases were found to be significantly associated with the dataset, all of which pertain to cancer (see Figure 1). Three of the cancers are reproductive in nature (breast, prostate, and endometrial), while two are gastrointestinal (colorectal and pancreatic).

Table 1. Profiling of high scores in overlapping genes for autism and cancer-associated diseases.

Score	Disease	Disease Categories	Number of Matched Genes (% of 138 Overlapping Genes)
33.84	Colorectal cancer	Gastrointestinal diseases, genetic diseases, rare diseases, cancer diseases	44 (32%)
30.70	Breast cancer	Reproductive diseases, genetic diseases, rare diseases, cancer diseases	39 (28%)
24.13	Prostate cancer	Reproductive diseases, genetic diseases, rare diseases, cancer diseases	31 (22%)
19.01	Lung cancer	Respiratory diseases, genetic diseases, cancer diseases	25 (18%)
18.43	Endometrial cancer	Reproductive diseases, genetic diseases, rare diseases, cancer diseases	19 (14%)
13.94	Leukemia, acute myeloid	Immune diseases, blood diseases, genetic diseases, rare diseases, cancer diseases	15 (11%)
13.64	Pancreatic cancer	Gastrointestinal diseases, endocrine diseases, genetic diseases, rare diseases, cancer diseases	15 (11%)

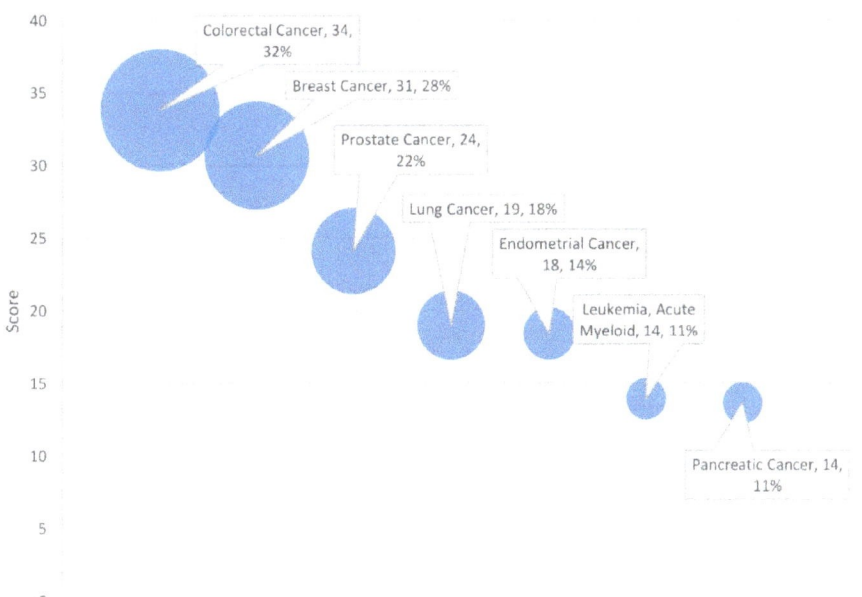

Figure 1. Diseases ranked by score and match rate (size of circle).

Super-pathways were likewise ranked and scored based on degree of association with the gene set. Top-scoring super-pathways are presented with matching rates in Table 2, restricted to the top 30 of 371 significant entries ($p < 0.05$). These included ubiquitous signaling super-pathways such as GPCR (score = 166, 54% match with gene set) and ERK (score = 146, 38% match). Numerous additional signaling super-pathways were found to be significantly associated with the combined gene set, including AKT, HGF development, CREB, cAMP-dependent PKA, fMLP, P70S6K, RET, TGF-β, PEDF induced, MTOR, and PI3K/AKT. Cancer-specific super-pathways, including "glioma" and "pathways in cancer", were also implicated at a statistically significant level ($p < 0.05$) (see Figure 2).

Table 2. Profiling of high scores in overlapping genes for autism and cancer-associated super-pathways.

Score	Super-Pathways	Number of Total Genes	Number of Super-Pathway Matched Genes	% of 138 Overlapping Genes
166.10	Elk-related tyrosine kinase (ERK) signaling	1177	74	54%
145.73	glioma	313	44	32%
131.74	G-protein coupled receptor (GPCR) pathway	708	53	38%
122.48	Pathways in cancer	395	42	30%
116.32	Signaling by GPCR	2601	80	58%
113.29	Phospholipase-C pathway	498	43	31%
98.91	Human immune-deficiency virus (HIV) life cycle	865	48	35%
97.32	NANOG in mammalian embryonic stem cell pluripotency	533	40	29%
95.18	Apoptotic pathways in synovial fibroblasts	725	44	32%
95.13	AKT murine thymoma viral oncogene homolog (AKT) signaling	681	43	31%
94.06	Development HGF signaling	234	30	22%
90.05	CAMP response element-binding protein (CREB) pathway	528	38	28%
81.54	Integrated breast cancer pathway	154	24	17%
81.30	Proteoglycans in cancer	203	26	19%
80.40	Nuclear factor of activated (NFAT) T cells and cardiac hypertrophy	326	30	22%
78.97	Integrin pathway	568	36	26%
78.26	Development of vascular endothelial growth factor (VEGF) signaling via VEGFR2, generic cascades	147	23	17%
77.70	Activation of cyclic adenosine monophosphate (CAMP)-dependent protein kinase A (PKA)	628	37	27%
77.43	Formyl peptide receptor (FMLP) pathway	317	29	21%
77.00	P70S6K signaling	390	31	22%
74.95	Rearranged during transfection (RET) signaling	974	43	31%
72.42	Transforming growth factor (TGF)-beta pathway	652	36	26%
72.03	Glioblastoma multiforme	111	20	14%
71.00	Pigment epithelium-deprived factor (PEDF) induced signaling	721	37	27%
70.30	P21-activated kinase (PAK) pathway	682	36	26%
69.39	Endometrial cancer	122	20	14%
67.08	Mechanistic target of rapamycin (MTOR) signaling pathway (KEGG)	209	23	17%
66.63	PI3K/AKT signaling pathway	342	27	20%
66.33	Developmental biology	1079	42	30%
65.44	Focal adhesion	283	25	18%

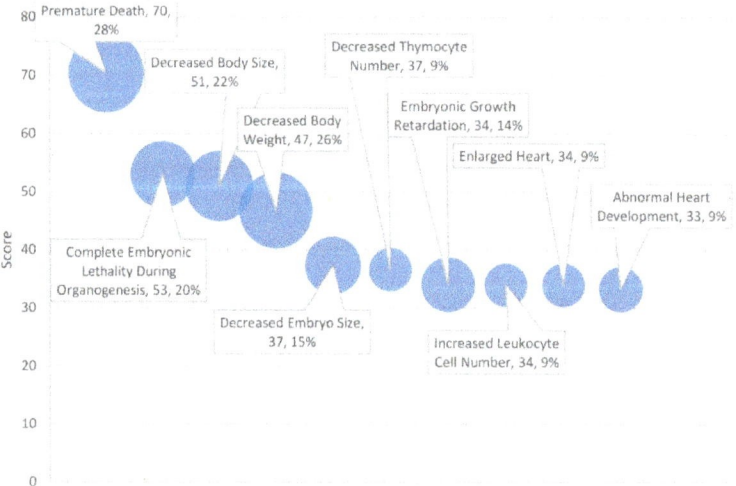

Figure 2. Phenotypes ranked by score and match rate (size of circle) for top ten phenotypes.

Statistically significant Gene Ontology (GO) biological processes are presented in Table 3, which are limited to the top 30 of 153 total high-scoring matches. The top three entries directly relate to the regulation of gene expression. These include "positive regulation of transcription, DNA-templated", "positive regulation of transcription from RNA polymerase II promoter", and "positive regulation of gene expression", which exhibited matching rates of 21%, 25%, and 15%, respectively, with the combined 138 overlapping gene set (see Figure 3).

Table 3. Profiling of high scores in overlapping genes for autism and cancer-associated Gene Ontology (GO) biological processes.

Score	GO Biological Processes	Number of Total Genes	Number of Matched Genes	% of 138 Overlapping Genes
53.00	Positive regulation of transcription, DNA-templated	596	29	21%
46.66	Positive regulation of transcription from RNA polymerase II promoter	1016	34	25%
44.49	Positive regulation of gene expression	346	21	15%
44.10	Heart development	232	18	13%
42.44	Negative regulation of cell proliferation	419	22	16%
41.44	Nervous system development	535	24	17%
39.38	Intracellular signal transduction	467	22	16%
39.37	Protein phosphorylation	629	25	18%
39.02	Positive regulation of apoptotic process	330	19	14%
37.45	Positive regulation of protein phosphorylation	155	14	10%
36.52	Apoptotic process	690	25	18%
36.16	Positive regulation of sequence-specific DNA-binding transcription factor activity	105	12	9%
34.58	Positive regulation of cell proliferation	500	21	15%
34.22	Negative regulation of apoptotic process	507	21	15%
33.45	Phosphorylation	700	24	17%
31.65	Canonical Wnt signaling pathway	80	10	7%
31.62	Cell adhesion	620	22	16%
31.02	Phosphatidylinositol-mediated signaling	112	11	8%
30.96	Signal transduction	2032	40	29%
29.94	Response to drug	323	16	12%
29.83	Thymus development	44	8	6%
29.33	Visual learning	46	8	6%
28.92	Extracellular matrix organization	203	13	9%
28.09	Protein autophosphorylation	173	12	9%
27.55	Negative regulation of transcription from RNA polymerase II promoter	724	22	16%
27.40	Cell-cycle arrest	143	11	8%
27.05	Regulation of phosphatidylinositol 3-kinase signaling	82	9	7%
26.20	Substrate adhesion-dependent cell spreading	39	7	5%
25.00	Negative regulation of cysteine-type endopeptidase activity involved in apoptotic process	68	8	6%
24.79	Peptidyl-tyrosine phosphorylation	171	11	8%

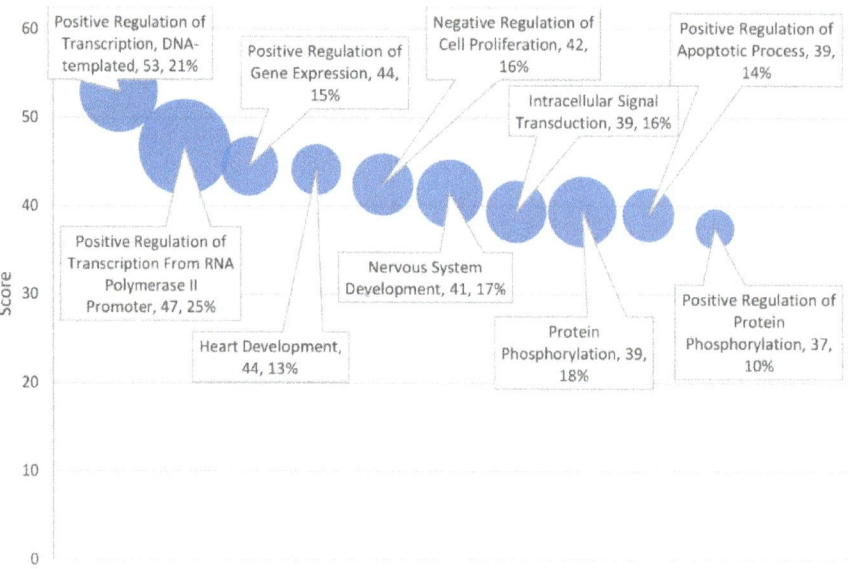

Figure 3. Gene Ontology (GO) biological processes ranked by score and match rate (size of circle) for top ten processes.

The top 30 significant GO molecular functions, of 41 total significant entries, are delineated in Table 4. Prominent entries include protein (score = 67, 83% match rate), enzyme (score = 43, 15% match rate), and β-catenin binding (score = 36, 8% match rate). Kinases and phosphatases were well represented in the analysis as well, with several obtaining high scores, including "protein kinase activity", "kinase activity", "TRK activity", "protein kinase binding", "protein tyrosine kinase activity", and "protein phosphatase binding" (see Figure 4).

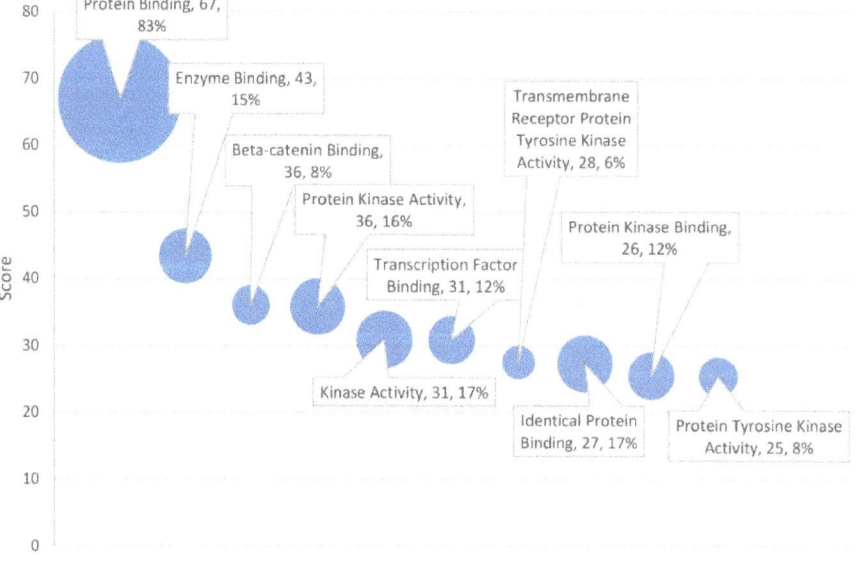

Figure 4. GO molecular function ranked by score and match rate (size of circle) for top ten functions.

Table 4. Profiling of high scores in overlapping genes for autism and cancer-associated GO molecular functions.

Score	GO Molecular Functions	Number of Total Genes	Number of Matched Genes	% of 138 Overlapping Genes
66.97	Protein binding	9013	115	83%
43.40	Enzyme binding	360	21	15%
36.09	β-Catenin binding	80	11	8%
35.87	Protein kinase activity	530	22	16%
30.98	Kinase activity	698	23	17%
30.91	Transcription factor binding	308	16	12%
27.55	Transmembrane receptor protein tyrosine kinase activity	54	8	6%
27.38	Identical protein binding	797	23	17%
25.54	Protein kinase binding	402	16	12%
25.40	Protein tyrosine kinase activity	164	11	8%
23.70	Transcription regulatory region DNA binding	229	12	9%
21.10	Phosphatidylinositol-4,5-bisphosphate 3-kinase activity	66	7	5%
20.68	Protein phosphatase binding	69	7	5%
20.58	RNA polymerase II Core promoter proximal region sequence-specific DNA binding	336	13	9%
20.43	Protein C-terminus binding	185	10	7%
19.66	Ubiquitin protein ligase binding	299	12	9%
18.88	Transcriptional activator activity, RNA polymerase II core promoter proximal region sequence-specific binding	260	11	8%
17.81	Repressing transcription factor binding	34	5	4%
17.69	Protein homodimerization activity	758	18	13%
17.69	Chromatin binding	404	13	9%
17.45	Cell adhesion molecule binding	63	6	4%
17.27	C–X3–C chemokine binding	5	3	2%
16.82	Protein heterodimerization activity	495	14	10%
16.48	Nitric-oxide synthase regulator activity	6	3	2%
16.19	Androgen receptor binding	43	5	4%
15.95	Protein domain specific binding	264	10	7%
15.57	Transferase activity	1759	28	20%
15.54	Receptor binding	398	12	9%
15.50	Nuclear hormone receptor binding	23	4	3%
15.28	Transcription factor activity, sequence-specific DNA binding	1029	20	14%

The 30 top scoring phenotypes, of 145 significant matches, are outlined in Table 5. Phenotypes reflect the importance of ASD and cancer-associated genes in growth and development-related processes (see Figure 5). The top phenotypes include "premature death" (score = 70, 28% match rate), "complete embryonic lethality during organogenesis" (score = 53, 20% match rate), and "decreased body size" (score = 51, 22% match rate).

Table 5. Profiling of high scores in overlapping genes for autism and cancer-associated phenotypes.

Score	Phenotypes	Number of Total Genes	Number of Matched Genes	% of 138 Overlapping Genes
70.49	Premature death	832	39	28%
53.00	Complete embryonic lethality during organogenesis	540	28	20%
51.00	Decreased body size	742	31	22%
46.85	Decreased body weight	1144	36	26%
37.37	Decreased embryo size	450	21	15%
36.64	Decreased thymocyte number	102	12	9%
34.08	Embryonic growth retardation	404	19	14%
33.98	Increased leukocyte cell number	120	12	9%
33.98	Enlarged heart	120	12	9%
33.25	Abnormal heart development	158	13	9%
33.05	Decreased B-cell number	196	14	10%
29.78	Partial embryonic lethality during organogenesis	234	14	10%
29.60	Partial postnatal lethality	546	20	14%
29.50	Increased tumor incidence	124	11	8%
28.15	Enlarged spleen	256	14	10%
27.97	Abnormal sensory neuron innervation pattern	52	8	6%
27.76	Abnormal rostral–caudal axis patterning	53	8	6%
27.60	Complete prenatal lethality	264	14	10%
27.18	Partial perinatal lethality	225	13	9%
27.13	Hyperactivity	271	14	10%
27.09	Abnormal blood vessel morphology	146	11	8%
27.04	Increased mammary adenocarcinoma incidence	20	6	4%
26.94	Complete lethality throughout fetal growth and development	186	12	9%
26.90	Abnormal response/metabolism to endogenous compounds	83	9	7%
26.76	Complete postnatal lethality	378	16	12%
25.78	Abnormal B-cell differentiation	91	9	7%
25.38	Abnormal definitive hematopoiesis	94	9	7%
24.21	Abnormal heart morphology	178	11	8%
24.05	Decreased sensory neuron number	14	5	4%
23.89	Partial prenatal lethality	274	13	9%

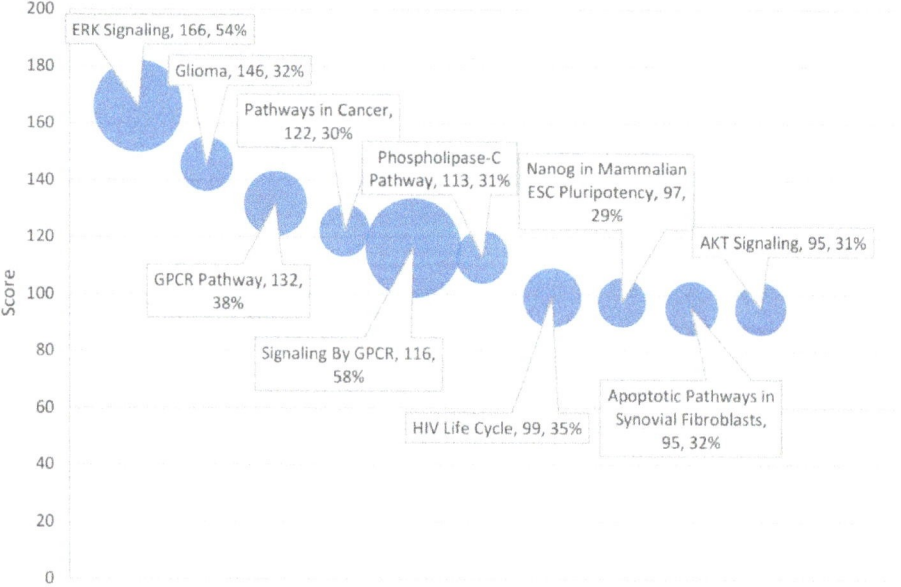

Figure 5. Pathways ranked by score and match rate (size of circle) for top ten pathways.

3. Discussion

As anticipated in our examination of gene data and profiling, the diseases found most in common with the combined autism and malignancy gene set did pertain to cancer. Moreover, colorectal cancer accounted for 32% of overlapping genes, followed by breast and prostate cancer (see Table 1). Two notable exceptions of our own cut-off criteria that may deserve further inspection include Alzheimer disease and amyotrophic lateral sclerosis (ALS), both of which approached but did not attain significance in their association with the gene set, achieving medium scores. Alzheimer disease and ALS are progressive neurodegenerative diseases [23–25]. Alzheimer disease and ALS exhibited 11% and 8% overlap with the ASD and cancer gene set, which is a small, though not trivial connection. Enrichment of genes associated with neurodegenerative illnesses among the autism and cancer gene set may be indicative of shared disturbances in neurological growth and development which could contribute to the divergent morphology of autism, cancer, Alzheimer disease, and ALS.

Regarding diseases cited in Table 1, one unusual observation was the lack of representation of brain and neurological diseases. Of the seven high-score matches and six selected borderline (medium-score) matches, only medulloblastoma qualified as a cancer of the brain and nervous system. Reproductive cancers (breast, prostate, and endometrial) and gastrointestinal cancers (colorectal, pancreatic, and hepatocellular carcinoma) were more prevalent. Notably, most of the cancers listed in Table 1 tend to be acquired diseases with a genetic diathesis (e.g., breast and prostate), as opposed to congenital diseases that arise early in development (medulloblastoma). It should also be noted that tumors of the ectoderm and endoderm were disproportionately represented relative to the mesoderm. This may reflect the tissue-specific nature of neural development in the onset of autism. Of note, ASD did not achieve statistical significance with the shared dataset, despite being a requisite for selection and receiving a relatively high-scoring entry. This may be a testament to the complexity of autism spectrum disorder. Even though the gene set was filtered by ASD connection, collectively, the combined genes were more diagnostic of cancer than ASD.

Overall, the highest-scoring super-pathways correlated more strongly with the autism and cancer combined gene set (as evidenced by the higher scores), compared to GO biological processes and GO molecular functions, which were not as strongly correlated, as reflected by their lower scores. The majority of super-pathways (see Table 2) in the top 30 reported entries in the high-scoring category achieved a match rate of at least 20% with the gene set, indicating the relative importance of these super-pathways in the autism and cancer connection. The GeneAnalytics output of the highest scores strongly implicated the ERK signaling pathway in shared pathogenesis based on super-pathway analysis, with a score of 166 and a match rate of 54%, followed by the GPCR pathway at 38%. The MAPK/ERK signaling pathway occupies a key role in mitogen signaling and cell growth with survival [26]. Disturbances in the ERK pathway can disrupt the cell cycle, leading to anomalous cell proliferation and malignant growth. Gene mutations or aberrant functioning in the pathway during early development could contribute to abnormal neuronal growth in ASD. Alterations in GPCR signaling could further contribute to the onset of ASD through aberrant cell signaling and neurotransmitter dysregulation, both of which might lead to changes in cognitive functioning characteristic of ASD.

For GO biological processes, the three highest-scoring entries pertain to the regulation of gene expression. The outcome of the analysis suggests that an important mechanism in the mutual pathology of autism and cancer may be attributed to variation in transcription factors and nongenic sequences and, hence, differences in the regulation and rate of gene expression. Processes involved in the growth, development, and death of cells were found to be highly associated with the gene set. Indeed, "positive regulation of apoptotic process", "apoptotic process", and "negative regulation of apoptotic process" were each flagged as biological processes significantly associated with the combined gene set, with scores of 39 (matching rate of 14%), 37 (18%), and 34 (15%), respectively. Additional growth and death biological processes were also found to be enriched in the gene set, including "heart development", "negative regulation of cell proliferation", "nervous system development", "positive regulation of cell proliferation", and the "canonical Wnt signaling pathway".

In terms of the GO molecular functions underlying cancer and autism pathology, the results strongly implicate "protein binding", which exhibited a score of 67, over 20 points larger than the second, less inclusive entry, "enzyme binding". Furthermore, 83% of the autism and cancer gene set with 115 out of 138 matched genes was associated with protein binding, suggesting that dysfunction in protein binding may play a significant role in the shared autism and cancer diathesis. In many respects, this paradigm is reflective of the pivotal role of protein binding in the diverse metabolic processes underlying growth and survival. There was a substantial disparity between the high matching rate of protein binding (83%) and that of enzyme binding specifically (15%). The remaining 68% of protein binding that is not explained by enzyme binding and activation by kinase pathways may be attributed to structural protein and signal–receptor binding. This may suggest that structural and signaling mechanisms are disproportionately involved in the shared pathology of cancer and autism as noted previously. MAPK and calcium signaling pathways in genes associated with autism are found in other disorders including cancer [19]. Enzymes may play more of a peripheral role. Enzyme binding overlaps with kinase pathways, many of which are involved in enzyme activation. Kinase and phosphatase activities were also prevalent among the high-scoring entries. Ten of the 30 highest-scoring molecular functions pertain to kinase or phosphatase activity. Both protein binding and kinase activities align with "protein kinase binding".

The report also implicated β-catenin binding (score of 36; 8% matching rate); β-catenin functions as both a moderator of gene transcription and as an agent of intercellular adhesion [27]. Overexpression of β-catenin, which is encoded by the *CTNNB1* gene, is well characterized as a candidate in the pathogenesis of numerous cancers, as well as heart disease (this may serve as a potential link to the high-scoring GO biological process of "heart development") (score = 44; match rate = 13%) [28]. The relationship between β-catenin signaling and autism was reported, as β-catenin is dependent on the absence of Wnt [29,30]. Its role in mediating cell adhesion and cellular development suggests it may be a candidate in the pathogenesis of both autism and cancer.

The two highest-scoring phenotypes, "premature death" and "complete embryonic lethality during organogenesis", reflect the delicacy of neurogenesis and embryonic development. It is likely that only certain combinations of mutations inherited from the autism and cancer gene set can be tolerated and that, at a certain genetic burden, dysfunction in pathways associated with these genes results in irretrievable failure to develop. Designated decreased body size and body weight may also reflect the vital importance of these genes in mediating development, early cell division and number, and the potential consequences of dysfunction.

Three functional pathways are potentially involved, which include genes and pathways for chromatin remodeling, (e.g., *CHD7*, *MECP2*, *DNMT3A*, and *PHF2*), Wnt (e.g., *CHD8*, *PAX5*, and *ATRX*), and other signaling super-pathways (e.g., GPCR, ERK, RET, and AKT) and mitochondrial dysfunction in ASD (e.g., Reference [30]). Theoretically, drugs could be targeted to treat ASD. By developing a rank-ordered list of functional categories significantly associated with autism and cancer using GeneAnalytics pathways and profiling of shared autism and cancer genes, we identified potentially high-impact pathways and common mechanisms which may serve as therapeutic targets in future studies.

The interconnected relationship between autism and cancer invites further investigation in the pathogenesis of the two seemingly unrelated disorders, and it warrants a pharmacological basis of treatment. *PTEN* is an example of a shared gene for autism and cancer and the direct and indirect subject of several formally approved cancer therapeutics including cisplatin, erlotinib, everolimus, cetuximab, and estradiol. For example, cisplatin circumscribes DNA synthesis, activates caspase-3, and facilitates apoptosis, thus rescuing the function of mutant *PTEN* [31]. Considering the role of cisplatin in complementing *PTEN* function, strategic application of the drug could potentially address the autism-associated symptoms arising from *PTEN* dysfunction. Another drug example is everolimus, which behaves as an inhibitor of the mammalian target of rapamycin, and it could impact cancer predisposition and possibly autism development in a manner similar to cisplatin [32].

Although invasive drugs and treatments exist for many types of cancer, a drug is yet to be successfully developed to prevent the onset or progression of ASD symptomology. The unexpected shared etiology with overlapping genes between cancer and autism, particularly those involved in cell-signaling pathways such as MAPK and calcium signaling [19], encourages cautious speculation that, as our knowledge of the staging and mechanisms of ASD improves and applied to animal model testing, the leverage of anti-cancer drugs at minimal dosages could be postulated. For example, the 16p11.2 chromosome deletion is one of the most common copy number variants linked to autism in humans and reportedly involves the *ERK1* gene and other related genes converging in the ERK/MAP kinase pathway. This pathway was the most recognized super-pathway found in our profiling analysis of autism and cancer genes (see Table 2). Perturbations of this pathway can contribute to neuropsychiatric disorders, cell growth, and malignancy; therefore, treatment could lessen these manifestations. To investigate whether pharmacological approaches could be helpful, researchers used a 16p11.2 equivalent deletion mouse model with the *ERK1* gene deleted, and they found that pharmacological inhibitions of ERK signaling (i.e., RB1 and RB3 peptides) rescued cortical cytoarchitecture abnormalities and the abnormal behavioral phenotype associated with this deletion, providing evidence for a potential targeted therapeutic intervention for autism [33]. Hypothetically, treatment could lessen the effects of autism when recognized early and during brain plasticity.

Furthermore, genetic analysis linked autism with mutations in tumor suppression genes and other cancer-associated genes and pathways reflected in our gene profiling analysis. Important candidate genes (e.g., *PTEN*, *NF1*, and *BRCA2*) are found meeting criteria clearly associated with predisposition to cancer such as colorectal, other gastrointestinal tumors, and breast reported in the top seven autism and cancer-associated diseases (see Table 1). For example, mutations in the *PTEN* gene are linked to colorectal, thyroid, head, neck, prostate, skin, breast, and lung cancer and about 10% of children with autism have *PTEN* gene mutations, making this an important gene to target regarding therapeutic intervention for autism with predisposition to cancer. ASDs and cancer overlap extensively in signal transduction pathways as illustrated by our study, involving metabolic processes; these areas should be targeted by treatment strategies. Such insights may enable more accurate gene-informed cancer risk assessment for targeted therapeutic and medical management.

To date, there were a few preclinical models tested with anticancer medication on ASD symptoms. For example, Kilincaslan et al. [34] reported the beneficial effects of everolimus on autism and attention-deficit hyperactivity disorder (ADHD) symptoms in a group of patients with tuberous sclerosis complex (TSC). This drug inhibits mTOR, one of the top 30 super-pathways identified with high scores when comparing shared autism and cancer genes. It is a treatment for TSC in which autism is a finding, along with renal angiomyolipomas and astrocytomas. The drug reduced tumor growth, decreased seizures, and improved autistic, ADHD, and depression symptoms. However, there is a paucity of studies on the effects of this drug on neuro-psychiatric symptoms, which merit further consideration. Treatment would be a new avenue to pursue and further explore, particularly in those with ASD, the involvement of shared autism and cancer-related genes.

4. Materials and Methods

Shared genetic architecture between cancer and ASD was examined firstly using VarElect, a sequence phenotyper affiliated with GeneAnalytics (Alameda, CA, USA) [35,36]. A reported list of 792 clinically relevant, susceptible, or known genes for ASD, summarized previously by Butler et al. [37], and over 3500 recognized cancer genes found in the GeneAnalytics databases were entered into the VarElect phenotyper program to identify overlapping genes.

The ASD genes were filtered by their association with the query "cancer" and limited to those with established pathways. Based on the above parameters, VarElect produced 138 genes with known connections to both cancer and ASD. The refined list of 138 genes was then entered into GeneAnalytics, a gene set analytical tool which uses GeneCards, an integrated genomic database, to parse genes and their relationships, as previously reported [22,38–40].

The GeneAnalytics program produces a report containing seven categories: diseases, pathways, tissues and cells, phenotypes, Gene Ontology (GO) molecular functions, GO biological processes, and compounds related to the query of interest (i.e., cancer and ASD gene). Each entry in these functional categories was sorted with the GeneAnalytics proprietary matching and scoring algorithm following protocols published previously in the study of psychiatric, behavior, and obesity-related genes by our research group [22,39,40]. Only those genes with the highest calculated scores were further analyzed for each of the seven GeneAnalytics categories. In addition to scoring fields based on their relevance to the gene set, fields were subdivided into three categories, "high-score matches", "medium-score matches", and "low-score matches". High-score matches exhibited a corrected p-value of less than 0.05, while medium-score matches exhibited a corrected p-value between 0.05 and 0.1. For the purposes of this investigation, medium- and low-score matches were excluded from the results. The reporting of high-score matches was restricted to the top 30 entries, in instances where more than 30 were found to be significant ($p < 0.05$). Corrections were made based on multiple testing (Bonferroni correction).

Author Contributions: M.G.B. and A.M.M. conceived and designed the study; A.P.G., A.M.M., and M.G.B. analyzed the data; A.P.G., A.M.M., and M.G.B. wrote the manuscript.

Funding: The authors acknowledge support from the National Institute of Child Health and Human Development (NICHD) and grant number HD02528.

Acknowledgments: We thank Charlotte Weber for help with manuscript preparation and Humaira Masoud for assistance in data collection.

Conflicts of Interest: The authors declare no conflicts of interest.

Abbreviations

ASD	Autism spectrum disorders
GWAS	Genome-wide association studies
RNA	Ribonucleic acid
DNA	Deoxyribonucleic acid
GO	Gene ontology
KEGG	Kyoto Encyclopedia of Genes and Genomes
NICHD	National Institute of Child Health and Human Development

References

1. American Psychiatric Association. *Diagnostic and Statistical Manual of Mental Disorders*, 4th ed.; American Psychiatric Association Press: Washington, DC, USA, 2013.
2. Colvert, E.; Tick, B.; McEwen, F.; Stewart, C.; Curran, S.R.; Woodhouse, E.; Gillan, N.; Hallett, V.; Lietz, S.; Garnett, T.; et al. Heritability of autism spectrum disorder in a UK population-based twin sample. *JAMA Psychiatry* **2015**, *72*, 415–423. [CrossRef] [PubMed]
3. Hua, X.; Thompson, P.M.; Leow, A.D.; Madsen, S.K.; Caplan, R.; Alger, J.R.; O'Neill, J.; Joshi, K.; Smalley, S.L.; Toga, A.W.; et al. Brain growth rate abnormalities visualized in adolescents with autism. *Hum. Brain Mapp.* **2013**, *34*, 425–436. [CrossRef] [PubMed]
4. Phillips, M.; Pozzo-Miller, L. Dendritic spine dysgenesis in autism related disorders. *Neurosci. Lett.* **2015**, *601*, 30–40. [CrossRef] [PubMed]
5. Butler, M.G.; Dasouki, M.J.; Zhou, X.; Talebizadeh, Z.; Brown, M.; Takahashi, T.N.; Miles, J.H.; Wang, C.H.; Stratton, R.; Pilarski, R.; et al. Subset of individuals with autism spectrum disorders and extreme macrocephaly associated with germline PTEN tumour suppressor gene mutations. *J. Med. Genet.* **2005**, *42*, 318–321. [CrossRef] [PubMed]

6. Marsh, D.J.; Kum, J.B.; Lunetta, K.L.; Bennett, M.J.; Gorlin, R.J.; Ahmed, S.F.; Bodurtha, J.; Crowe, C.; Curtis, M.A.; Dasouki, M.; et al. PTEN mutation spectrum and genotype-phenotype correlations in Bannayan-Riley-Ruvalcaba syndrome suggest a single entity with Cowden syndrome. *Hum. Mol. Genet.* **1999**, *8*, 1461–1472. [CrossRef] [PubMed]
7. Cristofano, A.D.; Pandolfi, P.P. The multiple roles of PTEN in tumor suppression. *Cell* **2000**, *100*, 387–390. [CrossRef]
8. Goffin, A.; Hoefsloot, L.H.; Bosgoed, E.; Swillen, A.; Fryns, J.P. PTEN mutation in a family with Cowden syndrome and autism. *Am. J. Med. Genet.* **2001**, *105*, 521–524. [CrossRef] [PubMed]
9. Yonan, A.L.; Alarcon, M.; Cheng, R.; Magnusson, P.K.; Spence, S.J.; Palmer, A.A.; Grunn, A.; Juo, S.H.; Terwilliger, J.D.; Liu, J.; et al. A genomewide screen of 345 families for autism-susceptibility loci. *Am. J. Hum. Genet.* **2003**, *73*, 886–897. [CrossRef] [PubMed]
10. Yu, T.W.; Chahrour, M.H.; Coulter, M.E.; Jiralerspong, S.; Okamura-Ikeda, K.; Ataman, B.; Schmitz-Abe, K.; Harmin, D.A.; Adli, M.; Malik, A.N.; et al. Using whole exome sequencing to identify inherited causes of autism. *Neuron* **2013**, *77*, 259–273. [CrossRef] [PubMed]
11. Butler, M.G.; Rafi, S.K.; Hossain, W.; Stephan, D.A.; Manzardo, A.M. Whole exome sequencing in females with autism implicates novel and candidate genes. *Int. J. Mol. Sci.* **2015**, *15*, 1312–1335. [CrossRef] [PubMed]
12. Zhang, Y.; Yuan, X.; Wang, Z.; Li, R. The canonical Wnt signaling pathway in autism. *CNS Neurol. Disord. Drug Targets* **2014**, *13*, 765–770. [CrossRef] [PubMed]
13. Crawley, J.N.; Heyer, W.D.; LaSalle, J.M. Autism and cancer share risk genes, pathways, and drug targets. *Trends Genet.* **2016**, *32*, 139–146. [CrossRef] [PubMed]
14. Darbro, B.W.; Singh, R.; Zimmerman, M.B.; Mahajan, V.B.; Bassuk, A.G. Autism linked to increased oncogene mutations but decreased cancer rate. *PLoS ONE* **2016**, *11*, e0149041. [CrossRef] [PubMed]
15. Blatt, J.; Deal, A.M.; Mesibov, G. Autism in children and adolescents with cancer. *Pediatr. Blood Cancer* **2010**, *54*, 144–147. [CrossRef] [PubMed]
16. Crespi, B. Autism and cancer risk. *Autism. Res.* **2011**, *4*, 302–310. [CrossRef] [PubMed]
17. Dhillon, A.S.; Hagan, S.; Rath, O.; Kolch, W. MAP kinase signalling pathways in cancer. *Oncogene* **2007**, *26*, 3279–3290. [CrossRef] [PubMed]
18. Pópulo, H.; Lopes, J.M.; Soares, P. The mTOR signalling pathway in human cancer. *Int. J. Mol. Sci.* **2012**, *13*, 1886–1918. [CrossRef] [PubMed]
19. Wen, Y.; Alshikho, M.J.; Herbert, M.R. Pathway network analyses for autism reveal multisystem involvement, major overlaps with other diseases and convergence upon MAPK and calcium signaling. *PLoS ONE* **2016**, *11*, e0153329. [CrossRef] [PubMed]
20. Wen, Y.; Herbert, M.R. Connecting the dots: Overlaps between autism and cancer suggest possible common mechanisms regarding signaling pathways related to metabolic alterations. *Med. Hypotheses* **2017**, *103*, 118–123. [CrossRef] [PubMed]
21. Varga, E.A.; Pastore, M.; Prior, T.; Herman, G.E.; Mcbride, K.L. The prevalence of PTEN mutations in a clinical pediatric cohort with autism spectrum disorders, developmental delay, and macrocephaly. *Genet. Med.* **2009**, *11*, 111–117. [CrossRef] [PubMed]
22. Sundararajan, T.; Manzardo, A.M.; Butler, M.G. Functional analysis of schizophrenia genes using GeneAnalytics program and integrated databases. *Gene* **2018**, *641*, 25–34. [CrossRef] [PubMed]
23. Wenk, G.L. Neuropathologic changes in Alzheimer's disease. *J. Clin. Psychiatry* **2003**, *64*, 7–10. [PubMed]
24. Tiraboschi, P.; Hansen, L.A.; Thal, L.J.; Corey-Bloom, J. The importance of neuritic plaques and tangles to the development and evolution of AD. *Neurology* **2004**, *62*, 1984–1989. [CrossRef] [PubMed]
25. Zarei, S.; Carr, K.; Reiley, L.; Diaz, K.; Guerra, O.; Altamirano, P.F.; Pagani, W.; Lodin, D.; Orozco, G.; Chinea, A. A comprehensive review of amyotrophic lateral sclerosis. *Surg. Neurol. Int.* **2015**, *6*, 171. [CrossRef] [PubMed]
26. Meloche, S.; Pouysségur, J. The ERK1/2 mitogen-activated protein kinase pathway as a master regulator of the G1- to S-phase transition. *Oncogene* **2007**, *26*, 3227–3239. [CrossRef] [PubMed]
27. MacDonald, B.T.; Tamai, K.; He, X. Wnt/beta-catenin signaling: Components, mechanisms, and diseases. *Dev. Cell* **2009**, *17*, 9–26. [CrossRef] [PubMed]
28. Morin, P.J. Beta-catenin signaling and cancer. *BioEssays* **1999**, *21*, 1021–1030. [CrossRef]

29. Yi, J.J.; Paranjape, S.R.; Walker, M.P.; Choudhury, R.; Wolter, J.M.; Fragola, G.; Emanuele, M.J.; Major, M.B.; Zylka, M.J. The autism-linked UBE3A T485A mutant E3 ubiquitin ligase activates the Wnt/?-catenin pathway by inhibiting the proteasome. *J. Biol. Chem.* **2017**, *292*, 12503–12515. [CrossRef] [PubMed]
30. Bae, S.M.; Hong, J.Y. The Wnt signaling pathway and related therapeutic drugs in autism spectrum disorder. *Clin. Psychopharmacol. Neurosci.* **2018**, *16*, 129–135. [CrossRef] [PubMed]
31. Dasari, S.; Tchounwou, P.B. Cisplatin in cancer therapy: Molecular mechanisms of action. *Eur. J. Pharmacol.* **2014**, *740*, 364–378. [CrossRef] [PubMed]
32. Hasskarl, J. Everolimus. Recent results. *Cancer Res.* **2014**, *201*, 373–392.
33. Pucilowska, J.; Vithayathil, J.; Pagani, M.; Kelly, C.; Karlo, J.C.; Robol, C.; Morella, I.; Gozzi, A.; Brambilla, R.; Landreth, G.E. Pharmacological inhibition of ERK signaling rescues pathophysiology and behavioral phenotype associated with 16p11.2 chromosomal deletion in mice. *J. Neurosci.* **2018**, *38*, 6640–6652. [CrossRef] [PubMed]
34. Kilincaslan, A.; Kok, B.E.; Tekturk, P.; Yalcinkaya, C.; Ozkara, C.; Yapici, Z. Beneficial effects of everolimus on autism and attention-deficit/hyperactivity disorder symptoms in a group of patients with tuberous sclerosis complex. *J. Child Adolesc. Psychopharmacol.* **2017**, *27*, 383–388. [CrossRef] [PubMed]
35. Stelzer, G.; Plaschkes, I.; Oz Levi, D.; Alkelai, A.; Olender, T.; Zimmerman, S.; Twik, M.; Belinky, F.; Fishilevich, S.; Nudel, R.; et al. VarElect: The phenotype—Based variation prioritizer of the GeneCards suite. *BMC Genom.* **2016**, *17*, 444. [CrossRef] [PubMed]
36. Stelzer, G.; Rosen, R.; Plaschkes, I.; Zimmerman, S.; Twik, M.; Fishilevich, S.; Stein, T.; Nudel, R.; Lieder, I.; Mazor, Y.; et al. The GeneCards suite: From gene data mining to disease genome sequence analysis. *Curr. Protoc. Bioinform.* **2016**, *54*, 1–30.
37. Butler, M.G.; Rafi, S.K.; Manzardo, A.M. High-resolution chromosome ideogram representation of currently recognized genes for autism spectrum disorders. *Int. J. Mol. Sci.* **2015**, *16*, 6464–6495. [CrossRef] [PubMed]
38. Ben-Ari Fuchs, S.; Lieder, I.; Stelzer, G.; Mazor, Y.; Buzhor, E.; Kaplan, S.; Bogoch, Y.; Plaschkes, I.; Shitrit, A.; Rappaport, N.; et al. GeneAnalytics: An integrative gene set analysis tool for Next generation sequencing, RNAseq and microarray data. *OMICS* **2016**, *20*, 139–151. [CrossRef] [PubMed]
39. Gabrielli, A.P.; Manzardo, A.M.; Butler, M.G. Exploring genetic susceptibility to obesity through genome functional pathway analysis. *Obesity* **2017**, *25*, 1136–1143. [CrossRef] [PubMed]
40. Khanzada, N.S.; Butler, M.G.; Manzardo, A.M. GeneAnalytics pathway analysis and genetic overlap among autism spectrum disorder, bipolar disorder and schizophrenia. *Int. J. Mol. Sci.* **2017**, *18*, 527. [CrossRef] [PubMed]

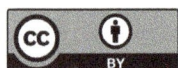

© 2019 by the authors. Licensee MDPI, Basel, Switzerland. This article is an open access article distributed under the terms and conditions of the Creative Commons Attribution (CC BY) license (http://creativecommons.org/licenses/by/4.0/).

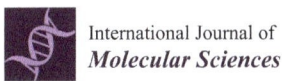

Article

Parent-of-Origin Effects in 15q11.2 BP1-BP2 Microdeletion (Burnside-Butler) Syndrome

Kyle W. Davis [1,*], Moises Serrano [1], Sara Loddo [2], Catherine Robinson [1], Viola Alesi [2], Bruno Dallapiccola [2], Antonio Novelli [2] and Merlin G. Butler [3]

1. Lineagen, Inc., Salt Lake City, UT 84109, USA; mserrano@lineagen.com (M.S.); k.mullin.robinson@gmail.com (C.R.)
2. Laboratory of Medical Genetics, Bambino Gesù Children's Hospital, IRCCS, Rome 00165, Italy; sara.loddo@opbg.net (S.L.); viola.alesi@opbg.net (V.A.); bruno.dallapiccola@opbg.net (B.D.); antonio.novelli@opbg.net (A.N.)
3. Departments of Psychiatry & Behavioral Sciences and Pediatrics, University of Kansas Medical Center, Kansas City, KS 66160, USA; mbutler4@kumc.edu
* Correspondence: kyle.walter.davis@gmail.com; Tel.: 1+801-931-6189

Received: 15 February 2019; Accepted: 21 March 2019; Published: 22 March 2019

Abstract: To identify whether parent-of-origin effects (POE) of the 15q11.2 BP1-BP2 microdeletion are associated with differences in clinical features in individuals inheriting the deletion, we collected 71 individuals reported with phenotypic data and known inheritance from a clinical cohort, a research cohort, the DECIPHER database, and the primary literature. Chi-squared and Mann-Whitney U tests were used to test for differences in specific and grouped clinical symptoms based on parental inheritance and proband gender. Analyses controlled for sibling sets and individuals with additional variants of uncertain significance (VOUS). Among all probands, maternal deletions were associated with macrocephaly ($p = 0.016$) and autism spectrum disorder (ASD; $p = 0.02$), while paternal deletions were associated with congenital heart disease (CHD; $p = 0.004$). Excluding sibling sets, maternal deletions were associated with epilepsy as well as macrocephaly ($p < 0.05$), while paternal deletions were associated with CHD and abnormal muscular phenotypes ($p < 0.05$). Excluding sibling sets and probands with an additional VOUS, maternal deletions were associated with epilepsy ($p = 0.019$) and paternal deletions associated with muscular phenotypes ($p = 0.008$). Significant gender-based differences were also observed. Our results supported POEs of this deletion and included macrocephaly, epilepsy and ASD in maternal deletions with CHD and abnormal muscular phenotypes seen in paternal deletions.

Keywords: 15q11.2 BP1-BP2 microdeletion (Burnside-Butler) syndrome; imprinting; parent-of-origin effects; phenotype-genotype correlation; autism; developmental delays; motor delays

1. Introduction

The 15q11.2 BP1-BP2 microdeletion syndrome (or Burnside-Butler syndrome; OMIM # 615656) is a neurodevelopmental disorder with clinical findings reported in hundreds of individuals [1,2]. This condition includes the deletion of four genes thought to be nonimprinted (*TUBGCP5, CYFIP1, NIPA1, NIPA2*), located between two distinct proximal 15q11.2 breakpoints (BP1 and BP2) and separated by about 500 kilobases (kb). Summarized findings from a large cohort of patients presenting for genetic services found that 0.41% of patients (69 of ~17,000) had a deletion of the proximal 15q11.2 BP1-BP2 region [3]. In a review of over 10,000 clinically affected individuals tested with ultra-high-resolution chromosome microarrays, the 15q11.2 BP1-BP2 microdeletion was the leading cytogenetic finding of those presenting with autism spectrum disorder (ASD) alone or ASD and other clinical features [4].

This condition can present with a wide range of clinical findings including cognitive deficits, language and/or motor delays, ASD, behavioral disturbances, poor coordination, ataxia, attention disorders, seizures, and dysmorphic or congenital anomalies [2]. Psychiatric findings can include schizophrenia, obsessive compulsive disorder, and oppositional defiant disorder. Dyscalculia, dyslexia and structural brain changes in both grey and white matter have been reported commonly in individuals with this deletion syndrome [5].

About 80% of children identified with the 15q11.2 BP1-BP2 microdeletion inherit it from a parent, who may or may not be clinically affected. Therefore, this susceptibility locus shows incomplete penetrance with variable expressivity. Approximately 30% of the parents ascertained through genetic testing with a clinically affected child due to the 15q11.2 BP1-BP2 microdeletion will have clinical findings or involvement [2].

Deletions can range from approximately 320 kb to 500 kb, though all four genes within this 320-kb region are highly conserved and, when disturbed, are associated with or cause neurological, motor, intellectual, and behavioral problems. For example, specific missense variants of the *NIPA1* (non-imprinted in PWS/AS 1; OMIM # 608145) gene are known to cause autosomal dominant hereditary spastic paraplegia and postural disturbance; repeat expansions have recently been associated with amyotrophic lateral sclerosis [6,7]. The NIPA1 protein is known to mediate magnesium transport and is highly expressed in the brain [8,9]. The *NIPA2* (non-imprinted in PWS/AS 2; OMIM # 608146) gene is also involved in magnesium transport and childhood absence epilepsy reported in a Han Chinese cohort [10]. However, this association has not been replicated in other cohorts and pathogenicity is unclear [11]. The third gene in the 15q11.2 BP1-BP2 region is *TUBGCP5* (tubulin gamma complex associated protein 5; OMIM # 608147) and is associated with attention-deficit hyperactivity disorder (ADHD) and obsessive-compulsive behavior. A recent publication associated biallelic loss of this gene with primary microcephaly [12]. Lastly, the *CYFIP1* (cytoplasmic fragile X mental retardation 1 *FMR1* interacting protein 1; OMIM # 606322) gene encodes a protein that interacts with FMRP, the protein produced by the *FMR1* (Fragile X Mental Retardation 1; OMIM # 309550) gene and in which triplet-repeat expansion causes fragile X syndrome, the most common cause of inherited cognitive disabilities in families [13]. The *CYFIP1* gene also interacts with the protein from the *RAC1* (RAS-related c3 botulinum toxin substrate 1; OMIM # 602048) gene, disruption of which causes an autosomal dominant form of intellectual disability [14]. Recent research has also shown that reduced *CYFIP1* expression leads to dysregulation of schizophrenia- and epilepsy-associated gene networks [15]. Mouse models have found that *CYFIP1* regulates development, function, and plasticity of presynaptic neurons [16].

Although these genes have previously been reported as non-imprinted, recent research found a methylated site within this chromosome 15 region in human DNA samples [17] and unequal gene expression in mice [18]. Using blood samples from individuals with maternal or paternal disomy 15, a maternally methylated CpG island near the promoter of the *TUBGCP5* gene was identified [17]. Additionally, mouse models heterozygous for maternal *or* paternal loss of the *CYFIP1* gene found unequal parental expression in the cortex, with different behavioral outcomes depending on parental inheritance patterns [18].

Several possible explanations may exist for the incomplete penetrance and variable expressivity observed in this condition. First, clinically affected individuals may have two hits, such as the cytogenetic microdeletion and a pathogenic variant of one or more of the genes in the 15q11.2 BP1-BP2 region or other developmentally important genes, while the clinically unaffected parent may have only the microdeletion. Second, a parent or their child may be mildly affected and not seek medical attention (i.e. ascertainment bias). A third possibility is that unequal parental expression of one or more genes causes specific phenotypes.

Given new data about *CYFIP1* gene expression and the maternally methylated region found near the *TUBGCP5* gene promoter, supported by previous expression studies showing parental bias in this region from lymphoblasts [19], deletions of these genes may show a parent-of-origin effect (POE).

For further investigation, we sought to determine if such an effect could be observed by analyzing reported clinical features in probands and the specific parental inheritance patterns of the deletion.

2. Results

2.1. Cohort Characteristics

Our cohort included 71 individuals, mostly male probands ($N = 42$, 1.4 male-to-female ratio), had an average age of testing at 6.9 years for males and 9.4 years for females (7.9 years among all individuals), and most were unrelated (i.e., not siblings; $N = 55$, 77%). This age distribution and male-to-female ratio is similar to a previous study of 52 individuals with a 15q11.2 BP1-BP2 microdeletion [20], which found a 1.7 male-to-female ratio and average age of testing at 8.6 years. Statistically significant differences were noted between male and female carriers of the 15q11.2 BP1-BP2 microdeletion using two-tailed t-tests, as males had significantly more clinical features as well as non-physical features (Table 1).

Table 1. Descriptive statistics of clinical features by gender in those with the 15q11.2 BP1-BP2 microdeletion.

Variable	Female Probands ($N = 29$)				Male Probands ($N = 42$)				
	Avg	SD	Med	Range	Avg	SD	Med	Range	p
Age (Years)	9.4	8.2	7.0	0.08–27	6.9	5.2	6.0	0.25–24	0.130
Total Symptoms	3.4	2.4	2.0	1–10	4.9	2.2	4.5	1–10	0.020
Physical Features	0.9	1.0	1.0	0–3	1.0	0.9	1.0	0–3	0.610
Non-physical Features	2.5	2.4	2.0	0–9	3.95	2.1	4.0	0–8	0.009

Avg: average; Med: median; t-test; p-values (significance $p < 0.05$); compares differences in average age or symptoms in male and female probands with the 15q11.2 BP1-BP2 microdeletion.

However, within paternally- and maternally-inherited deletions, the male-to-female ratio differed from that of the full group. For paternally-inherited deletions, we observed a 1.1 male-to-female ratio (19 males vs. 18 females), whereas in maternally-inherited deletions we observed a 2.1 male-to-female ratio (23 males vs. 1 females). Using these ratios in chi-squared testing, we found that there is a statistically significant difference in the male-to-female ratio between paternally- and maternally-inherited deletions ($p = 0.03$).

Using chi-squared testing with the 1.7 male-to-female ratio reported by Vanlerberghe et al. [20] to derive an "expected" ratio of males-to-females within each parental deletion group, we found that neither male-to-female distribution was significantly different from 1.7. For paternal deletions, we used our observed ratio of 1.1 (19 males and 18 females) versus an expected ratio of 1.64 (23 males and 14 females, $p = 0.48$). For maternal deletions, we again used our observed ratio of 2.1 (23 males vs. 11 females) versus and expected ratio of 1.62 (21 males vs. 13 females, $p = 0.8$).

Loss of the 15q11.2 BP1-BP2 region was slightly more often paternally than maternally inherited ($N = 37$ and 34, respectively). No differences were observed regarding the parental origin of the deletion in relation to the proband's average age at genetic testing, the total number of clinical features, total physical symptoms, or total non-physical symptoms (Table 2). When analyzing our cohort by specific clinical features, the most common findings were speech and motor delays ($N = 35$, 49% for both) followed by facial dysmorphisms ($N = 30$, 42%). See Table 3 for the frequency of individual clinical features found in this set of probands.

Table 2. Descriptive statistics of parental inheritance of individuals with the 15q11.2 BP1-BP2 microdeletion.

Variable	Maternal (N = 34)				Paternal (N = 37)				
	Avg	SD	Med	Range	Avg	SD	Med	Range	P
Age (Years)	8.7	7.1	6.5	1.5–27	7.1	6.2	5.3	0.08–24	0.33
Total Symptoms	4.7	2.2	5.0	1–9	3.9	2.8	3.0	1–10	0.18
Physical Features	0.8	0.9	1.0	0–3	1.0	0.9	1.0	0–3	0.35
Non-physical Features	3.9	2.1	4.0	0–8	2.9	2.5	2.0	0–9	0.07

Avg: average; Med: median; *t*-test; *p*-values (significance $p < 0.05$); compares differences in average age or symptoms based on parental inheritance of the 15q11.2 BP1-BP2 microdeletion.

Table 3. Frequency of clinical features in the 71 probands with the 15q11.2 BP1-BP2 microdeletion.

Clinical Feature	Percentage	Total Individuals
Speech Delay	49	35
Motor Delay	49	35
Facial Dysmorphisms	42	30
Developmental Delay	37	26
Behavioral Differences	37	26
Intellectual Disability	35	25
Muscular Problems	31	22
Learning Difficulties	30	21
Psychiatric Diagnosis	30	21
Epilepsy	24	17
Microcephaly	20	14
ASD	18	13
Short Stature	14	10
Congenital Heart Condition	11	8
Macrocephaly	7	5

Arranged in descending order of frequency.

2.2. Differences in Clinical Features by Parent-of-Origin of the 15q11.2 BP1-BP2 Microdeletion

When analyzing for differences using the entire cohort (N = 71), we found statistically significant differences in several clinical features based on the parental inheritance of the 15q11.2 BP1-BP2 microdeletion (Table 4). Using chi-squared analyses, we found paternal but not maternal deletions to be significantly associated with congenital heart disease (CHD; 22% vs. 0%, $p = 0.004$). However, maternally inherited deletions were significantly associated with macrocephaly (15% vs. 0%, $p = 0.016$) and ASD (29% vs. 8%, $p = 0.02$).

Several clinical features remained significantly associated with specific parental inheritance when controlling for sibling sets and other genetic variants (a VOUS). In the cohort without sibling sets (N = 55), CHD was still significantly more likely in individuals with paternal deletions compared with maternal deletions (19% vs. 0%, $p = 0.013$); muscle-related clinical findings (e.g., hypotonia) were also associated with paternal deletions (50% vs. 24%, $p = 0.047$). Maternal deletions were significantly associated with macrocephaly (17% vs. 0%, $p = 0.026$) and associated with epilepsy (34% vs. 12%, $p = 0.046$). In the cohort without sibling sets and/or individuals with an additional VOUS (N = 44), the association between CHD and paternal deletions became non-significant (10% vs. 0%, $p = 0.113$), while muscle-related clinical features in paternal deletions strengthened (55% vs. 17%, $p = 0.008$); epilepsy remained significantly associated with maternal deletions (42% vs. 10%, $p = 0.019$).

Mann-Whitney U-test revealed marginally statistically significant differences among the entire cohort between maternally and paternally inherited deletions in the non-physical features group variable. Maternally inherited deletions had a higher median number of clinical features than paternally inherited alleles ($p = 0.04$). However, this difference was not observed when removing sibling sets or probands with an additional VOUS.

Table 4. Differences in clinical features in the proband by parental origin and gender of the 15q11.2 BP1-BP2 microdeletion.

	Clinical Feature	Parent-of-Origin Differences						Gender Differences					
		Full Cohort (N = 71)		No Siblings (N = 55)		No Siblings and/or VOUS (N = 44)		Full Cohort (N = 71)		No Siblings (N = 55)		No Siblings and/or VOUS (N = 44)	
		% Mat	% Pat	% Mat	% Pat	% Mat	% Pat	% F	% M	% F	% M	% F	% M
Grouped Clinical Features	Any Behavior	62	41	59	42	50	45	31	64 **	36	61	32	60
	Any Delays	65	68	62	77	54	75	48	79 **	55	79	47	76 *
	Any Non-physical	97	92	97	92	96	95	90	98	91	97	89	100
	Any Physical	56	65	59	73	54	65	55	64	59	70	53	64
Specific Clinical Features	ASD	29	8 *	24	8	21	5	17	19	18	15	11	16
	CHD	0	22 ***	0	19 **	0	10	17	7	14	6	11	0
	DD	41	32	41	38	38	40	24	45	32	45	26	48
	Difficult Behaviors	47	27	45	27	38	25	24	45	27	42	21	40
	Epilepsy	29	19	34	12 *	42	10 **	38	14 *	32	18	32	24
	Facial Dysmorphisms	47	38	48	46	42	45	38	45	45	48	42	44
	ID	44	27	45	31	46	35	28	40	32	42	32	48
	LD	38	22	38	19	38	20	17	38	23	33	16	40
	Macrocephaly	15	0 *	17	0 *	13	0	7	7	9	9	5	8
	Microcephaly	15	24	10	27	13	25	17	21	18	18	16	20
	Motor Delay	53	46	48	54	50	55	28	64 ***	32	64 *	32	68 *
	Muscular Diagnosis	24	38	24	50 *	17	55 **	28	33	36	36	32	36
	Psychiatric Diagnosis	32	27	31	23	29	30	17	38	23	30	26	32
	Short Stature	9	19	10	19	13	20	10	17	14	15	16	16
	Speech Delay	56	43	52	54	46	50	38	57	41	61	32	60

Mat: maternal; Pat: paternal; F: female; M: male; Any Behavior: Any behavioral symptoms; Any Delays: speech, motor, or general developmental delays; Any Non-physical: Any non-physical feature noted; Any Physical: Any physical feature noted; ASD: autism spectrum disorder; CHD: congenital heart disease; DD: Developmental delays; ID: Intellectual disability; LD: Learning disorder/difficulties; Muscular Diagnosis: muscle-related phenotypes; Psychiatric Diagnosis: Psychiatric condition diagnosis. VOUS: variant of unknown significance by genetic testing (e.g., microarray analysis). chi-squared test; p-values (significance $p < 0.05$); * $p \leq 0.05$, ** $p \leq 0.01$, *** $p \leq 0.005$.

2.3. Differences in Clinical Features between Proband Gender

Given our unique and granular dataset, we also did exploratory analyses to determine if there were differences in clinical features based on an individual's gender, as a previous report found substantial differences in neurodevelopmental features between males and females with various genetic conditions [21]. Using chi-squared analyses, several statistically significant differences emerged in clinical features when analyzing the entire cohort between males and females with 15q11.2 BP1-BP2 microdeletions (Table 4).

When using the entire cohort ($N = 71$), we found males were significantly more likely than females to have motor delays (64% vs. 28%, $p = 0.002$), a behavioral phenotype (64% vs. 31%, $p = 0.006$), and any type of developmental delay (79% vs. 48%, $p = 0.008$). Additionally, learning difficulties and psychiatric diagnoses were marginally associated with males (both clinical features: 35% vs. 17%, $p = 0.058$). Only epilepsy was significantly associated with females (38% vs. 14%, $p = 0.022$).

In the cohort without sibling sets ($N = 55$), males were still significantly more likely than females to have motor delays (64% vs. 32%, $p = 0.021$), while males were marginally more likely to have any type of developmental delay (79% vs. 55%, $p = 0.057$) and receive genetic testing at a younger age (5.4 vs. 9.9 years of age, $p = 0.018$). In the cohort without sibling sets and/or individuals with an additional VOUS ($N = 44$), males were still significantly more likely than females to have motor delays (68% vs. 32%, $p = 0.017$), any type of developmental delay (76% vs. 47%, $p = 0.05$) and receive testing at a younger age (3.5 vs. 4.9 years of age, $p = 0.05$).

3. Discussion

Our study identified differences in specific clinical features depending on the parental inheritance of a 15q11.2 BP1-BP2 microdeletion. Several differences remained significant when removing sibling sets and other genetic variants from the analyses and provide evidence that POE exists in this deletion syndrome. Additionally, we observed an unequal male-to-female ratio between maternal verse paternal deletions. Neither paternal nor maternal deletions appeared to cause a more "severe phenotype" (i.e., more clinical features); however, unequal distribution of clinical features were found providing evidence for POE.

The basis for POE in this condition is buttressed by several pieces of data. First, a recent publication analyzing potential methylated regions in individuals with various regions of uniparental disomy found a maternally methylated region near the promoter of the *TUBGCP5* gene [17]. This methylated segment may act on the *TUBGCP5* gene, other genes in this cytogenetic region, or may act in a tissue-specific manner. However, previous studies of expression using blood samples have not found altered expression for genes within this deletion [22–24]. But, a second line of evidence supportive POE uses mouse models heterozygous for loss of the *CYFIP1* gene for either the maternal or paternal allele, which showed unequal and significant differences in expression in the brain cortex, which was correlated with differences in observed behaviors [18]. Another intriguing line of evidence is the differences in male-to-female ratios in maternal versus paternal deletions (2.1 vs. 1.1). Lastly, several genes in this broader region of chromosome 15 are methylated and known to cause genetic conditions with POEs, including Schaff-Yang syndrome (OMIM # 615547) with paternal loss of the imprinted *MAGEL2* gene; Angelman syndrome (OMIM # 105830) with maternal loss of the imprinted *UBE3A* gene; Prader-Willi syndrome (OMIM # 176270) due to paternal loss of imprinted genes and transcripts in the 15q11-q13 region such as *SNRPN*; and central precocious puberty 2 (OMIM # 615346) with paternal loss of the imprinted *MKRN3* gene. Given previous data, analysis of the literature and our findings, POE seems likely to exist for the 15q11.2 BP1-BP2 microdeletion with involvement of one or more genes within this region as described below.

Which gene or genes within the 15q11.2 BP1-BP2 region are undergoing POE is unknown at this time, as all four genes within this ~500 kb region are highly conserved, apparently biallelically expressed (at least in blood) and not thought to be imprinted [24,25]. However, Bittel and colleagues [19] reported unequal parental expression bias compared with controls for the SHGC-32610 transcript located proximal to the D15S1035, a standard marker in the 15q11.2 BP1-BP2 region at that time and significantly increased in expression in lymphoblastoid cell lines established from individuals with Prader-Willi syndrome having either maternal disomy 15 or the paternal 15q11-q13 deletion. Loss of the 15q11.2 BP1-BP2 region causes more severe behavioral symptoms and learning difficulties in individuals with Prader-willi syndrome or Angelman syndrome [1,24,26].

Of the genes in this region, certain pathogenic variants in the *NIPA1* gene causes an autosomal dominant form of spastic paraplegia and triplet repeat expansion within this gene is associated with a higher risk for amyotrophic lateral sclerosis [6,7]. Haploinsufficiency of this gene has not been reported to cause these conditions. Variants in the *NIPA2* gene are reported to cause childhood absence epilepsy [10,27]. Both the *NIPA1* and *NIPA2* genes regulate magnesium transport in neurons [9,27]. The *TUBGCP5* gene is expressed highly in the subthalamic nuclei of the brain and plays a role in formation and function of the centrosome [12,28]. A recent study proposed that biallelic loss of this gene may cause a form of microcephaly, as a rare missense variant in *TUBGCP5* was identified in *trans* with a microdeletion of 15q11.2 BP1-BP2 [12]. Variants in this gene have also been associated with ADHD and obsessive-compulsive disorder [29]. Lastly, the *CYFIP1* gene encodes a protein with multiple actions in the cell, including participating in maturation and stabilization of dendritic spines and organization of the actin cytoskeleton [30]. The CYFIP1 protein interacts with the FMR1 protein (and other proteins) to control neuronal mRNA transcription and translation [15]. Reduced expression of *FMR1* causes fragile X syndrome, the most common cause of familial intellectual disability [13]. Haploinsufficiency of *CYFIP1* can cause similar symptoms to fragile X syndrome in mice [25,31]. Additionally, the CYFIP1 protein is also a member of the WAVE regulatory complex, which plays a role in actin polymerization [32]. Reduced expression of the *CYFIP1* gene in model organisms and human blood samples correlates with reduced mRNA for WAVE regulatory complex members. Additionally, the *CYFIP1* gene has been found to be differentially expressed in the brain depending on the stage of embryonic development in mice, with the highest expression in the cortex and cerebellum [30].

Current and emerging evidence points to altered expression of the *CYFIP1* gene as the leading candidate for neuronal phenotypes and thus becomes a candidate for a potential POE. In the previous mouse model study of *CYFIP1* gene haploinsufficiency, maternal loss of *CYFIP1* (leading to only paternal allele expression) showed significantly higher expression in the mouse cerebral cortex than paternal loss of *CYFIP1*. Maternal loss and paternal expression of *CYFIP1* was 55%-57% relative to wild type, while paternal loss and maternal expression was 48%–52% ($p = 0.03$) [18]. No other differences were found in expression for other brain tissues studied, including the hippocampus, amygdala, and cerebellum. More recently, *CYFIP1* gene expression in murine brain tissue and expression patterns are dependent on the POE of the deletion. For example, paternal loss of the *CYFIP1* gene was associated with lower protein expression in the hypothalamus, while maternal loss was associated with lower expression in the nucleus accumbens [33]. In this study, the effect of certain *CYFIP2* variants was tested and the expression patterns were dependent on the gender of the mice. Given these studies, there is evidence that mild preferential expression for the paternal *CYFIP1* allele exists (at least in certain tissues), which would be expected if a maternally methylated region were acting in *cis* on the *CYFIP1* gene.

Previous work using human neural progenitor cells has found that reduced *CYFIP1* expression caused dysregulation in schizophrenia- and epilepsy-associated gene networks [15]. However, neither expression patterns nor a POE were studied. The *CYFIP1* gene is known to interact with the WAVE regulatory complex and proteins from two genes: *RAC1*, disruption of which causes an autosomal dominant form of intellectual disability, and *FMR1*, the causative gene for fragile X syndrome [14,16,31,34]. The CYFIP1-FMRP protein complex has been found to control both transcription and translation of mRNAs in neuronal cells [15]. Additionally, previous studies have noted that *CYFIP1* haploinsufficiency can generate features of the fragile X syndrome phenotype in mice [25,31], while a subgroup of individuals with fragile X syndrome have a Prader-Willi-like phenotype, but no specific cause for these phenotypes is known [35].

In terms of specific clinical features showing a potential POE, we found that CHD, macrocephaly, ASD, epilepsy and muscle-related phenotypes were statistically associated with a deletion from a specific parent. Although selection bias is a significant concern, and this region is known as a susceptibility region, previous work suggested that a POE does exist in CHD involving the 15q11.2 BP1-BP2 microdeletion as well as in well-characterized imprinting disorders such as Prader-Willi syndrome resulting from a paternal 15q11-q13 deletion or maternal uniparental disomy 15 [36]. Kuroda and colleagues [36] found seven individuals with CHD had paternal inheritance of the 15q11.2 BP1-BP2 microdeletion while only one individual with CDH was found when the deletion was from the mother. (Our dataset included two of these seven individuals with paternal deletions.) Our data further buttress this finding, as CHD was reported exclusively in individuals with paternally inherited deletions (8 vs. 0 including siblings, 5 vs. 0 omitting siblings). Although our sample size was too small to detect a statistical difference when omitting sibling sets and individuals with a VOUS, there were two individuals with CHD and paternal deletions and zero with maternal deletions.

Interestingly, the *CYFIP1* gene has the highest expression of the four genes in this chromosomal region in both heart muscle and vasculature [37]. For example, expression in four types of cardiac tissue from the Gene-Tissue Expression Project (GTEx) showed that, relative to other genes in this deletion, *CYFIP1* was expressed 2.9-8.8x higher in the aorta, 2.2-8.2x higher in the coronary artery, 1.1-5.0x higher in the left ventricle, and 1.2-4.2x higher in the atrial appendage. A previous study found that CHD was highly enriched in those individuals with the 15q11.2 BP1-BP2 microdeletion but the phenotype was not consistent involving both heart muscle and vasculature [38]. This lack of a phenotypic pattern appears consistent with the *CYFIP1* expression data, such that dysregulated expression could result in multiple different types of CHD.

A similar pattern for *CYFIP1* gene expression in heart muscle was also observed in the GTEx data for skeletal muscle, where *CYFIP1* has the second highest expression, at 1.8x higher than *TUBGCP5* and 6.2x higher than *NIPA1*, while being slightly lower than *NIPA2* expression. CHD and muscular phenotypes were both associated with paternally inherited 15q11.2 BP1-BP2 microdeletions, while mouse models showed a preference for paternal *CYFIP1* expression in various parts of the brain. Possibly, the paternal *CYFIP1* allele is preferentially expressed in other tissues as well, such as the heart or skeletal muscle and vasculature.

Our association for maternal deletions with ASD, macrocephaly, and epilepsy are intriguing. Only epilepsy remained significantly associated with maternal deletions when omitting siblings and probands with a VOUS finding. However, it should be noted that we lost statistical power from our small sample size to determine if a difference was present in these features when omitting these probands. Although our results were not statistically significant, ASD and macrocephaly were enriched in individuals with a maternal deletion (21% vs. 5% and 13% vs. 0%, respectively). This association may hold when omitting siblings and probands with a VOUS, but a larger sample size is needed.

Interestingly, clinical features of fragile X syndrome in humans can include the three features associated with maternal 15q11.2 BP1-BP2 microdeletions (ASD, seizures, and macrocephaly) [39]. *RAC1*-related intellectual disability also includes macrocephaly and one individual was reported to have ASD. One possibility for the associated phenotypes with a maternal POE is the maternal *CYFIP1* gene allele is preferentially expressed in different brain tissue(s) and a loss of the maternal allele is more detrimental than loss of the paternal allele in these tissues, which may somehow disrupt *FMR1* and/or *RAC1* activities or the WAVE regulatory complex. In one study using a mouse model, there was evidence for maternal expression of *CYFIP1* in the nucleus accumbens [33]. Further, Abekhoukh and colleagues [32] noted that previous studies found inconsistent neural spine phenotypes when observing *CYFIP1*-deficient mice. A POE was not assessed in either of these studies and could potentially explain these differences. Lastly, we cannot rule out that this association between maternal deletions and ASD, epilepsy, and macrocephaly could be spurious, influenced by ascertainment bias, or both.

Differences in clinical features between males and females has been noted in other neurodevelopmental conditions [21]. Our analyses between males and females are notable because we applied statistical testing to the distribution of clinical features based on gender, which has not been done in a previous, large case series [20]. Our findings indicate that females were more likely to have epilepsy, while males were more likely to have either motor or developmental delays. These differences may be due to distinct biological differences; however, it is also possible that these represent ascertainment bias and females received a medical examination and genetic testing when a more "severe" symptom was present, such as epilepsy, while milder clinical features may have been ignored or thought less important to investigate. Similarly, males with a developmental delay may have been more likely to receive an examination.

Several other points have been discussed in the literature regarding 15q11.2 BP1-BP2 microdeletions. First, one study suggested that this condition may show a "two-hit" model, such that individuals with additional genomic variants that impact neurodevelopment, as well as a 15q11.2 BP1-BP2 microdeletion, may be more likely to have clinical features or perhaps have more clinical features than individuals with only a 15q11.2 BP1-BP2 microdeletion [40]. Although we had a large sample size, the number of individuals with additional genomic alterations ($N = 12$) was too limited to determine if phenotypic differences existed between individuals with another genomic alteration; also, no individuals were reported to have a second alteration within one of the four genes in the 15q11.2 BP1-BP2 region. However, sequence variants were not routinely assessed in our cohort. Second, a recent paper identified a statistically significantly enrichment of the 15q11.2 BP1-BP2 microdeletion in three individuals with gender dysphoria (3 of 69 birth-assigned females; 4.3%) [41], suggesting that this deletion may influence gender identity. Of the 71 probands in our study, none were specifically noted to have gender dysphoria or other disorders of gender development. While we cannot rule out this deletion is associated with gender dysphoria, our data do not support the possibility that this is an additional clinical feature.

Lastly, we can assess the rate at which parents were identified with clinical features of 15q11.2 BP1-BP2 microdeletion syndrome. Previous studies have estimated that approximately 30% of parents are affected [2]. We found that when phenotype information was available, and in unrelated individuals to avoid double-counting parents with multiple children in our cohort, approximately 38% of parents (19 of 50) were found to have one or more clinical feature. Because some studies did not report on parental clinical features and other papers may not have assessed parental clinical or developmental history, we restricted our analysis to the two cohorts of individuals that represent a "high-confidence" group for detailed phenotyping. These cohorts included probands and their parents assessed by two different geneticists from the ongoing study of chromosomal 15 abnormalities and the group identified during routine clinical work-up ($N = 22$ when omitting sibling sets). In these groups, 50% of parents (11 of 22) were affected with one or more clinical feature. In contrast, the frequency reported in individuals from the primary literature was approximately 26% (7 of 27). Although our 50% rate may represent ascertainment bias of the parent's child, it is likely that more parents are more often affected (albeit mildly) and previous studies were not sensitive to this possibility or to the full phenotypic spectrum.

Our study had several strengths, including the large sample size, use of statistical analyses, granular analyses of clinical features, investigation of gender-based differences and parental penetrance, and our ability to control for other potentially confounding variables in clinical variability, such as siblings and additional genomic alterations. The authors encourage additional studies, both clinically and by genomic characterization to delineate this emerging microdeletion syndrome to gain a better understanding of the collection of clinical findings and their causation, specifically in view of our evidence presented on parent-of-origin effects.

Limitations in this study include likely ascertainment bias, variable quality in phenotypic information from disparate sources, that uncharacterized genes within larger BP1-BP2 deletions may play a role in one or more phenotype(s), and the fact that individuals in this cohort were not evaluated by the same observer(s). Indeed, the average number of reported symptoms in the probands assessed by the two geneticists were 5.6, while the average number of symptoms in probands from the primary literature was 3.4. Additionally, it is possible that some of these associations are spurious and will not be consistent in follow-up studies. Further studies analyzing POEs in this condition are warranted, especially gene expression studies and the presence of a maternally methylated region near the *TUBGCP5* gene. Lastly, it is possible, though unlikely, that a small percentage of individuals in this study were reported in multiple sources, such as the online database DECIPHER and later reported in a paper in the primary literature. Given the nature of this research, we cannot be absolutely sure we did not double-count individuals in our analyses. Regardless, this is most likely a small risk and unlikely to impact the main findings. Additional research with a deeply phenotyped cohort assessed by the same observer(s) would be helpful. Finally, many of these individuals were not reported to have undergone a next generation sequencing study (e.g., exome), and therefore, a second variant associated with neurodevelopmental findings cannot be ruled out and will require further studies.

4. Materials and Methods

We collected 71 reported individuals with known parental inheritance of a 15q11.2 BP1-BP2 microdeletion from four sources: (1) the medical literature (N = 43) [22,23,36,42–50], (2) the DECIPHER database (N = 1) [51], 3) a cohort of patients with 15q11.2 BP1-BP2 microdeletion syndrome obtained during routine genetic diagnostic procedures (N = 11), and 4) a genetics study of chromosome 15 abnormalities, including 15q11.2 BP1-BP2 microdeletions (N = 16). This study of chromosome 15 abnormalities was approved by the University of Kansas Medical Center IRB to study genotype-phenotype correlations (FWA#: 00003411). As all individuals in this study were either previously published or de-identified data was provided from families who gave consent to share data, our study did not require IRB approval or a waiver.

In order to standardize this cohort for analysis of the potential POEs, we omitted individuals with an additional known, abnormal genetic diagnoses (e.g., Williams syndrome) and reports of *de novo* 15q11.2 BP1-BP2 microdeletions. All clinical features were categorized as a specific feature (e.g., microcephaly) when possible or a general clinical finding if the symptom noted was non-specific (e.g., "delays" versus speech delay or motor delay). We also grouped clinical features into overarching categories. Individual and grouped symptom-related variables were coded categorically (present vs. absent). For example, the variable "Psychiatric diagnosis" was classified as being present if an individual had specific diagnoses, such as anxiety or obsessive-compulsive disorder. Similarly, the variable "Behavioral differences" included individuals with "difficult" or "odd" behaviors, such as aggression or skin picking.

The four grouped variables included: (1) "any behavioral features" and included the categories of ASD diagnosis, psychiatric diagnoses, and any behavioral difference; (2) "any physical features", which included CHD or malformations, short stature, micro/macrocephaly, and dysmorphisms; (3) "non-physical features" and included developmental delays, muscular features, intellectual disability, epilepsy, ASD, learning difficulties, psychiatric diagnoses, and behavioral differences and lastly (4) "any delays" which included speech delays, motor delays, global developmental delays, and any mention of non-specific delays. The only variable that was not categorical was "Total clinical features", which added the described clinical features for an individual into a continuous variable. For example, if an individual was noted to have dysmorphic facial features, obsessive-compulsive disorder, ADHD, and ASD, this would count as three total clinical features because these features fall into three general categories (dysmorphisms, psychiatric diagnoses, and an ASD diagnosis).

In primary analyses, we used chi-squared tests to ascertain differences between individuals reported with a specific clinical symptom and the parent of origin for the deletion (maternal vs. paternal). Mann-Whitney U-tests were used to determine differences in grouped clinical features, as the distribution of these variables was non-normal. In sub-analyses, we performed chi-squared and Mann-Whitney U-tests on groups that omitted (1) sibling sets and (2) sibling sets and individuals with one or more additional VOUS. This was done to control for the fact that (1) shared genetic variants between siblings that may cause or contribute to certain clinical features and (2) a VOUS finding may be pathogenic and also cause or contribute to clinical features. In secondary analyses, we also used two-sided *t*-tests to determine if cohort characteristics differed between gender (e.g., age of diagnosis), as well as chi-squared to tests differences in specific clinical findings and Mann-Whitney U-test to determine differences between grouped symptoms (e.g., physical features). All findings were considered significant when $p \leq 0.05$.

Lastly, these analyses were conceived and conducted solely by the authors; the original contributors to the DECIPHER Database bear no responsibility for this analysis or interpretation.

5. Conclusions

The findings from the literature and survey reports add further clinical evidence to the previous molecular findings that the 15q11.2 BP1-BP2 microdeletion (Burnside-Butler) syndrome may exhibit POEs. Several gender-based differences in clinical features were reported in individuals with the 15q11.2 BP1-BP2 microdeletion. These findings, if replicated, may help prognosis and in counseling families identified with a 15q11.2 BP1-BP2 microdeletion to further expand the clinical phenotype of this emerging syndrome, now recognized as the most common cytogenetic finding in those presenting with ASD with or without congenital anomalies and developmental delays.

Author Contributions: Conceptualization, K.W.D. and M.S.; methodology, K.W.D., M.S., C.R. and M.G.B.; formal analysis, K.W.D., C.R. and M.G.B.; data curation, K.W.D., M.G.B., S.L, V.A., B.D., and A.N.; writing—original draft preparation, K.W.D.; writing—review and editing, K.W.D., MS, S.L., and M.G.B.; project administration, K.W.D.; Supervision, K.W.D. and M.G.B.

Funding: This research received no external funding.

Acknowledgments: We would like to thank Rena Vanzo for her valuable feedback on this study. This study makes use of data generated by the DECIPHER Consortium. A full list of centers who contributed to the generation of the data is available from https://decipher.sanger.ac.uk/ and via email from decipher@sanger.ac.uk. Funding for the DECIPHER project was provided by the Wellcome Trust. We acknowledge the Smith Intellectual and Developmental Disabilities Research Center (NIH U54 HD 090216), Molecular Regulation of Cell Development and Differentiation—COBRE (5P20GM104936-10), NIH S10 High-End Instrumentation Grant (NIH S10OD021743), KUMC Research Institute Clinical Pilot Research Program, University of Kansas Medical Center Grant (Y6B00030) Kansas City, KS 66160 and Prayer-Will Support PWS Organization (Family & Friends of Kyleigh Ellington).

Conflicts of Interest: This study was partially funded by Lineagen, Inc., where three of the authors (Kyle Davis, Catherine Robinson, and Moises Serrano) are currently or were previously employed be and hold stock options in Lineagen, Inc. The study design, data collection, analyses, interpretation, and the writing of the manuscript, were done by members of Lineagen, Inc. All other authors have no conflicts to declare.

Abbreviations

ASD	Autism spectrum disorder
ADHD	Attention-deficit hyperactivity disorder
BP1-BP2	Breakpoint 1–Breakpoint 2
CHD	Congenital heart disease
DECIPHER	DatabasE of genomiC varIation and Phenotype in Humans using Ensembl Resources
GTEx	Gene-Tissue Expression Project
OMIM	Online Mendelian Inheritance in Man
POE	Parent-of-origin effect
VOUS	Variant of uncertain (clinical) significance

References

1. Butler, M.G. Clinical and genetic aspects of the 15q11.2 BP1-BP2 microdeletion disorder. *J. Intellect. Disabil. Res.* **2017**, *61*, 568–579. [CrossRef] [PubMed]
2. Cox, D.M.; Butler, M.G. The 15q11.2 BP1-BP2 microdeletion syndrome: A review. *Int. J. Mol. Sci.* **2015**, *16*, 4068–4082. [CrossRef]
3. Burnside, R.D.; Pasion, R.; Mikhail, F.M.; Carroll, A.J.; Robin, N.H.; Youngs, E.L.; Gadi, I.K.; Keitges, E.; Jaswaney, V.L.; Papenhausen, P.R.; et al. Microdeletion, microduplication of proximal 15q11.2 between BP1 and BPP2: A susceptibility region for neurological dysfunction including develpomental and language delay. *Hum. Genet.* **2011**, *130*, 517–528. [CrossRef] [PubMed]

4. Ho, K.S.; South, S.T.; Lortz, A.; Hensel, C.H.; Sdano, M.R.; Vanzo, R.J.; Martin, M.M.; Peiffer, A.; Lambert, C.G.; Calhoun, A.; et al. Chromosomal microarray testing identifies a 4p terminal region associated with seizures in Wolf-Hirschhorn syndrome. *J. Med. Genet.* **2016**, *53*, 256–263. [CrossRef] [PubMed]
5. Ulfarsson, M.O.; Walters, G.B.; Gustafsson, O.; Steinberg, S.; Silva, A.; Doyle, O.M.; Brammer, M.; Gudbjartsson, D.F.; Arnarsdottir, S.; Jonsdottir, G.A.; et al. 15q11.2 CNV affects cognitive, structural and functional correlates of dyslexia and dyscalculia. *Transl. Psychiatry* **2017**, *7*, e1109. [CrossRef]
6. Arkadir, D.; Noreau, A.; Goldman, J.S.; Rouleau, G.A.; Alcalay, R.N. Pure hereditary spastic paraplegia due to a de novo mutation in the NIPA1 gene. *Eur. J. Neurol.* **2014**, *21*, e2. [CrossRef] [PubMed]
7. Tazelaar, G.H.P.; Dekker, A.M.; van Vugt, J.; van der Spek, R.A.; Westeneng, H.J.; Kool, L.; Kenna, K.P.; van Rheenen, W.; Pulit, S.L.; McLaughlin, R.L.; et al. Association of NIPA1 repeat expansions with amyotrophic lateral sclerosis in a large international cohort. *Neurobiol. Aging* **2018**, *74*, 234.e9–234.e15. [CrossRef] [PubMed]
8. Uddin, M.; Tammimies, K.; Pellecchia, G.; Alipanahi, B.; Hu, P.; Wang, Z.; Pinto, D.; Lau, L.; Nalpathamkalam, T.; Marshall, C.R.; et al. Brain-expressed exons under purifying selection are enriched for de novo mutations in autism spectrum disorder. *Nat. Genet.* **2014**, *46*, 742–747. [CrossRef] [PubMed]
9. Goytain, A.; Hines, R.M.; El-Husseini, A.; Quamme, G.A. NIPA1(SPG6), the basis for autosomal dominant form of hereditary spastic paraplegia, encodes a functional Mg2+ transporter. *J. Biol. Chem.* **2007**, *282*, 8060–8068. [CrossRef] [PubMed]
10. Jiang, Y.; Zhang, Y.; Zhang, P.; Zhang, F.; Xie, H.; Chan, P.; Wu, X. NIPA2 mutations are correlative with childhood absence epilepsy in the Han Chinese population. *Hum. Genet.* **2014**, *133*, 657–676. [CrossRef] [PubMed]
11. Hildebrand, M.S.; Damiano, J.; Mullen, S.A.; Bellows, S.T.; Scheffer, I.E.; Berkovic, S.F. Does variation in NIPA2 contribute to genetic generalized epilepsy? *Hum. Genet.* **2014**, *133*, 673–674. [CrossRef] [PubMed]
12. Maver, A.; Cuturilo, G.; Kovanda, A.; Miletic, A.; Peterlin, B. Rare missense TUBGCP5 gene variant in a patient with primary microcephaly. *Eur. J. Med. Genet.* **2018**. [CrossRef] [PubMed]
13. Hagerman, R.J.; Berry-Kravis, E.; Hazlett, H.C.; Bailey, D.B., Jr.; Moine, H.; Kooy, R.F.; Tassone, F.; Gantois, I.; Sonenberg, N.; Mandel, J.L.; et al. Fragile X syndrome. *Nat. Rev. Dis. Primers* **2017**, *3*, 17065. [CrossRef] [PubMed]
14. Reijnders, M.R.F.; Ansor, N.M.; Kousi, M.; Yue, W.W.; Tan, P.L.; Clarkson, K.; Clayton-Smith, J.; Corning, K.; Jones, J.R.; Lam, W.W.K.; et al. RAC1 Missense Mutations in Developmental Disorders with Diverse Phenotypes. *Am. J. Hum. Genet.* **2017**, *101*, 466–477. [CrossRef] [PubMed]
15. Nebel, R.A.; Zhao, D.; Pedrosa, E.; Kirschen, J.; Lachman, H.M.; Zheng, D.; Abrahams, B.S. Reduced CYFIP1 in Human Neural Progenitors Results in Dysregulation of Schizophrenia and Epilepsy Gene Networks. *PLoS ONE* **2016**, *11*, e0148039. [CrossRef] [PubMed]
16. Hsiao, K.; Harony-Nicolas, H.; Buxbaum, J.D.; Bozdagi-Gunal, O.; Benson, D.L. Cyfip1 Regulates Presynaptic Activity during Development. *J. Neurosci.* **2016**, *36*, 1564–1576. [CrossRef] [PubMed]
17. Joshi, R.S.; Garg, P.; Zaitlen, N.; Lappalainen, T.; Watson, C.T.; Azam, N.; Ho, D.; Li, X.; Antonarakis, S.E.; Brunner, H.G.; et al. DNA Methylation Profiling of Uniparental Disomy Subjects Provides a Map of Parental Epigenetic Bias in the Human Genome. *Am. J. Hum. Genet.* **2016**, *99*, 555–566. [CrossRef] [PubMed]
18. Chung, L.; Wang, X.; Zhu, L.; Towers, A.J.; Cao, X.; Kim, I.H.; Jiang, Y.H. Parental origin impairment of synaptic functions and behaviors in cytoplasmic FMRP interacting protein 1 (Cyfip1) deficient mice. *Brain Res.* **2015**, *1629*, 340–350. [CrossRef] [PubMed]
19. Bittel, D.; Kibiryeva, N.; Talebizadeh, Z.; Butler, M. Microarray analysis of gene/transcript expression in Prader-Willi syndrome: Deletion versus UPD. *J. Med. Genet.* **2003**, *40*, 568–574. [CrossRef]
20. Vanlerberghe, C.; Petit, F.; Malan, V.; Vincent-Delorme, C.; Bouquillon, S.; Boute, O.; Holder-Espinasse, M.; Delobel, B.; Duban, B.; Vallee, L.; et al. 15q11.2 microdeletion (BP1-BP2) and developmental delay, behaviour issues, epilepsy and congenital heart disease: A series of 52 patients. *Eur. J. Med. Genet.* **2015**, *58*, 140–147. [CrossRef] [PubMed]
21. Polyak, A.; Rosenfeld, J.A.; Girirajan, S. An assessment of sex bias in neurodevelopmental disorders. *Genome Med.* **2015**, *7*, 94. [CrossRef] [PubMed]
22. Picinelli, C.; Lintas, C.; Piras, I.S.; Gabriele, S.; Sacco, R.; Brogna, C.; Persico, A.M. Recurrent 15q11.2 BP1-BP2 microdeletions and microduplications in the etiology of neurodevelopmental disorders. *Am. J. Med. Genet. Part B Neuropsychiatry Genet.* **2016**, *171*, 1088–1098. [CrossRef]

23. Madrigal, I.; Rodriguez-Revenga, L.; Xuncla, M.; Mila, M. 15q11.2 microdeletion and FMR1 premutation in a family with intellectual disabilities and autism. *Gene* **2012**, *508*, 92–95. [CrossRef]
24. BIttel, D.C.; Kibiryeva, N.; Butler, M.G. Expression of 4 Genes Between Chromosome 15 Breakpoints 1 and 2 and Behavioral Outcomes in Prader-Willi Syndrome. *Pediatrics* **2006**, *118*, e1276–e1283. [CrossRef]
25. De Rubeis, S.; Bagni, C. Regulation of molecular pathways in the Fragile X Syndrome: Insights into Autism Spectrum Disorders. *J. Neurodev. Disord.* **2011**, *3*, 257–269. [CrossRef]
26. Butler, M.G.; Bittel, D.C.; Kibiryeva, N.; Talebizadeh, Z.; Thompson, T. Behavioral differences among subjects with Prader-Willi syndrome and type I or type II deletion and maternal disomy. *Pediatrics* **2005**, *113*, 565–573. [CrossRef]
27. Xie, H.; Zhang, Y.; Zhang, P.; Wang, J.; Wu, Y.; Wu, X.; Netoff, T.; Jiang, Y. Functional study of NIPA2 mutations identified from the patients with childhood absence epilepsy. *PLoS ONE* **2014**, *9*, e109749. [CrossRef]
28. Nagase, T.; Kikuno, R.; Ohara, O. Prediction of the coding sequences of unidentified human genes. XXI. The complete sequences of 60 new cDNA clones from brain which code for large proteins. *DNA Res.* **2001**, *8*, 179–187. [CrossRef]
29. De Wolf, V.; Brison, N.; Devriendt, K.; Peeters, H. Genetic counseling for susceptibility loci and neurodevelopmental disorders: The del15q11.2 as an example. *Am. J. Med. Genet. Part A* **2013**, *161A*, 2846–2854. [CrossRef]
30. Bonaccorso, C.M.; Spatuzza, M.; Di Marco, B.; Gloria, A.; Barrancotto, G.; Cupo, A.; Musumeci, S.A.; D'Antoni, S.; Bardoni, B.; Catania, M.V. Fragile X mental retardation protein (FMRP) interacting proteins exhibit different expression patterns during development. *Int. J. Dev. Neurosci.* **2015**, *42*, 15–23. [CrossRef]
31. Bozdagi, O.; Sakurai, T.; Dorr, N.; Pilorge, M.; Takahashi, N.; Buxbaum, J.D. Haploinsufficiency of Cyfip1 produces fragile X-like phenotypes in mice. *PLoS ONE* **2012**, *7*, e42422. [CrossRef]
32. Abekhoukh, S.; Sahin, H.B.; Grossi, M.; Zongaro, S.; Maurin, T.; Madrigal, I.; Kazue-Sugioka, D.; Raas-Rothschild, A.; Doulazmi, M.; Carrera, P.; et al. New insights into the regulatory function of CYFIP1 in the context of WAVE- and FMRP-containing complexes. *Dis. Models Mech.* **2017**, *10*, 463–474. [CrossRef]
33. Babbs, R.K.; Ruan, Q.T.; Kelliher, J.C.; Beierle, J.A.; Chen, M.M.; Feng, A.X.; Kirkpatrick, S.L.; Benitez, F.A.; Rodriguez, F.A.; Pierre, J.; et al. Cyfip1 haploinsufficiency increases compulsive-like behavior and modulates palatable food intake: Implications for Prader-Willi Syndrome. *bioRxiv* **2018**. [CrossRef]
34. Napoli, I.; Mercaldo, V.; Boyl, P.P.; Eleuteri, B.; Zalfa, F.; De Rubeis, S.; Di Marino, D.; Mohr, E.; Massimi, M.; Falconi, M.; et al. The Fragile X Syndrome Protein Represses Activity-Dependent Translation through CYFIP1, a New 4E-BP. *Cell* **2008**, *134*, 1042–1054. [CrossRef] [PubMed]
35. de Vries, B.B.; Fryns, J.P.; Butler, M.G.; Canziani, F.; Wesby-van Swaay, E.; van Hemel, J.O.; Oostra, B.A.; Halley, D.J.; Niermeijer, M.F. Clinical and molecular studies in fragile X patients with a Prader-Willi-like phenotype. *J. Med. Genet.* **1993**, *30*, 761–766. [CrossRef] [PubMed]
36. Kuroda, Y.; Ohashi, I.; Naruto, T.; Ida, K.; Enomoto, Y.; Saito, T.; Nagai, J.I.; Yanagi, S.; Ueda, H.; Kurosawa, K. Familial total anomalous pulmonary venous return with 15q11.2 (BP1-BP2) microdeletion. *J. Hum. Genet.* **2018**, *63*, 1185–1188. [CrossRef] [PubMed]
37. Carithers, L.J.; Ardlie, K.; Barcus, M.; Branton, P.A.; Britton, A.; Buia, S.A.; Compton, C.C.; Deluca, D.S.; Peter-demchok, J.; Gelfand, E.T.; et al. A Novel Approach to High-Quality Postmortem Tissue Procurement: The GTEx Project. *Biopreserv. Biobank.* **2015**, *13*, 311–319. [CrossRef] [PubMed]
38. Soemedi, R.; Wilson, I.J.; Bentham, J.; Darlay, R.; Topf, A.; Zelenika, D.; Cosgrove, C.; Setchfield, K.; Thornborough, C.; Granados-riveron, J.; et al. Contribution of Global Rare Copy-Number Variants to the Risk of Sporadic Congenital Heart Disease. *Am. J. Hum. Genet.* **2012**, *91*, 489–501. [CrossRef] [PubMed]
39. Rajaratnam, A.; Shergill, J.; Salcedo-arellano, M.; Saldarriaga, W.; Duan, X.; Hagerman, R. Fragile X syndrome and fragile X-associated disorders. *F1000 Res.* **2017**, *6*, 2112. [CrossRef]
40. Girirajan, S.; Rosenfeld, J.A.; Coe, B.; Parikh, S.; Friedman, N.; Goldstein, A.; Filipink, R.A.; Mcconnell, J.S.; Angle, B.; Meschino, W.S.; et al. Phenotypic Heterogeneity of Genomic Disorders and Rare Copy-Number Variants. *N. Engl. J. Med.* **2012**, *367*, 1321–1331. [CrossRef]
41. Pang, K.C.; Feldman, D.; Oertel, R.; Telfer, M. Molecular Karyotyping in Children and Adolescents with Gender Dysphoria. *Transgender Health* **2018**, *3*, 147–153. [CrossRef] [PubMed]

42. Doornbos, M.; Sikkema-Raddatz, B.; Ruijvenkamp, C.A.; Dijkhuizen, T.; Bijlsma, E.K.; Gijsbers, A.C.; Hilhorst-Hofstee, Y.; Hordijk, R.; Verbruggen, K.T.; Kerstjens-Frederikse, W.S.; et al. Nine patients with a microdeletion 15q11.2 between breakpoints 1 and 2 of the Prader-Willi critical region, possibly associated with behavioural disturbances. *Eur. J. Med. Genet.* **2009**, *52*, 108–115. [CrossRef] [PubMed]
43. Murthy, S.K.; Nygren, A.O.H.; El Shakankiry, H.M.; Schouten, J.P.; Al Khayat, A.I.; Ridha, A.; Al Ali, M.T. Detection of a novel familial deletion of four genes between BP1 and BP2 of the Prader-Willi/Angelman syndrome critical region by oligo-array CGH in a child with neurological disorder and speech impairment. *Cytogenet. Genome Res.* **2007**, *116*, 135–140. [CrossRef]
44. von der Lippe, C.; Rustad, C.; Heimdal, K.; Rodningen, O.K. 15q11.2 microdeletion—Seven new patients with delayed development and/or behavioural problems. *Eur. J. Med. Genet.* **2011**, *54*, 357–360. [CrossRef] [PubMed]
45. Chen, C.P.; Lin, S.P.; Lee, C.L.; Chern, S.R.; Wu, P.S.; Chen, Y.N.; Chen, S.W.; Wang, W. Familial transmission of recurrent 15q11.2 (BP1-BP2) microdeletion encompassing NIPA1, NIPA2, CYFIP1, and TUBGCP5 associated with phenotypic variability in developmental, speech, and motor delay. *Taiwan J. Obstetr. Gynecol.* **2017**, *56*, 93–97. [CrossRef] [PubMed]
46. Sempere Perez, A.; Manchon Trives, I.; Palazon Azorin, I.; Alcaraz Mas, L.; Perez Lledo, E.; Galan Sanchez, F. 15q11.2 (BP1-BP2) microdeletion, a new syndrome with variable expressivity. *An. Pediatr. (Barc.)* **2011**, *75*, 58–62. [CrossRef]
47. Jahn, J.A.; von Spiczak, S.; Muhle, H.; Obermeier, T.; Franke, A.; Mefford, H.C.; Stephani, U.; Helbig, I. Iterative phenotyping of 15q11.2, 15q13.3 and 16p13.11 microdeletion carriers in pediatric epilepsies. *Epilepsy Res.* **2014**, *108*, 109–116. [CrossRef]
48. Abdelmoity, A.T.; LePichon, J.-B.; Nyp, S.S.; Soden, S.E.; Daniel, C.A.; Yu, S. 15q11.2 Proximal Imbalances Associated With a Diverse Array of Neuropsychiatric Disorders and Mild Dysmorphic Features. *J. Dev. Behav. Pediatr.* **2012**, *33*, 570–576. [CrossRef] [PubMed]
49. Mullen, S.A.; Carvill, G.L.; Bellows, S.; Bayly, M.A.; Berkovic, S.F.; Dibbens, L.M.; Scheffer, I.E.; Mefford, H.C. Copy number variants are frequent in genetic generalized epilepsy with intellectual disability. *Neurology* **2013**, *81*, 1507–1514. [CrossRef]
50. Usrey, K.M.; Williams, C.A.; Dasouki, M.; Fairbrother, L.C.; Butler, M.G. Congenital Arthrogryposis: An Extension of the 15q11.2 BP1-BP2 Microdeletion Syndrome? *Case Rep. Genet.* **2014**, *2014*, 127258. [CrossRef] [PubMed]
51. Firth, H.V.; Richards, S.M.; Bevan, A.P.; Clayton, S.; Corpas, M.; Rajan, D.; Van Vooren, S.; Moreau, Y.; Pettett, R.M.; Carter, N.P. DECIPHER: Database of Chromosomal Imbalance and Phenotype in Humans Using Ensembl Resources. *Am. J. Hum. Genet.* **2009**, *84*, 524–533. [CrossRef] [PubMed]

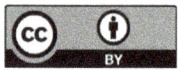

© 2019 by the authors. Licensee MDPI, Basel, Switzerland. This article is an open access article distributed under the terms and conditions of the Creative Commons Attribution (CC BY) license (http://creativecommons.org/licenses/by/4.0/).

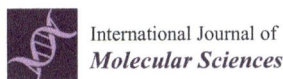

Article

Altered Intestinal Morphology and Microbiota Composition in the Autism Spectrum Disorders Associated SHANK3 Mouse Model

Ann Katrin Sauer [1], Juergen Bockmann [2], Konrad Steinestel [3], Tobias M. Boeckers [2] and Andreas M. Grabrucker [1,4,5,*]

1. Cellular Neurobiology and Neuro-Nanotechnology lab, Dept. of Biological Sciences, University of Limerick, V94PH61 Limerick, Ireland; Ann.Katrin.Sauer@ul.ie
2. Institute for Anatomy and Cell Biology, Ulm University, 89081 Ulm, Germany; juergen.bockmann@uni-ulm.de (J.B.); tobias.boeckers@uni-ulm.de (T.M.B.)
3. Gerhard-Domagk-Institute of Pathology, Muenster University Medical Center, 48149 Münster, Germany; Konrad.Steinestel@ukmuenster.de
4. Health Research Institute (HRI), University of Limerick, V94PH61 Limerick, Ireland
5. Bernal Institute, University of Limerick, V94PH61 Limerick, Ireland
* Correspondence: andreas.grabrucker@ul.ie; Tel.: +353-61-237-756

Received: 27 February 2019; Accepted: 28 April 2019; Published: 30 April 2019

Abstract: Autism spectrum disorders (ASD) are a group of neurodevelopmental disorders characterized by deficits in social interaction and communication, and repetitive behaviors. In addition, co-morbidities such as gastro-intestinal problems have frequently been reported. Mutations and deletion of proteins of the SH3 and multiple ankyrin repeat domains (*SHANK*) gene-family were identified in patients with ASD, and *Shank* knock-out mouse models display autism-like phenotypes. SHANK3 proteins are not only expressed in the central nervous system (CNS). Here, we show expression in gastrointestinal (GI) epithelium and report a significantly different GI morphology in *Shank3* knock-out (KO) mice. Further, we detected a significantly altered microbiota composition measured in feces of *Shank3* KO mice that may contribute to inflammatory responses affecting brain development. In line with this, we found higher *E. coli* lipopolysaccharide levels in liver samples of *Shank3* KO mice, and detected an increase in Interleukin-6 and activated astrocytes in *Shank3* KO mice. We conclude that apart from its well-known role in the CNS, SHANK3 plays a specific role in the GI tract that may contribute to the ASD phenotype by extracerebral mechanisms.

Keywords: microbiome; gut; ProSAP2; Phelan McDermid Syndrome; gut–brain interaction; leaky gut; IL-6; SHANK

---

1. Introduction

SHANK3 (SH3 and multiple ankyrin repeat domains 3, also known as proline-rich synapse-associated protein 2 (ProSAP2)) is a known scaffolding protein of the postsynaptic density (PSD) of glutamatergic excitatory synapses [1–3] that has been associated with autism spectrum disorders (ASD) [4–7]. Further, the Phelan McDermid Syndrome (PMDS/22q13.3 deletion syndrome) is a rare genetic disorder associated with a heterozygous loss of SHANK3 in the majority of patients. Individuals with PMDS show symptoms of the autism spectrum along with mental retardation and muscular hypotonia, and can suffer from seizures and gastrointestinal (GI) problems [8–10]. Besides the CNS, SHANK3 is expressed in different levels in many tissues, such as liver, heart, kidney, skeletal muscle [8], and epithelial cells of the GI tract [11,12].

A growing number of studies indicate a role of abnormal development and function of the gastro-intestinal (GI) system as a factor in ASD, with many patients having symptoms associated with

GI disorders [13]. Research indicates a link between the dysfunctions associated with ASD and GI problems such as abnormal trace metal uptake, alterations in the microbiome, and immune dysfunction and inflammatory processes [13,14]. In line with this, we have reported expression of SHANK3 in human enterocytes, where SHANK3 was functionally linked to zinc (Zn) transporter levels mediating Zn absorption [12].

The gut harbors a complex community of microbes—the microbiome—that is able to influence, among others, the development of the central nervous system (CNS) [15]. Recently, a study identified a dysregulation of several genera and species of bacteria in the gut and colon of *Shank3* KO mice [16] and the treatment of *Shank3* KO mice with *L. reuteri* led to the attenuation of some ASD-associated behaviors [16]. However, the underlying factors of the altered microbiota composition are currently not well understood.

Thus, here, we made use of a *Shank3αβ* knock-out mouse line that was reported to display ASD-like behavior with abnormal ultrasonic vocalization, repetitive self-grooming, and reduced interest in novel mice in nonsocial versus novel social pairing in the three-chamber test [17,18]. In these animals we performed a detailed analysis of the GI tract including further analyses determining microbiota composition. Our results confirm expression of SHANK3 in the GI epithelium. Further, *Shank3αβ* knock-out mice display an altered GI morphology and, in line with published data [16] we can confirm changes in gut microbiota composition. Altered GI morphology and microbiota composition lead to exaggerated responses to bacterial metabolites and compounds eliciting an immune response [19]. An increase of inflammatory markers has been reported in individuals with ASD and animal models [20,21]. Especially the cytokine Interleukin-6 (IL-6) has been proposed as a biomarker for autism [22] and was shown to be mechanistically linked to the development of autistic behaviors in mice [23–25]. Intriguingly, we detected an increase in IL-6 levels in *Shank3αβ* knock-out mice along with increased activation of astrocytes in the frontal cortex of *Shank3αβ* knock-out mice. Astrocyte activation has previously been linked to ASD [26].

2. Results

2.1. SHANK3 is Expressed in GI Epithelium of Mice

In the first set of experiments, we investigated the GI system of *Shank3αβ* KO mice that have been characterized in the lab previously [27]. Using the method described by Nik and Carlsson [28], we separated intestinal epithelium from mesenchyme. The purity of the lysate was confirmed by Western Blot analysis of the expression of Vimentin, whose presence would indicate unsuccessful separation of the epithelium, and Cytokeratin 7, which should be found in epithelium but not in mesenchymal cells of the submucosa (Figure S1). Apart from the expression of many ASD-associated genes [29] normally found at synapses in the CNS, we detected mRNA of SHANK family proteins and their "synaptic" interaction partners in GI epithelium (Figure 1A).

On protein level, in wildtype animals, only expression of SHANK2 and SHANK3, but not SHANK1 was found in GI epithelium in mice (Figure 1B). Further, in gut epithelium obtained from *Shank3αβ* KO mice, gene expression of *Shank2* and *Shank3* was decreased in comparison to wild type controls (Figure 1C). Knock-out animals do not show a total loss of *Shank3* due to the expression of the *Shank3γ* isoform that is detected by qRT-PCR primers.

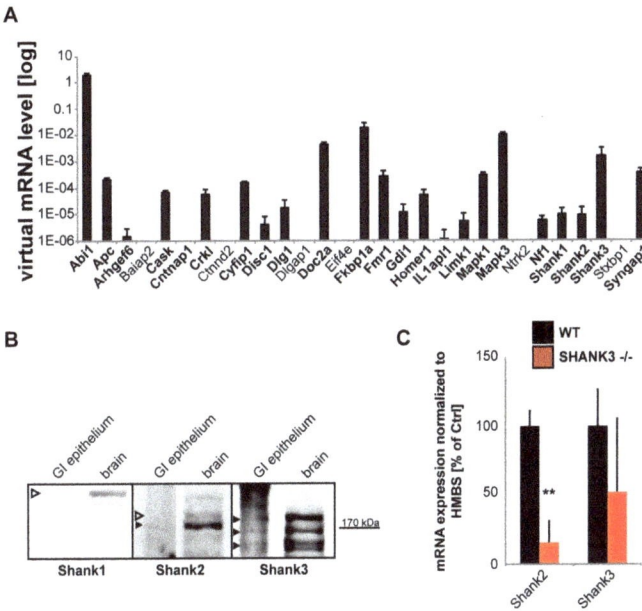

Figure 1. Expression of autism spectrum disorder (ASD)-associated postsynaptic density (PSD) proteins in gut epithelial cells. Several further ASD-associated PSD proteins are expressed in gut epithelial cells. (**A**) Screening of lysate from wild type mice ($n = 5$; used in technical triplicates) from isolated gut epithelium for the expression of "synaptic" ASD-associated genes using qRT-PCR. The genes were selected based on their occurrence at excitatory postsynapses and a reported association with ASD. On mRNA level, expression of all SH3 and multiple ankyrin repeat domains (*Shank*) family members was detected, as well as the expression of several direct interacting proteins such as *Abi1* (Abelson interactor 1), and *Homer1* (Homer protein homolog 1). Furthermore, the expression of *Apc* (Adenomatous-polyposis-coli), *Arhgef6* (Rac/Cdc42 Guanine Nucleotide Exchange Factor (GEF) 6, Alpha-PIX), *Cask* (Calcium/Calmodulin-Dependent Serine Protein Kinase), *Cntnap1* (Contactin Associated Protein 1), *Crkl* (V-Crk Avian Sarcoma Virus CT10 Oncogene Homolog-Like), *Cyfip1* (Cytoplasmic FMR1 Interacting Protein 1), *Disc1* (Disrupted In Schizophrenia 1), *Dlg1* (Discs, Large Homolog 1), *Doc2a* (Double C2-Like Domains, Alpha), *Fkbp1a* (FK506 Binding Protein 1A), *Fmr1* (Fragile X Mental Retardation 1), *Gdi1* (GDP Dissociation Inhibitor 1), *Il1apl1*, *Limk1* (LIM Domain Kinase 1), *Mapk1* and *Mapk3* (Mitogen-Activated Protein Kinase 1 and 3), *Nf1* (Neurofibromin 1), and *Syngap1* (Synaptic Ras GTPase Activating Protein 1) was detected. (**B**) Western Blot analysis for the expression of SHANK family members SHANK1, SHANK2, and SHANK3 using GI epithelium and brain tissue from wild-type mice. Only expression of SHANK2 and SHANK3 was detected on protein level in GI epithelium (full arrows). (**C**) Expression-analysis *Shank2* and *Shank3* in wildtype and *Shank3αβ* KO mice. Significantly lower expression of *Shank2* was found in *Shank3αβ* KO mice (t-test, 3 technical replicates from 3 animals per group; *Shank2* $p = 0.0067$ ($n = 3$); ** $p < 0.01$).

2.2. Shank3 KO Mice Show Abnormal GI Morphology

Shank3αβ KO mice did not show signs of diarrhea, stool blood, weight loss, or increased mortality. However, the analysis of the GI tract of *Shank3αβ* KO mice revealed significantly altered gut morphology (Figure 2A–D). Using paraffin-embedded sections from intestine, we performed histological and morphometric analyses. *Shank3αβ* KO mice show a significantly decreased length, but not width, of small intestinal villi compared to wild type mice (Figure 2B,C). Given that the crypt depth remains unchanged in *Shank3αβ* KO mice (Figure 2D), the ratio between villi length and crypt depth, which is considered normal in a range between 3 and 5, is reduced to below 3 in *Shank3αβ* KO mice.

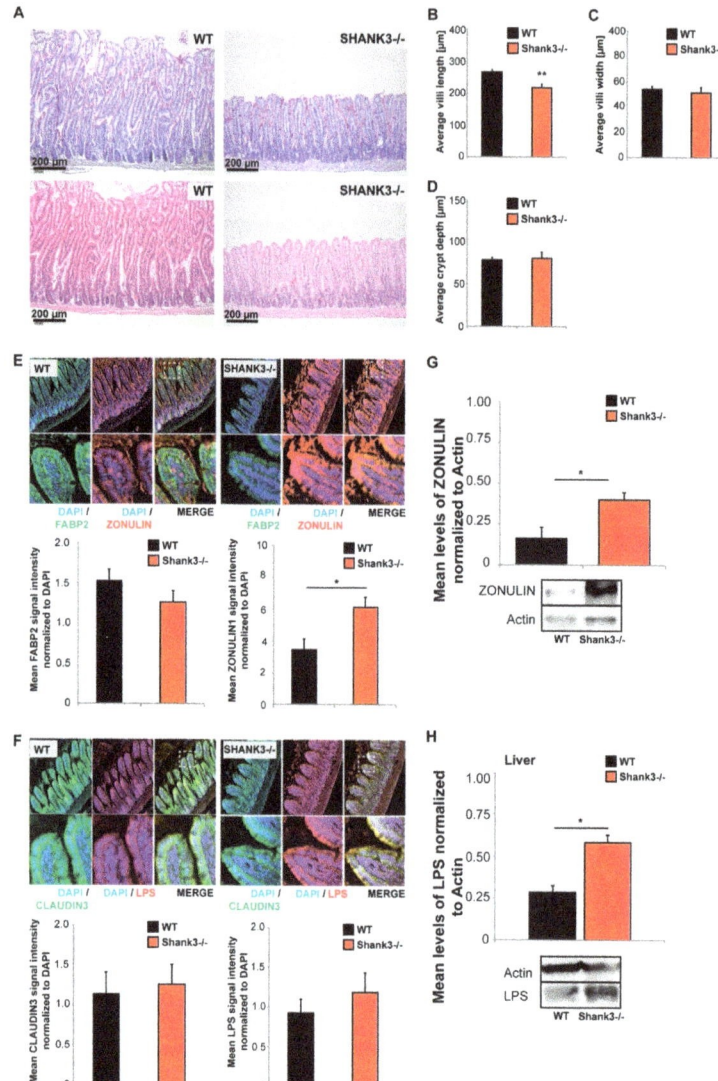

Figure 2. Altered gut morphology in *Shank3αβ* knock-out (KO) mice. (**A–D**) Histological evaluation of GI tract from wild type and *Shank3αβ* KO mice. (**A**) Longitudinal cross sections of *Shank3αβ* KO mice and wild type (WT) mice were stained with hematoxylin/eosin (HE) (upper panels) and periodic acid schiff (PAS) reaction (lower panels). Exemplary images are shown. (**B–D**) Morphological analysis of (**B**) villi length and (**C**) width, and (**D**) crypt depth reveals a significantly decreased villi length (Mann-Whitney *U*-test, $p = 0.009$; $n = 5$ animals per group) but not width ($p = 0.534$), and normal crypt depth ($p = 0.983$) in *Shank3αβ* KO mice. (**E,F**) Immunohistochemistry was performed on 5 mice per group and 5 optic fields of view each from 3 sections per mouse were analyzed. (**E**) A slight but non-significant decrease in FABP2 signal intensity was observed in *Shank3αβ* KO mice compared to wild types (left panel). Significantly higher ZONULIN-1 levels were found in *Shank3αβ* KO mice (right panel) (*t*-test, $p = 0.0413$). (**F**) The levels of CLAUDIN3 and lipopolysaccharide (LPS) were not significantly different between *Shank3αβ* KO mice and wild types in gut epithelium. (**G**) Significantly

higher ZONULIN-1 levels in *Shank3αβ* KO mice were confirmed by western blotting using gut epithelium protein lysate (*t*-test, $p = 0.0434$, $n = 3$ per group). (**H**) Protein lysate from liver tissue from WT and *Shank3αβ* KO mice ($n = 3$ per group) were analyzed for *E. coli* LPS levels using Western Blotting. The results show significantly higher LPS levels in the liver of *Shank3αβ β* KO mice (*t*-test, $p = 0.0452$). * $p < 0.05$, ** $p < 0.01$.

Further analyses of the GI epithelium using immunohistochemistry and protein biochemistry revealed further alterations. We selected three markers, FABP2 (Intestinal fatty acid-binding protein 2), CLAUDIN3, and ZONULIN1 (Figure 2E,F). FABP2 is a cytosolic protein found in small intestine epithelial cells where it participates in the uptake, intracellular metabolism, and transport of long chain fatty acids. CLAUDIN3 is a cell adhesion protein found at tight junctions between gut epithelial cells. ZONULIN1 is a modulator of tight junctions and alterations in the ZONULIN-regulated pathways have been associated with both intestinal and extra-intestinal inflammatory disorders [30]. Especially a decrease in FABP2 and increase in ZONULIN1 have been proposed as markers of gut dysbiosis and gut permeability integrity [31]. Protein levels were assessed measuring fluorescence intensities. The results reveal slight but not significantly lower levels of FABP2 in *Shank3αβ* KO mice. In contrast, the levels of ZONULIN1 were significantly higher in *Shank3αβ* KO mice compared to wild types (Figure 2E). This result was confirmed using gut epithelial protein lysate and western blotting (Figure 2G). No significant differences were found in CLAUDIN3 levels (Figure 2F).

A loss of intestinal barrier function was reported secondary to upregulation of ZONULIN, which is, to our knowledge, the only known physiological modulator of intercellular tight junctions [32]. Increased intestinal permeability may be responsible for increased translocation of bacterial components and metabolites into the systemic circulation [33]. Given the observed abnormalities in GI epithelium, we therefore investigated next whether the abnormal GI morphology of *Shank3αβ* KO mice facilitates the enrichment of bacterial compounds in the host system.

Lipopolysaccharide (LPS) levels from bacterial origin were not significantly different in the GI epithelium between *Shank3αβ* KO and wild type mice (Figure 2F). Detoxification and degradation of microbial products from gut-derived microbiota is a function of the liver. In the liver, hepatocytes mediate the clearance of endotoxin of intestinal origin [34]. Interestingly, when we analyzed liver samples regarding the levels of bacterial (*E. coli*) LPS, we found a significant increase in liver LPS in *Shank3αβ* KO mice (Figure 2G), hinting at increased LPS absorption (leakiness) of the GI system.

2.3. The Microbiome of Shank3 KO Mice Is Altered

Abnormalities in the GI system might translate into persistent changes that may affect several processes and features such as microbiota composition and may cause chronic inflammatory activity. Altered composition of gut microbiota has been reported before in Shank3 KO mice [16]. Thus, in the next set of experiments, we assessed the microbiome of *Shank3αβ* KO mice to confirm the presence of alterations in our mice. Feces from 10 weeks old *Shank3αβ* KO mice were collected and compared to age and gender matched controls. Housing conditions of the mice (bedding material, nesting material, number of animals per cage) were the same between groups and animals were housed side by side in wire cages. DNA was extracted from feces from four mice and pooled to one sample and three samples per group were analyzed using 16s microbiome profiling (Figure 3). The results show significant alterations in the microbiome of *Shankaβ* KO mice compared to Controls (Figure S2A,B). The amount of *Actinobacteria* was significantly higher in feces from *Shank3αβ* KO mice (Figure 3A). While the amount of *Bacteroidetes* (Figure 3B) was not altered, significantly higher levels of *Firmicutes* (Figure 3C) were detected in *Shank3αβ* KO mice. Further, only in *Shank3αβ* KO mice, *Deferribacteres* (Figure 3D), *Tenericutes* (Figure 3F), and *Chlamydiae* (Figure 3H) were found. In contrast, significantly lower levels of *Proteobacteria* (Figure 3E) and *Verrucomicrobia* (Figure 3G) were detected. In general, the phyla *Firmicutes* and *Proteobacteria* dominate the microbiome of control mice, while a shift towards *Firmicutes* and *Actinobacteria* occurs in *Shank3αβ* KO mice (Figure 3I).

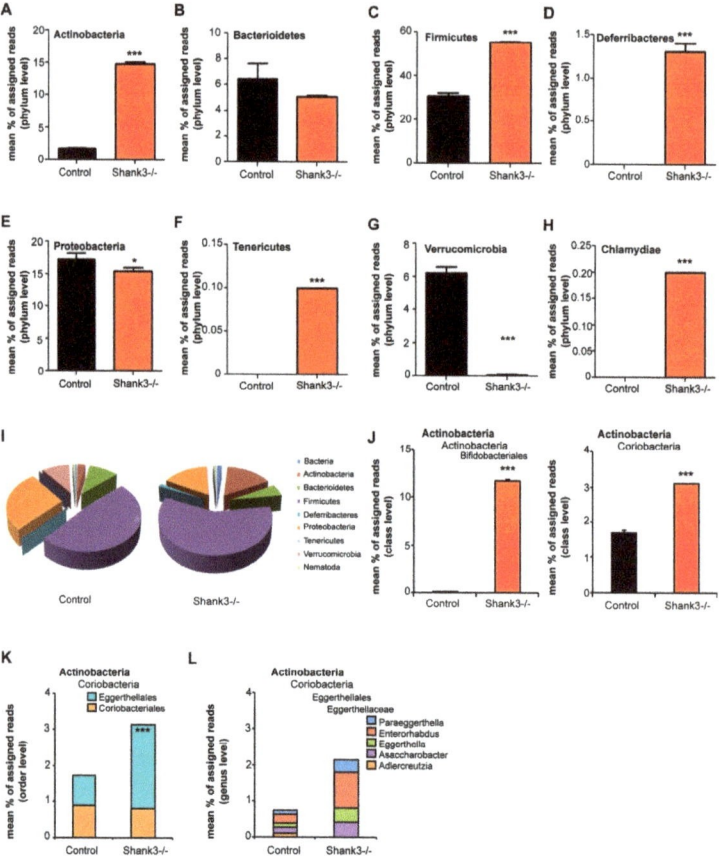

Figure 3. Altered microbiome in *Shank3αβ* KO mice. DNA was extracted from feces from 10 weeks old animals and microbiome analysis was performed using 16S Microbiome Profiling. Feces from four different animals were pooled per sample and three samples per group were analyzed. (**A**) The amount of *Actinobacteria* is significantly higher in feces from *Shank3αβ* KO mice. (**B**) The amount of *Bacterioidetes* is not significantly different between control and *Shank3αβ* KO mice. (**C**) A significant increase in Firmicutes was found in *Shank3αβ* KO mice. (**D**) Bacteria of the phylum *Deferribacteres* were only found in *Shank3αβ* KO mice. (**E**) Significantly reduced levels of Proteobacteria were detected in *Shank3αβ* KO mice. (**F**) Bacteria of the phylum *Tenericutes* were only found in *Shank3αβ* KO mice. (**G**) The amount of *Verrucomicrobia* was significantly lower in *Shank3αβ* KO mice. (**H**) Bacteria of the phylum *Chlamydiae* were only found in *Shank3αβ* KO mice. (**I**) Overview of the identified relative frequencies of different phyla found in control and *Shank3αβ* KO mice. (**J**) The increase in *Actinobacteria* is caused by a significant increase in both classes *Actinobacteria* (order *Bifidobacteriales*) (t-test, $p < 0.0001$) and *Coriobacteria* (t-test, $p < 0.0001$). (**K**) *Coriobacteria* increase due to a significant higher levels in the order *Eggerthellales*, but not *Coriobacteriales*. (**L**) Within the family *Eggerthellaceae*, *Adlercreutzia* did not show an increase. The genera *Asaccharobacter*, *Eggerthella*, *Enterorhabdus*, and *Paraeggerthella* show significant increase. * $p < 0.05$, *** $p < 0.001$.

Given that an increase in Actinobacteria in the gut of *Shank3* KO mice has been reported before [16], we closer investigated the alterations within this phylum. The increase in *Actinobacteria* was caused by a significant increase in the order *Bifidobacteriales* (class *Actinobacteria*) and *Eggerthellales* (class *Coriobacteria*) (Figure 3J,K). Both orders consist of one detected family, *Bifidobacteriaceae* and *Eggerthellaceae*, respectively. Within the family *Bifidobacteriaceae*, only bacteria of the genus Bifidobacterium were detected. Within the family *Eggerthellaceae*, the genus *Adlercreutzia* did not show an increase, while bacteria of the genus *Asaccharobacter*, *Eggerthella*, *Enterorhabdus*, and *Paraeggerthella* increased in abundance (Figure 3L). In particular, the bacteria species *Bifidobacterium pseudolongum*, *Assacharobacter WCA-131-CoC-2*, *Eggerthella YY7918*, and *Enterorhabdus caecimuris* were drivers of this increase (Figure S2C), which have been associated with inflammation and infection of the gastrointestinal tract [35,36]. However, classification on species level using 16S RNA sequencing cannot be done with a high level of confidence and needs to be confirmed by more detailed studies in the future. Another limitation of the performed analysis is that mice have been pooled into three samples, which obscures inter-individual differences. For analysis, we assumed a normal distribution of data. While pooled samples within one group showed great homogeneity, high levels of variability on individual level are not uncommon for microbiota composition.

2.4. Altered GI Morphology and Microbiome of Shank3 KO Mice May Be Linked to Increased Inflammatory Marker Expression

One hypothesis that has been proposed for ASD is that GI pathologies such as a "leaky gut" will expose the host to epitopes from microbiota that reside within the gut in altered composition, and thereby produce an immune activation leading to inflammatory responses, which may contribute to CNS pathologies during certain time-windows in development. Altered inflammatory cytokine levels have been reported recently in *Shank3* KO mice [16].

Therefore, next, to investigate whether higher intestinal barrier dysfunction of *Shank3αβ* KO mice might translate into increased expression of inflammatory markers, we analyzed the expression of Glial fibrillary acidic protein (GFAP), a marker for astrogliosis, in the cortex of WT and *Shank3αβ* KO mice using immunohistochemistry. Our results reveal a significantly increased number of GFAP positive cells in *Shank3αβ* KO mice (Figure 4A). Further, because of its importance in relation to ASD, we analyzed IL-6 levels in brain sections of *Shank3αβ* KO mice. IL-6 signals resulted from diffuse staining of neural tissue and signals from blood vessels. The immunofluorescence of IL-6 was slightly, but not significantly, higher in neural tissue of *Shank3αβ* KO mice compared to WT (Figure 4B). In contrast, signals in blood vessels were significantly increased in *Shank3αβ* KO mice (Figure 4B) hinting at a systemic increase of IL-6 as previously reported in individuals with ASD.

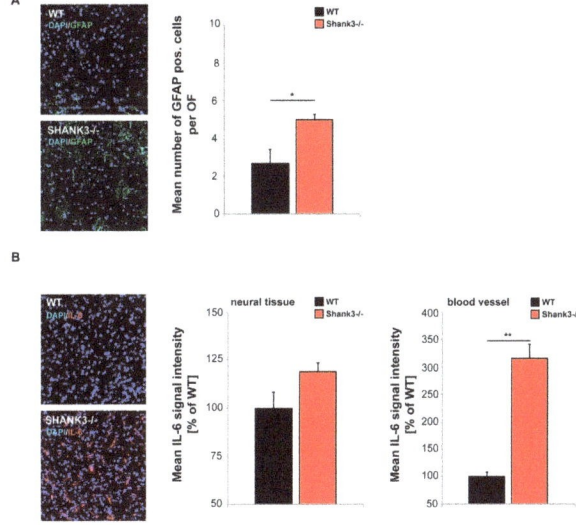

Figure 4. Confocal microscopy images with same acquisition time taken from frontal cortex of brain sections from WT and *Shank3αβ* KO mice (*n* = 3 animals per group) were used to assess the number of

activated astrocytes labeled by Glial fibrillary acidic protein (GFAP), and IL-6 levels in neural tissue and blood vessels. DAPI staining was used to visualize cell nuclei. (**A**) Optic fields (OF) of view were analyzed and the number of GFAP positive cells per OF measured. The results show a significantly higher number of activated astrocytes in *Shank3αβ* KO mice (t-test, $p = 0.0407$). (**B**) The immunofluorescence of IL-6 was slightly higher in *Shank3αβ* KO mice compared to WT (t-test, $p = 0.1164$) in neural tissue and significantly higher in blood vessels (t-test, $p = 0.0014$). * $p < 0.05$, ** $p < 0.01$.

3. Discussion

A growing amount of research reveals abnormalities in the GI system of ASD patients with many of them having symptoms associated with GI disorders. It is likely that these extracerebral alterations contribute to and modify the pathology of ASD. Here, we investigated *Shank3αβ* KO mice and found significant GI abnormalities that translated into altered microbiota composition, increased accumulation of bacterial LPS in liver, and signs of increased immune activation in the periphery and the brain.

The structural and functional integrity of the gastrointestinal mucosal barrier is important for protection from various luminal agents such as acids, enzymes, bacteria, viruses, and toxins. The abnormal GI morphology may lead to downstream effects resulting in the often-reported GI-related symptoms and co-morbidities in ASD [13]. One frequently reported GI alteration in ASD is an altered microbiome. In mammals, intestinal microbiota have a marked influence on health status via gut–brain–microbiota interactions [37,38]. In humans, stool was shown to contain a high bacterial composition, with >90% of sequence data belonging to bacteria [39], with predominately bacteria belonging to two phyla, *Firmicutes* and *Bacteriodetes* [39]. Interestingly, feces of mice also showed mostly bacteria from the phyla *Firmicutes* and *Bacteriodetes* in our analyses. The dysbiosis we observed in *Shank3αβ* KO mice is marked by an increase in microbiota of the phylum *Actinobacteria* and *Firmicutes*, and bacteria from the phylum *Tenericutes*, *Deferribacteres*, and *Chlamydiae* were only present in *Shank3αβ* KO mice, while the mount of *Proteobacteria* and *Verrucomicrobia* was lower. Interestingly, in humans, a significant increase in the *Actinobacterium* phylum was found in patients with ASD [40]. Our results are also in line with the previous reported alterations in gut microbiota of *Shank3* KO mice [16], where similar to our results, an increase in *Actinobacteria* was reported. The consistent increase in *Actinobacteria* in two distinct *Shank3* KO models housed in different animal facilities therefore arises as consistent pattern with relation to ASD in humans.

On genus level, we found a significant increase in *Enterorhabdus* and *Mucispirillum* in *Shank3αβ* KO mice. Both genera contain species that have been associated with both inflammatory markers and active colitis [36,41]. In particular, *Mucispirillum* expansion has been observed during intestinal inflammation [41]. In addition, we observed an increase in the *Clostridium* genus. Bacteria of this genus are major producers of toxins and an increase has been reported in ASD [40,42]. Further, *Shank3αβ* KO mice show significantly higher levels of *Parasutterella*. *Parasutterella* were reported to be characteristic for patients with Crohn's disease [43] but they also emerged as significantly associated with children with Autism and functional gastrointestinal disorders that experience abdominal pain [44]. Among the genera significantly decreased in *Shank3αβ* KO mice were *Akkermansia*. *Akkermansia* (e.g., *Akkermansi muciniphila*) were found low in feces of children with autism [45]. In general, a picture emerges where the observed alterations in the microbiota composition of *Shank3αβ* KO mice support a model of increased inflammation.

In ASD, dysbiosis of microbiota has been associated with a disruption of the mucosal barrier leading to alteration in the intestinal permeability [46], which may cause a change in the inflammatory status of mice, a major process in the interaction between gut and brain. In our study, we could confirm the previously reported expression of *Shank3* in gut epithelial cells [12]. Loss of *Shank3αβ* in mice not only produces a phenotype in nervous tissue. Here, we report abnormal GI morphology. The length of villi was reduced in *Shank3αβ* KO mice and ZONULIN expressed at significantly higher level.

Increased intestinal permeability has been recently proposed to play a key role in the pathogenesis of chronic inflammatory diseases [32], such as irritable bowel syndrome [47], but also ASD [48]. Since the intestinal epithelium provides the interface between host and environment, inappropriate antigen trafficking through the intestinal mucosa may occur upon increased intestinal permeability. While under normal physiological conditions, the majority of antigens passes through the transcellular pathway, where lysosomal degradation produces small non-immunogenic peptides, only ~10% of proteins cross the epithelium through the paracellular pathway as full intact proteins or partially digested peptides. This results in antigenic tolerance, which can be severely affected in case this ratio changes [32]. Intestinal permeability in turn is tightly connected to microbiota composition. ZONULIN is a major regulator of intestinal permeability and an increase in ZONULIN as observed here in *Shank3αβ* KO mice has been associated with increased permeability [49].

In line with this, we could show that bacterial LPS accumulates in significantly higher amount in the liver of *Shank3αβ* KO mice. Together, these results hint towards a disruption of the mucosal barrier.

We could further confirm the increased expression of inflammatory markers in *Shank3* KO mice. In particular, we observed significantly higher IL-6 levels in the capillary network within the brain of *Shank3αβ* KO mice, likely reflecting higher systemic IL-6 levels. Increased serum cytokine levels in autistic patients have previously been modeled in mice by maternal immune activation (MIA). MIA results in the production of inflammatory cytokines leading to neurological and immunological disturbances in the offspring resulting in autism-like behavioral deficits. These studies have pointed towards IL-6 as a key cytokine involved in these events [25]. During inflammation, IL-6 was shown to induce the expression of other cytokines and immune regulatory genes. In addition, IL-6 can initiate the transcription of neural regulatory genes [25]. Intriguingly, administration of an anti-IL-6 antibody in MIA mice rescued some of the behavioral deficits.

The increased levels of IL-6 were accompanied by significantly increased number of GFAP positive cells in the brain of *Shank3αβ* KO mice. GFAP expression is a marker for astrogliosis [50] and increased levels of GFAP expression in cortex were also reported in some human individuals with ASD [51].

Taken together, in line with our previous report on SHANK3 in the GI tract [12] the presence of other "synaptic" proteins in the GI epithelium makes the existence of a protein complex similar to the one described at excitatory postsynapses in enterocytes more than likely. The loss of this complex may lead to morphological and functional abnormalities in the GI tract, ultimately resulting in alterations in the microbiome and the passage of bacterial metabolites and compounds into the host animal. While our data shows correlation and not causation, these molecules may act as trigger for immune responses leading to increased levels of cytokines, among them IL-6 causing an inflammatory response that ultimately will affect brain development and function, e.g., via the activation of astrocytes. Thus, the contribution of extracerebral factors to the phenotype of SHANK3 deficient mice and humans is likely. The possibility of specific interventions to alter the microbiome may provide new vistas for novel therapeutic approaches such as dietary manipulations in ASD.

4. Materials and Methods

4.1. Materials

Paraformaldehyde was purchased from Merck and D-Saccharose was from Roth, Karlsruhe, Germany. Alexa Fluor conjugated secondary antibodies and ProLong® Gold antifade reagent from Invitrogen/Life Technologies Europe, Darmstadt, Germany. Zonulin 1 antibody was purchased from Thermo Fisher Scientific (Invitrogen) (Waltham, MA, USA); Claudin3 antibody from Abcam (Berlin, Germany); FABP2 antibody from Thermo Fisher Scientific (Invitrogen); LPS antibody from Origene (Rockville, MD, USA); and IL6 antibody was purchased from Cell signaling Technologies (Danvers, MA, USA); GFAP antibody was purchased from Sigma Aldrich (St. Louis, MO, USA); Cytokeratin and Vimentin antibody from Abcam. For SHANK3 western blotting in-house polyclonal rabbit SHANK3 antibodies were used that have been described previously [27,52]. iScriptTM cDNA Synthesis Kit,

SSoAdvanced Universal SYBR® Green Supermix and customized PrimePCR plates were purchased from Bio-Rad, Hercules, CA, USA. QuantiTect Primer Assays, RNeasy Mini Kit and QuantiFastTM SYBR_Green RT-PCR kit were purchased from Qiagen, Hilden, Germany. Unless otherwise indicated, all other chemicals were obtained from Sigma-Aldrich.

4.2. Animals

Shank3αβ mutants were published and characterized before and raised on a C57BL/6 background [27]. All animal experiments were performed in compliance with the guidelines for the welfare of experimental animals issued by the Federal Government of Germany and approved by the Regierungspraesidium Tuebingen and the local ethics committee (Ulm University) (project code - O.103, date of approval May 12th 2016). Both wild type and *Shank3αβ* KO mice received the same standard laboratory diet (ssniff GmbH, Germany) and consumed similar amounts of food and water that was accessed ad libitum.

4.3. Microbiome Analysis

DNA extraction—DNA extraction of murine fecal samples was performed using the Mo Bio PowerFecal DNA Isolation Kit (Qiagen, Hilden, Germany) according to the manufacturer´s protocol. After elution, the resulting DNA concentration was measured on the Nanodrop 2000 (Thermo Fisher Scientific, Waltham, MA, USA). Purity was assessed by calculating the measured A260/A280 ratio using a Nanodrop. DNA samples with an A260/A280 ratio in between 1.7 to 2.0 were considered pure and used for MiSeq.

Pyrosequencing of 16S rDNA region V3 to V5—Primers were designed to target conserved sequences around the variable region 3 to 5 (V3 to V5) of bacterial 16S rDNA. 16s Microbiome Profiling with MiSeq was performed by Eurofins Genomics (Ebersberg, Germany).

Pyrosequencing data processing and taxonomic classification—Data processing and taxonomic classification was performed by Eurofins Genomics. In brief, after removing all reads with errors, the remaining reads were processed using minimum entropy decomposition (MED), thereby partitioning the marker gene dataset into OTUs (Operational Taxonomic Units). Taxonomic information was assigned to each OTU by BLAST alignments of representative cluster sequences to the NCBI database. A specific taxonomic assignment for each OUT was transferred from a set of best-matching reference sequences. Only reference sequences with an 80% sequence identity across at least 80% of the sequence were considered for reference purposes. Sequences were not assigned to an OTU if they were considered as noise according to the OTU picking algorithm (including potential chimeric sequences and singletons). OTU and taxonomic assignments were further processed with the QIIME software package (version 1.8.0, http://qiime.org/). Normalization after Angly [53] of bacterial and archaea taxonomic assignment abundance with lineage specific copy numbers of marker genes was performed for estimate improvement. Therefore, the number of reads assigned to one species was divided by a known or assumed number of marker regions/genes.

Statistical analysis was performed testing for significance without correction for multiple comparisons due to the low number of simultaneous tested hypotheses. Correction for multiple comparisons does not alter results reported in the manuscript with the exception of differences observed for Proteobacteria on phylum level.

4.4. Immunohistochemistry

Paraffin-embedded sections of small intestine were cut at 4.5 to 5 µm thickness. Afterwards, sections were treated with Xylene 2× for 5 min each and submerged in 100%, 90%, 70% Ethanol and H_2O for 5 min each. Sections were treated in 10 mM sodium citrat buffer pH 6.0 for 15 min around boiling point (Microwave at 600 W). The slides were cooled down to room temperature (RT) for approximately 30 min und washed two times in PBS for 2 min each. The tissue on each slide was surrounded with a fat tissue stick. To avoid unspecific antibody binding the tissue was blocked with blocking solution

(BS) (10% FBS in 1× PBS) for 1 h at RT. Subsequently, the tissue was incubated with primary antibody diluted in BS for 2 h at RT in a humid chamber. After washing 3× with PBS for 5 min, the tissue was incubated with secondary antibody, diluted in BS, for 1 h in a humid chamber, followed by a wash step with PBS for 5 min. The tissue was counterstained with DAPI (4′,6-Diamidin-2-phenylindol).

Frozen brain sections were cut at 14 µm thickness. After cryosections were thawed for 20 min in a hydrated staining chamber, sections were fixed in 4% paraformaldehyde (PFA)/4% sucrose/PBS for 20 min and washed three times in PBS for 5 min each. Subsequently, sections were treated with 1× PBS with 0.2% Triton X-100 for 20 min at RT and 1× PBS with 0.05% Triton X-100 for 10 min at RT. To avoid unspecific antibody binding blocking was performed with blocking solution (BS) (10% FBS in 1× PBS) for 1 h at RT. Afterwards, the tissue was incubated with primary antibody diluted in BS overnight at 4 °C in a humid chamber. The following day after washing with 1× PBS with 0.05% Triton X-100 for 10 min, the tissue was incubated with secondary antibody coupled to alexa488 or alexa568, diluted in BS, for 2 h at 37 °C in a dark humid chamber, followed by a 3× wash steps with 1× PBS with 0.05% Triton X-100 for 5 min each and a 5 min wash step with 1× PBS. The tissue was counterstained with DAPI (4′,6-Diamidin-2-phenylindol) for 5 min at RT, washed with aqua bidest before being mounted with Vecta Mount. Fluorescence images were obtained using an inverted confocal microscope (Zeiss LSM710, Göttingen, Germany) and an ImageXpress Micro Spinning Disc Confocal High-Content Imaging System (Molecular Devices, San Jose, CA, USA), and analyses of signal intensities were performed with ImageJ 1.48r.

4.5. Histology

Paraffin-embedded sections from intestine were obtained of small intestine from adult mice (10 weeks of age). From each intestine, 4 cm were fixed in 4% buffered formalin. Per sample, three small parts were embedded in paraffin wax longitudinally (for cross sections) and horizontally (for longitudinal sections). For morphological analyses, small intestinal sections were cut at 2 µm and stained with Haematoxylin/Eosin (HE) or the periodic acid–Schiff (PAS)-reaction. Immunohistochemistry staining of 4.5 to 5 µm sections was performed using the Benchmark XT Autostainer (Ventana Medical systems, Tucson, USA). All required reagents were purchased from Ventana. Dilution of primary antibodies was done according to the respective manufacturer's recommendations. For detection of primary antibody the OptiView DAB IHC Detection Kit or the ultra universal Alkaline Phosphatase Red Kit was used. Additionally, sections were washed in water, lightly counterstained with Haematoxylin, dehydrated, and mounted. Images were obtained using the Mirax Desk scanner and the MIRAX Viewer 1.12.22.0 software (Zeiss, Göttingen, Germany).

4.6. qRT-PCR

Total RNA was isolated with the RNeasy Mini Kit according to the manufacturer's protocol. All of the optional purification steps were performed and RNA eluted with sterile RNAse-free water.

cDNA synthesis of pooled RNAs was performed with the iScript™ cDNA Synthesis Kit (Bio-Rad) according to the manufacturer's protocol in a total reaction volume of 20 µL and a maximum of 1 µg RNA/reaction. Quantitative real-time-PCR was performed using the SSoAdvanced Universal SYBR® Green Supermix (Bio-Rad) and customized PrimePCR plates in 96 well format with immobilized primers (Bio-Rad) according to the manufacturer's protocol with a final reaction volume of 20 µL and 2 ng cDNA/well. Resulting data were analyzed using the hydroxymethylbilane synthase (*HMBS*) or Glyceraldehyde 3-phosphate dehydrogenase (*GAPDH*) gene as an internal standard to normalize transcript levels. Cycle threshold (*ct*) values were calculated by the CFX Manager (Bio-Rad, version 3.1, Hercules, CA, USA).

Alternatively, first strand synthesis and quantitative real-time-PCR amplification were performed in a one-step, single-tube format using the QuantiFast™ SYBR_Green RT-PCR kit from Qiagen according to the manufacturer's protocol in a total volume of 20 µL. Thermal cycling and fluorescent detection were performed using the Rotor-Gene Q real-time PCR machine (model 2-Plex HRM)

(Qiagen, Hilden, Germany). The SYBR Green I reporter dye signal was measured. Resulting data were analyzed using the *HMBS* gene as an internal standard to normalize transcript levels. Cycle threshold (*ct*) values were calculated by the Rotor-Gene Q Software (Qiagen, version 2.0.2, Hilden, Germany). All quantitative real-time PCR reactions were run in technical triplicates and mean *ct*-values for each reaction were taken into account for calculations.

4.7. Protein Biochemistry

To obtain homogenate from GI tissue, small intestinal epithelium was isolated from mesenchyme following a protocol after Nik and Carlsson [28]. In brief, small intestine was cut into 4–5 cm long pieces. Gut mucus was removed by gently squeezing it out of the intestine with the blunt point of tweezers. Each piece was inverted by inserting a rod, securing the intestine at one end with a suture and pulling the rod back. The rod with the inverted piece was inserted into a pipet tip (1000 µL) and one end of the intestine pulled onto the tip. After careful removal of the rod, the second end of the intestinal piece is pinched off with a suture. The inverted intestine with the attached pipet tip was submerged in cell recovery solution and repeatedly inflated and reflated with air over the course of at least 30 min per piece. During this time the epithelium is separated from the other intestinal layers. For lysis, RIPA buffer + PI (Complete EDTA-free Protease Inhibitor Cocktail tablets; Roche, Mannheim, Germany) is applied to the collected mouse tissue. To disrupt the epithelium a sonicator was used (4 pulses, lasting 1 s each). Afterwards the lysate was incubated for 2 h at 4 °C on a rotator followed by centrifugation for 20 min at 4 °C at 11,700 rpm. Protein concentration was determined by Bradford protein assay.

To obtain homogenate from liver tissue, tissue was immersed in Hepes Sucrose buffer (10 mM Hepes, 0.32 M Sucrose) and disrupted using a sonicator (fisherbrand sonic dismembranator 120, Fisher scientific, Hampton, NH, USA). Proteins were separated by SDS-PAGE and blotted onto nitrocellulose membranes (GE Healthcare). Immunoreactivity was visualized using horseradish peroxidase (HRP)-conjugated secondary antibodies and the SuperSignal detection system (Pierce, Thermo Fisher, Waltham, MA, USA).

4.8. Statistic

Statistical analysis was performed using Graph Pad Prism 5 (La Jolla, CA, USA), and tested for significance using *t* tests. All values were normally distributed. In experiments using pooled samples or three replicates, normal distribution was not tested but assumed as the most likely scenario. Statistical tests were two tailed with a significance level of $\alpha \leq 0.05$. Significances are stated with *p* values <0.05 *; <0.01 **; <0.001 ***.

qRT PCR quantification—Relative quantification is based on internal reference genes to determine virtual mRNA levels of target genes. Cycle threshold (ct) values were calculated by the Rotor-Gene Q Software (version 2.0.2, Qiagen, Hilden, Germany). Ct values were transformed into virtual mRNA levels according to the formula: Virtual mRNA level = $10 * ((ct_{(target)} - ct_{(standart)})/\text{slope of standard curve})$.

Western blot quantification—Evaluation of bands from Western blots (WBs) was performed using ImageJ. Three independent experiments were performed and blots imaged using a UVITEC Alliance Q9 Advanced system (Cleaver scientific, Rugby, UK). The individual bands were selected and the integrated density was measured. All WB bands were normalized to β-Actin and the ratios averaged and tested for significance.

Supplementary Materials: Supplementary materials can be found at http://www.mdpi.com/1422-0067/20/9/2134/s1.

Author Contributions: Conceptualization, A.M.G.; Data curation, A.K.S.; Formal analysis, A.K.S. and A.M.G.; Funding acquisition, T.M.B. and A.M.G.; Investigation, A.K.S., K.S. and A.M.G.; Methodology, A.K.S., J.B. and K.S.; Resources, J.B. and T.M.B.; Supervision, T.M.B. and A.M.G.; Writing—original draft, A.M.G.; Writing—review & editing, A.K.S. and T.M.B.

Funding: T.M.B. has received support from the DFG (SFB1149, A02), the Else Kröner-Fresenius Stiftung, the Helmholtz Society (DZNE, Ulm Site), and the Innovative Medicines Initiative (IMI) Joint Undertaking (AIMS-2-Trials) under grant agreement n°777394, resources of which are composed of financial contribution from the European Union and EFPIA companies' in kind contribution. A.M.G. was supported by the Else Kröner-Fresenius Stiftung (214_A251).

Acknowledgments: The authors gratefully acknowledge the technical assistance of Katharina Mangus, Claudia Schlosser and the Department of Pathology of the Bundeswehrkrankenhaus Ulm.

Conflicts of Interest: The authors declare that they have no competing interests. The funders had no role in the design of the study; in the collection, analyses, or interpretation of data; in the writing of the manuscript; or in the decision to publish the results.

References

1. Boeckers, T.M.; Bockmann, J.; Kreutz, M.R.; Gundelfinger, E.D. ProSAP/SHANK proteins—A family of higher order organizing molecules of the postsynaptic density with an emerging role in human neurological disease. *J. Neurochem.* **2002**, *81*, 903–910. [CrossRef]
2. Lim, S.; Naisbitt, S.; Yoon, J.; Hwang, J.; Suh, P.; Sheng, M.; Kim, E. Characterization of the SHANK Family of Synaptic Proteins. *J. Biol. Chem.* **1999**, *274*, 29510–29518. [CrossRef] [PubMed]
3. Naisbitt, S.; Kim, E.; Tu, J.C.; Xiao, B.; Sala, C.; Valtschanoff, J.; Weinberg, R.J.; Worley, P.F.; Sheng, M. SHANK, a novel family of postsynaptic density proteins that binds to the NMDA receptor/PSD-95/GKAP complex and cortactin. *Neuron* **1999**, *23*, 569–582. [CrossRef]
4. Bourgeron, T. A synaptic trek to autism. *Curr. Opin. Neurobiol.* **2009**, *19*, 231–234. [CrossRef]
5. Delorme, R.; Ey, E.; Toro, R.; Leboyer, M.; Gillberg, C.; Bourgeron, T. Progress toward treatments for synaptic defects in autism. *Nat. Med.* **2013**, *19*, 685–694. [CrossRef] [PubMed]
6. Grabrucker, A.M.; Schmeisser, M.J.; Schoen, M.; Boeckers, T.M. Postsynaptic ProSAP/SHANK scaffolds in the cross-hair of synaptopathies. *Trends Cell. Biol.* **2011**, *21*, 594–603. [CrossRef]
7. Guilmatre, A.; Huguet, G.; Delorme, R.; Bourgeron, T. The emerging role of *SHANK* genes in neuropsychiatric disorders. *Dev. Neurobiol.* **2014**, *74*, 113–122. [CrossRef]
8. Bonaglia, M.C.; Giorda, R.; Borgatti, R.; Felisari, G.; Gagliardi, C.; Selicorni, A.; Zuffardi, O. Disruption of the ProSAP2 gene in a t(12;22)(q24.1;q13.3) is associated with the 22q13 deletion syndrome. *Am. J. Hum. Genet.* **2001**, *69*, 261–268. [CrossRef] [PubMed]
9. Kolevzon, A.; Angarita, B.; Bush, L.; Wang, A.T.; Frank, Y.; Yang, A.; Rapaport, R.; Saland, J.; Srivastava, S.; Farrell, C.; et al. Phelan-McDermid syndrome: A review of the literature and practice parameters for medical assessment and monitoring. *J. Neurodev. Disord.* **2014**, *6*, 39. [CrossRef]
10. Wong, A.C.; Ning, Y.; Flint, J.; Clark, K.; Dumanski, J.P.; Ledbetter, D.H.; McDermid, H.E. Molecular characterization of a 130-kb terminal microdeletion at 22q in a child with mild mental retardation. *Am. J. Hum. Genet.* **1997**, *60*, 113–120. [PubMed]
11. Huett, A.; Leong, J.M.; Podolsky, D.K.; Xavier, R.J. The cytoskeletal scaffold SHANK3 is recruited to pathogen-induced actin rearrangements. *Exp. Cell Res.* **2009**, *315*, 2001–2011. [CrossRef]
12. Pfaender, S.; Sauer, A.K.; Hagmeyer, S.; Mangus, K.; Linta, L.; Liebau, S.; Bockmann, J.; Huguet, G.; Bourgeron, T.; Boeckers, T.M.; et al. Zinc deficiency and low enterocyte zinc transporter expression in human patients with autism related mutations in SHANK3. *Sci. Rep.* **2017**, *7*, 45190. [CrossRef]
13. Vela, G.; Stark, P.; Socha, M.; Sauer, A.K.; Hagmeyer, S.; Grabrucker, A.M. Zinc in gut–brain interaction in Autism and neurological disorders. *Neural Plast.* **2015**, *2015*, 972791. [CrossRef]
14. Hughes, H.; Ko, E.M.; Rose, D.; Ashwood, P. Immune Dysfunction and Autoimmunity as Pathological Mechanisms in Autism Spectrum Disorders. *Front. Cell. Neurosci.* **2018**, *12*, 405. [CrossRef]
15. Mulle, J.G.; Sharp, W.G.; Cubells, J.F. The gut microbiome: A new frontier in autism research. *Curr. Psychiatry Rep.* **2013**, *15*, 337. [CrossRef]
16. Tabouy, L.; Getselter, D.; Ziv, O.; Karpuj, M.; Tabouy, T.; Lukic, I.; Maayouf, R.; Werbner, N.; Ben-Amram, H.; Nuriel-Ohayon, M.; et al. Dysbiosis of microbiome and probiotic treatment in a genetic model of autism spectrum disorders. *Brain Behav. Immun.* **2018**, *73*, 310–319. [CrossRef]
17. Jiang, Y.H.; Ehlers, M.D. Modeling autism by SHANK gene mutations in mice. *Neuron* **2013**, *78*, 8–27. [CrossRef]

18. Yoo, J.; Bakes, J.; Bradley, C.; Collingridge, G.L.; Kaang, B.K. SHANK mutant mice as an animal model of autism. *Philos. Trans. R. Soc. B Biol. Sci.* **2014**, *369*, 20130143. [CrossRef]
19. Wang, M.; Zhou, J.; He, F.; Cai, C.; Wang, H.; Wang, Y.; Lin, Y.; Rong, H.; Cheng, G.; Xu, R.; Zhou, W. Alteration of gut microbiota-associated epitopes in children with autism spectrum disorders. *Brain Behav. Immun.* **2018**, *75*, 192–199. [CrossRef]
20. Gumusoglu, S.B.; Stevens, H.E. Maternal Inflammation and Neurodevelopmental Programming: A Review of Preclinical Outcomes and Implications for Translational Psychiatry. *Biol. Psychiatry* **2018**, *85*, 107–121. [CrossRef]
21. Boulanger-Bertolus, J.; Pancaro, C.; Mashour, G.A. Increasing Role of Maternal Immune Activation in Neurodevelopmental Disorders. *Front. Behav. Neurosci.* **2018**, *12*, 230. [CrossRef]
22. Yang, C.J.; Liu, C.L.; Sang, B.; Zhu, X.M.; Du, Y.J. The combined role of serotonin and interleukin-6 as biomarker for autism. *Neuroscience* **2015**, *2015*. *284*, 290–296. [CrossRef]
23. Gumusoglu, S.B.; Fine, R.S.; Murray, S.J.; Bittle, J.L.; Stevens, H.E. The role of IL-6 in neurodevelopment after prenatal stress. *Brain Behav. Immun.* **2017**, *65*, 274–283. [CrossRef]
24. Wei, H.; Alberts, I.; Li, X. Brain IL-6 and autism. *Neuroscience* **2013**, *252*, 320–325. [CrossRef]
25. Parker-Athill, E.C.; Tan, J. Maternal immune activation and autism spectrum disorder: Interleukin-6 signaling as a key mechanistic pathway. *Neurosignals* **2010**, *18*, 113–128. [CrossRef]
26. Petrelli, F.; Pucci, L.; Bezzi, P. Astrocytes and Microglia and Their Potential Link with Autism Spectrum Disorders. *Front. Cell. Neurosci* **2016**, *10*, 21. [CrossRef] [PubMed]
27. Schmeisser, M.J.; Ey, E.; Wegener, S.; Bockmann, J.; Stempel, A.V.; Kuebler, A.; Janssen, A.-L.; Udvardi, P.T.; Shiban, E.; Spilker, C.; et al. Autistic-like behaviours and hyperactivity in mice lacking ProSAP1/SHANK2. *Nature* **2012**, *486*, 256–260. [CrossRef]
28. Nik, A.M.; Carlsson, P. Separation of intact intestinal epithelium from mesenchyme. *Biotechniques* **2013**, *55*, 42–44. [CrossRef] [PubMed]
29. Huguet, G.; Ey, E.; Bourgeron, T. The genetic landscapes of autism spectrum disorders. *Annu. Rev. Genom. Hum. Genet.* **2013**, *14*, 191–213. [CrossRef]
30. Fasano, A. Zonulin and its regulation of intestinal barrier function: The biological door to inflammation, autoimmunity, and cancer. *Physiol Rev.* **2011**, *91*, 151–175. [CrossRef]
31. Stevens, B.R.; Goel, R.; Seungbum, K.; Richards, E.M.; Holbert, R.C.; Pepine, C.J.; Raizada, M.K. Increased human intestinal barrier permeability plasma biomarkers zonulin and FABP2 correlated with plasma LPS and altered gut microbiome in anxiety or depression. *Gut.* **2018**, *67*, 1555–1557. [CrossRef] [PubMed]
32. Sturgeon, C.; Fasano, A. Zonulin, a regulator of epithelial and endothelial barrier functions, and its involvement in chronic inflammatory diseases. *Tissue Barriers* **2016**, *4*, e1251384. [CrossRef] [PubMed]
33. Szabo, G.; Bala, S.; Petrasek, J.; Gattu, A. Gut-liver axis and sensing microbes. *Dig. Dis.* **2010**, *28*, 737–744. [CrossRef]
34. Jirillo, E.; Caccavo, D.; Magrone, T.; Piccigallo, E.; Amati, L.; Lembo, A.; Kalis, C.; Gumenscheimer, M. The role of the liver in the response to LPS: Experimental and clinical findings. *J. Endotoxin Res.* **2002**, *8*, 319–327. [CrossRef] [PubMed]
35. Gardiner, B.J.; Tai, A.Y.; Kotsanas, D.; Francis, M.J.; Roberts, S.A.; Ballard, S.A.; Junckerstorff, R.K.; Korman, T.M. Clinical and microbiological characteristics of Eggerthella lenta bacteremia. *J. Clin. Microbiol.* **2015**, *53*, 626–635. [CrossRef]
36. Clavel, T.; Duck, W.; Charrier, C.; Wenning, M.; Elson, C.; Haller, D. *Enterorhabdus caecimuris* sp. nov., a member of the family *Coriobacteriaceae* isolated from a mouse model of spontaneous colitis, and emended description of the genus *Enterorhabdus* Clavel et al. 2009. *Int. J. Syst. Evol. Microbiol.* **2010**, *60*, 1527–1531. [CrossRef]
37. De Angelis, M.; Francavilla, R.; Piccolo, M.; de Giacomo, A.; Gobbetti, M. Autism spectrum disorders and intestinal microbiota. *Gut Microbes* **2015**, *6*, 207–213. [CrossRef]
38. Wang, Y.; Kasper, L.H. The role of microbiome in central nervous system disorders. *Brain Behav. Immun.* **2014**, *38*, 1–12. [CrossRef]
39. Arumugam, M.; Raes, J.; Pelletier, E.; Le Paslier, D.; Yamada, T.; Mende, D.R. Enterotypes of the human gut microbiome. *Nature* **2011**, *473*, 174–180. [CrossRef]

40. Finegold, S.M.; Dowd, S.E.; Gontcharova, V.; Liu, C.; Henley, K.E.; Wolcott, R.D.; Youn, E.; Summanen, P.H.; Granpeesheh, D.; Dixon, D.; et al. Pyrosequencing study of fecal microflora of autistic and control children. *Anaerobe* **2010**, *16*, 444–453. [CrossRef]
41. Loy, A.; Pfann, C.; Steinberger, M.; Hanson, B.; Herp, S.; Brugiroux, S.; Gomes Neto, J.C.; Boekschoten, M.V.; Schwab, C.; Urich, T.; et al. Lifestyle and Horizontal Gene Transfer-Mediated Evolution of Mucispirillum schaedleri, a Core Member of the Murine Gut Microbiota. *Msystems* **2017**, *2*, e00171-16. [CrossRef] [PubMed]
42. De Angelis, M.; Piccolo, M.; Vannini, L.; Siragusa, S.; de Giacomo, A.; Serrazzanetti, D.I.; Cristofori, F.; Guerzoni, M.E.; Gobbetti, M.; Francavilla, R. Fecal microbiota and metabolome of children with autism and pervasive developmental disorder not otherwise specified. *PLoS ONE* **2013**, *8*, e76993. [CrossRef]
43. Ricanek, P.; Lothe, S.M.; Frye, S.A.; Rydning, A.; Vatn, M.H.; Tønjum, T. Gut bacterial profile in patients newly diagnosed with treatment-naïve Crohn's disease. *Clin. Exp. Gastroenterol.* **2012**, *5*, 173–186. [CrossRef]
44. Luna, R.A.; Oezguen, N.; Balderas, M.; Venkatachalam, A.; Runge, J.K.; Versalovic, J.; Veenstra-VanderWeele, J.; Anderson, G.M.; Savidge, T.; Williams, K.C. Distinct Microbiome-Neuroimmune Signatures Correlate With Functional Abdominal Pain in Children With Autism Spectrum Disorder. *Cell Mol. Gastroenterol. Hepatol.* **2017**, *3*, 218–230. [CrossRef]
45. Wang, L.; Christophersen, C.T.; Sorich, M.J.; Gerber, J.P.; Angley, M.T.; Conlon, M.A. Low relative abundances of the mucolytic bacterium *Akkermansia muciniphila* and *Bifidobacterium* spp. in feces of children with autism. *Appl. Environ. Microbiol.* **2011**, *77*, 6718–6721. [CrossRef]
46. De Magistris, L.; Familiari, V.; Pascotto, A.; Sapone, A.; Frolli, A.; Iardino, P.; Garteni, M.; de Rosa, M.; Francavilla, R.; Riegler, G.; et al. Alterations of the intestinal barrier in patients with autism spectrum disorders and in their first-degree relatives. *J. Pediatr. Gastroenterol. Nutr.* **2010**, *51*, 418–424. [CrossRef] [PubMed]
47. Camilleri, M.; Gormyan, H. Intestinal permeability and irritable bowel syndrome. *Neurogastroenterol. Motil.* **2007**, *19*, 545–552. [CrossRef]
48. D'Eufemia, P.; Celli, M.; Finocchiaro, R.; Pacifico, L.; Viozzi, L.; Zaccagnini, M.; Cardi, E.; Giardini, O. Abnormal intestinal permeability in children with autism. *Acta Paediatr.* **1996**, *85*, 1076–1079. [CrossRef]
49. El Asmar, R.; Panigrahi, P.; Bamford, P.; Berti, I.; Not, T.; Coppa, G.V.; Catassi, C.; Fasano, A. Host-dependent zonulin secretion causes the impairment of the small intestine barrier function after bacterial exposure. *Gastroenterology* **2002**, *123*, 1607–1615. [CrossRef]
50. Dossi, E.; Vasile, F.; Rouach, N. Human astrocytes in the diseased brain. *Brain. Res. Bull.* **2018**, *136*, 139–156. [CrossRef]
51. Edmonson, C.; Ziats, M.N.; Rennert, O.M. Altered glial marker expression in autistic post-mortem prefrontal cortex and cerebellum. *Mol. Autism.* **2014**, *5*, 3. [CrossRef] [PubMed]
52. Grabrucker, S.; Jannetti, L.; Eckert, M.; Gaub, S.; Chhabra, R.; Pfaender, S.; Mangus, K.; Reddy, P.P.; Rankovic, V.; Schmeisser, M.J.; et al. Zinc deficiency dysregulates the synaptic ProSAP/SHANK scaffold and might contribute to autism spectrum disorders. *Brain* **2014**, *137*, 137–152. [CrossRef] [PubMed]
53. Angly, F.E.; Dennis, P.G.; Skarshewski, A.; Vanwonterghem, I.; Hugenholtz, P.; Tyson, G.W. CopyRighter: A rapid tool for improving the accuracy of microbial community profiles through lineage-specific gene copy number correction. *Microbiome* **2014**, *2*, 11. [CrossRef] [PubMed]

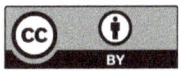

© 2019 by the authors. Licensee MDPI, Basel, Switzerland. This article is an open access article distributed under the terms and conditions of the Creative Commons Attribution (CC BY) license (http://creativecommons.org/licenses/by/4.0/).

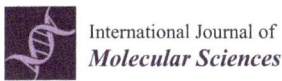

Review

Crmp4-KO Mice as an Animal Model for Investigating Certain Phenotypes of Autism Spectrum Disorders

Ritsuko Ohtani-Kaneko

Graduate School of Life Sciences, Toyo University, 1-1-1 Itakura, Oura 374-0193, Japan; r-kaneko@toyo.jp

Received: 24 April 2019; Accepted: 18 May 2019; Published: 20 May 2019

Abstract: Previous research has demonstrated that the collapsin response mediator protein (CRMP) family is involved in the formation of neural networks. A recent whole-exome sequencing study identified a de novo variant (S541Y) of collapsin response mediator protein 4 (CRMP4) in a male patient with autism spectrum disorder (ASD). In addition, *Crmp4*-knockout (KO) mice show some phenotypes similar to those observed in human patients with ASD. For example, compared with wild-type mice, *Crmp4*-KO mice exhibit impaired social interaction, abnormal sensory sensitivities, broader distribution of activated (c-Fos expressing) neurons, altered dendritic formation, and aberrant patterns of neural gene expressions, most of which have sex differences. This review summarizes current knowledge regarding the role of CRMP4 during brain development and discusses the possible contribution of CRMP4 deficiencies or abnormalities to the pathogenesis of ASD. *Crmp4*-KO mice represent an appropriate animal model for investigating the mechanisms underlying some ASD phenotypes, such as impaired social behavior, abnormal sensory sensitivities, and sex-based differences, and other neurodevelopmental disorders associated with sensory processing disorders.

Keywords: collapsin response mediator protein 4; autism spectrum disorder; neurodevelopmental disorder; whole-exome sequencing; animal model; sex different phenotypes

---

1. Introduction

The formation of neural networks is temporally and spatially regulated by numerous molecules, such as extracellular molecules regulating cell adhesion and axon guidance, and intracellular signaling molecules regulating axon elongation and the formation of dendrites, spines, and synapses. Collapsin response mediator proteins (CRMPs) are intracellular signaling molecules elicited by extracellular signals (e.g., semaphorin (Sema) 3A and reelin) during neuronal migration, differentiation, neurite network organization, and even remodeling [1–3]. Genome-wide studies, genetic linkage analyses, proteomic analyses, and translational approaches have revealed altered expression levels of CRMPs in neurodevelopmental disorders, such as schizophrenia, attention-deficit/hyperactivity disorder (ADHD), and autism spectrum disorder (ASD) [3–8]. Similar findings have been observed for neurological disorders such as Alzheimer's disease [9–11] and hyperalgesia syndrome [12–15]. Furthermore, during the past decade, many studies using knockout (KO) mice have demonstrated the role of CRMPs in the pathogenesis of neurodevelopmental disorders, as described in Section 3 below. In our recent whole-exome sequencing study, we identified a de novo variant of *CRMP4* in a male patient with ASD [8]. In this review, we discuss the functions of CRMP4 in the developing brain and the possible involvement of CRMP4 deficiencies and abnormalities in the pathogenesis of neurodevelopmental disorders.

2. Identification of CRMP4

Sema1A guides the growth cone in the proper direction during neural circuit formation in the developing brain. Sema1A was first identified as fasciclin IV in *Drosophila* [16] and subsequently identified as collapsin in chickens [17]. Since then, numerous members of the Sema family have been identified. Among them, Sema3A has been implicated in each step of neural circuit formation from axonal and dendritic development to synaptic assembly [18–21]. Goshima et al. [22] identified a CRMP with a relative molecular mass of 62 kDa (CRMP-62), now known as CRMP2, which is required for Sema3A-induced inward currents in the *Xenopus laevis* oocyte expression system. The authors further reported that introduction of anti-CRMP-62 antibodies into dorsal root ganglion neurons blocks Sema3A-induced growth cone collapse [22]. In 1995, Minturn et al. identified a 64-kDa protein in the rat embryo known as turned on after division 64 (TOAD-64), which was eventually classified as CRMP4 [23,24]. The CRMP family comprises five homologous cytosolic proteins (CRMP1 ~ 5) with high (50–70%) homology. CRMP4 is also referred to as TUC-4, unc-33-like phosphoprotein 1 (Ulip-1), dihydropyrimidase 3 (DRP3), and dihydropyrimidase-like 3 (DPYSL3) because those were found to be homologous to CRMP4 later [23–26]. These multiple names of CRMP4 have sometimes caused confusion.

3. The Regulatory Mechanisms Suggested for CRMP4

CRMPs regulate intercellular signaling pathways mediated through extracellular molecules such as Sema3A, reelin, neurotrophins, and myelin-associated inhibitors (MAIs) [22–28]. Through transduction of these extracellular cues, CRMPs have been reported to regulate various neurodevelopmental events including neuronal apoptosis, migration, axonal elongation, dendritic elongation and branching, spine development, and synaptic plasticity [27–31]. CRMP functions are controlled by the dynamic spatiotemporal regulation of phosphorylation status, which is mediated by kinases such as Cdk5, Rho/ROCK, and GSK3β, which alter CRMP binding to various cytoskeletal proteins such as actin, tubulin, and tau [32–36]. Cytoskeletal proteins regulate neuronal polarity, axonal and dendritic outgrowth, neuronal migration, synaptic formation, and other functions of neurons like transportation of neurotransmitters-containing vesicles. Therefore, effects on cytoskeletal dynamics promote neurodevelopmental responses mediated by CRMPs.

Numerous studies have focused on the relationship between CRMP phosphorylation and the roles of CRMPs. For example, MAIs regulate neurite extension via the phosphorylation of CRMP4, which is mediated by upstream phospho-inactivation of GSK3β [28]. Loss of GSK3β phosphorylation permits L-CRMP4–RhoA binding and suppresses neurite outgrowth. Therefore, MAI–CRMP4 signaling normally contributes to myelin-dependent growth inhibition [37]. Additionally, phosphorylation of CRMP2 and CRMP4 by Cdk5 is required for the proper positioning of Rohon–Beard primary sensory neurons and neural crest cells as well as caudal primary motor neurons in the zebrafish spinal cord during neurulation [38,39].

In addition to phosphorylation, truncation of CRMP4 by calpain-mediated cleavage is found in glutamate- and N-methyl-D-aspartate (NMDA) receptor-induced excitotoxicity and oxidative stress, both of which reduce cellar viability in primary cultured cortical neurons [40–42]. The similar regulatory mechanism of CRMP4 is also involved in potassium deprivation-induced apoptosis in cultured cerebellar granule cells [43].

Furthermore, CRMP4 is expressed as both a short isoform (CRMP4a) and a longer isoform (CRMP4b) [44,45]. Previous studies have indicated that these two isoforms exhibit opposing functions during neurite outgrowth [44,46], though the mechanisms regulating their expressions remain unclear.

4. Potential Involvement of CRMPs Including CRMP4 in Neurodevelopmental Disorders

CRMP family genes and proteins are abundantly expressed in the developing brain, strongly suggesting that they play important roles in neuronal circuit formation [23,47,48]. Furthermore, in situ hybridization experiments have revealed that there are regional differences in *Crmp4* mRNA expression during postnatal brain development [49]. In addition, while *Crmp4* mRNA expression is scarcely detectable in most areas of the adult brain, it remains considerably detectable in adult neurogenic regions containing immature neurons, such as the subgranular zone of the dentate gyrus and subventricular zone–olfactory bulb (OB) migratory pathway [49]. Such findings highlight the crucial role of CRMP4 in neuronal circuit formation.

Abnormal CRMP expression in the brain has been associated with several neurodevelopmental disorders. For example, patients with schizophrenia exhibit alterations in levels of CRMP1 and CRMP2 protein (for review, see [4], [7,50–52]. Liu et al. [53] suggested that reduced transcription and mTOR-regulated translation of certain DPYSL2 isoforms (i.e., genes encoding CRMP2) increase the risk of schizophrenia. Lee et al. [6] further reported that two functional single-nucleotide polymorphisms of the human DRYSL2 gene are associated with susceptibility to schizophrenia. Pham et al. [7] demonstrated that allelic variants of the di-nucleotide repeat at the 5′-untranslated repeat of *DPYSL2* change the interaction between CRMP2 and mTOR effector proteins. In addition, findings obtained from *Crmp1*- and *Crmp2*-KO mice suggest that impairments in CRMP1 and CRMP2 functions are involved in the pathogenesis of schizophrenia [5,54,55]. Furthermore, brain-specific *Crmp2*-KO mice display molecular, cellular, structural, and behavioral deficits, many of which are reminiscent of the features associated with schizophrenia [56].

In contrast to CRMP1 and CRMP2, relatively few studies have investigated the involvement of CRMP4 in neurodevelopmental disorders [8,57–59]. Miller et al. [57] suggested that microRNA (miR)-132, CREB-regulated miRNA associated with NMDAR signaling, is involved in the pathogenesis of schizophrenia and revealed that expressions of several genes including CRMP4 (DPYSL3) are regulated by miR-132, though the relation between CRMP4 and miR-132 and that between CRMP4 and schizophrenia remain unknown. A missense variant and four other de novo variants of the CRMP4 gene were identified in an ASD proband from the Simons Simplex Collection [58]. A recent whole-exome sequencing study also identified another likely pathogenic missense variant in the *CRMP4* gene (*CRMP4^{S541Y}*) in a male patient with ASD [8]. In addition, Tsutiya et al. [8] investigated the effect of *Crmp4* missense mutation, which was found in ASD patients, on dendritic extension. In their study, dendritic formation was compared among neurons from wild type (WT) mice (WT neurons) transfected with enhanced green fluorescent protein (pEGFP), and neurons from *Crmp4*-KO mice (*Crmp4*-KO neurons) transfected with either a pEGFP, pEGFP-WT *Crmp4* or pEGFP-*Crmp4^{S540Y}* (the site homologous to human S541) (Figure 1). *Crmp4*-KO neurons transfected with pEGFP had significantly longer dendrites with more branching points than WT-neurons transfected with pEGFP. *Crmp4*-KO neurons transfected with pEGFP-*Crmp4^{S540Y}* exhibited significantly greater numbers of dendritic branching points than *Crmp4*-KO neurons transfected with pEGFP-WT *Crmp4* (Figure 1). These results suggest that ASD-linked CRMP4 mutations alter dendritic morphology. Furthermore, accumulating evidence suggests that *Crmp4*-KO mice exhibit several phenotypes that resemble those observed in human patients with ASD (DSM-V [60]). In the following sections, we review the autism-like phenotypes observed in *Crmp4*-KO mice and other animal models of ASD.

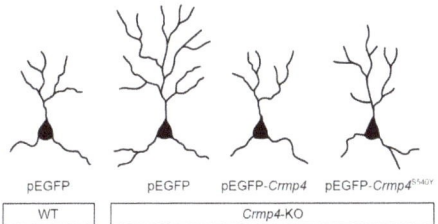

Figure 1. Schematic drawings showing dendritic arborization of cultured hippocampal pyramidal neurons differentially expressing CRMP4. The S540Y mutation in mouse *Crmp4* is homologous to S541Y in human *CRMP4*, which was observed in a patient with autism spectrum disorder (ASD). Representative drawings of cultured hippocampal cells from wildtype (WT) mice transfected with control (pEGFP) vector, *Crmp4*-knockout (KO) mice transfected with pEGFP vector, *Crmp4*-KO mice transfected with pEGFP-*Crmp4* vector, and *Crmp4*-KO mice transfected with pEGFP-*Crmp4^{S540Y}* vector. CRMP: collapsin response mediator protein.

5. Behavioral and Perceptual Abnormalities Observed in *Crmp4*-KO Mice

5.1. Impairments in Social Behavior

Tsutiya et al. [8,61] examined behavioral deficits in young or adolescent *Crmp4*-KO mice. Their open-field test and elevated plus maze results suggested that *Crmp4*-KO mice of both sexes exhibited locomotive activity and anxiety levels similar to those observed in WT mice. Similarly, the novel object recognition test revealed no significant differences in memory acquisition/retention between WT and *Crmp4*-KO mice of both sexes. However, the authors also utilized the three-chamber test for investigating social behavior, which compares time spent investigating (sniffing) a stranger mouse and a novel object. Male *Crmp4*-KO mice spent significantly more time in the "object side chamber" than in the "stranger side chamber", while WT mice of both sexes and female *Crmp4*-KO mice spent more time sniffing the stranger mouse. In addition, in the social interaction test, male *Crmp4*-KO mice spent significantly less time actively interacting with a stranger mouse than male WT littermates, although there were no significant differences in the amount of active interaction between WT and *Crmp4*-KO females. These findings indicate that male-dominant impairments in social behavior can be observed in *Crmp4*-KO mice [8].

5.2. Abnormalities in Sensory Perception

"Hyper-reactivity or hypo-reactivity to sensory input" is among the diagnostic criteria for ASD specified in the DSM-V. Recent studies have indicated that patients with ASD exhibit neural hyperactivity [62,63], which may account for abnormal sensory sensitivity. Neuronal hyperactivity is considered to result from membrane hyperexcitability and/or abnormal connectivity in neural circuits, such as recurrent excitation or a change in the balance between excitatory and inhibitory synaptic input. Altered neural activity has also been observed in animal models of ASD. For example, mice with null mutations in the *Fmr1* gene exhibit social deficits [64] and impaired sensory adaptation [65], which may be due to cortical hyper-excitability [66]. In addition, mice with null mutations of *Shank2* exhibit social deficits [67,68] and have been reported to exhibit hypo-excitability to mechanical and noxious heat stimuli as well as to inflammatory and neuropathic pain [69].

Several studies have examined sensory perception in *Crmp4*-KO mice. Tsutiya et al. [8,61] reported that *Crmp4*-KO pups exhibit alterations in temperature and olfactory perceptions when compared to WT mice. Infant mice produce ultrasonic vocalizations (UVs) as a normal response to sensory stimulation [70], and the number of UVs is usually used to evaluate the sensory perception ability.

The numbers of UVs emitted by WT and *Crmp4*-KO pups of both sexes are similar at room temperature (RT, 23 °C). However, when WT pups of both sexes and *Crmp4*-KO females were subjected to a 19 °C environment, they produced significantly more UVs. When moved from RT to 9 °C, both groups emitted significantly fewer UVs. Surprisingly, when *Crmp4*-KO males were moved from RT to a 19 °C environment, the authors observed no increases in the number of UVs emitted. However, the number of UVs significantly increased when *Crmp4*-KO males were moved from RT to 9 °C. These findings indicate that temperature perception markedly differs between *Crmp4*-KO males and WT mice of both sexes/*Crmp4*-KO females [8].

In addition, *Crmp4*-KO mice of both sexes demonstrate impaired olfactory sensitivity when compared to WTs [8,61]. In these previous studies, WT pups of both sexes produced more UVs during exposure to unfamiliar bedding than during exposure to familiar bedding. In contrast, there was no significant difference in the number of UVs emitted by *Crmp4*-KO pups of both sexes when exposed to the different smells.

Many people diagnosed with ASD have difficulty processing sensory information, which often manifests as hyper- or hypo-sensitivity to sensory stimuli. To examine whether *Crmp4* KO is associated with hyper- or hypo-sensitivity to olfactory stimuli, a previous study utilized immunohistochemical experiments to examine the expression of the neuronal activity marker c-Fos following exposure to the odorant ethyl acetate (EA) [61]. Cells positive for c-Fos were counted in each layer of the OB (glomerular layer (GL), external plexiform layer (EPL), mitral cell layer (MCL), granule cell layer (GCL)) and compared among male WT pups and *Crmp4*-KOs with or without EA exposure. In WT and *Crmp4*-KO males without EA stimulation, only a few c-Fos-positive cells were observed in sections of the OB. In accordance with a study by Van der Gucht et al. [71], who reported that c-Fos is expressed by neurons after sensory induction, many c-Fos-positive cells were detected after EA exposure. Research has indicated that specific odorants induce neuronal activity in a spatially restricted area known as the odorant map [72,73]. The study has reported that c-Fos-positive cells can be observed in restricted areas of the EPL, MCL, and GCL of WT pups after EA exposure, and that the distribution of these cells is similar for the previous work performed in adult WT mice exposed to EA [74]. In contrast, *Crmp4*-KO pups exhibited broad, dramatic increases in the number of c-Fos-positive cells in all OB layers following EA exposure. Therefore, the number of active neurons with c-Fos expression is much greater in *Crmp4*-KO pups than in WT pups after exposure to a single odorant (EA), suggesting that the altered olfactory perception observed in *Crmp4*-KO pups stems from neuronal hyperactivity in the OB and may be other brain areas related to perception.

6. Altered Dendritic Arborization in *Crmp4*-KO Mice and *Crmp4*-Knockdown (KD) Neurons

As shown in Section 3, transfection of cultured hippocampal *Crmp4* −/− neurons with mutated mouse CRMP4^{S540Y} (homologous to human CRMP4^{S541Y} found in a patient with ASD) increases dendritic branching when compared to transfection of WT *Crmp4*. Several studies have also reported altered dendritic involvement in other mouse models of ASD [75–78]. Indeed, animal models of ASD exhibit hippocampal and cortical pyramidal neurons with significantly longer apical and basal dendrites, as well as significantly greater branching, than WT neurons.

Recent studies have reported that dendritic morphology and axon elongation are altered in *Crmp4*-KO mice and *Crmp4*-knockdown (KD) cells [46,59,79–82]. Niisato et al. [79,80] revealed that deficiency of CRMP4 increases the bifurcation of pyramidal neuron apical dendrites in the mouse hippocampus and in primary cultures. Cha et al. [81] further reported that overexpression of the C-terminal actin-interacting site of CRMP4 facilitates dendritic growth in cultured hippocampal neurons. Using the DiI tracing method, Tsutiya et al. [8] reported that the extension of apical dendrites from OB mitral cells in vivo is enhanced in *Crmp4*-KO neonates, to those in WT animals [59]. Exaggerated elongation of neurites has also been observed in hippocampal neuronal cell line (HT22) cells transfected with *Crmp4* siRNA (*Crmp4*-KD HT22 cells) [59]. In addition, dendritic length and branching are greater in cultured hippocampal pyramidal neurons derived from *Crmp4*-KO neonates than in those derived from WT mice [8]. In contrast, overexpression of *Crmp4* suppresses dendritic elongation and branching in these cells [8]. Collectively, these results suggest that deficiencies in CRMP4 can increase dendritic elongation and branching in various types of neurons.

7. Altered Expressions of Genes Related to Excitatory and Inhibitory Synaptic Transmission in the Brain of *Crmp4*-KO Mice

ASD has been reported to be associated with alterations in the expression of several genes related to receptors, transporters, and synthesis enzymes for neurotransmitters such as glutamate, γ-aminobutyric acid (GABA), dopamine, serotonin, acetylcholine, and histamine (for review, see [83]). In addition, *Crmp4*-KO mice exhibit alterations in the expression of genes mainly related to the glutamatergic and GABAergic systems [8,61]. Since abnormalities in glutamate and GABA have been hypothesized to underlie ASD symptoms, recent translational proton magnetic resonance spectroscopy (MRS) studies have investigated levels of glutamate and GABA in adult humans with ASD as well as rodent ASD models. Such studies have reported that glutamate concentrations in the striatum are decreased in human patients with ASD and some animal models, although no such alterations in GABA levels were observed [84]. Glutamatergic abnormalities are well known to occur in models of ASD (for review, see [85]): For example, proline-rich synapse-associated protein 1 (ProSAP1/Shank2)-KO mice exhibit early, region-specific upregulation of ionotropic glutamate receptors at the synapse [67]. In addition, telomerase reverse transcriptase-overexpressing (TERT transgenic, TERT-tg) mice exhibit male-specific autism-like behaviors, as well as increases in the expression of the NMDA receptor NR2A and NR2B subunits and AMPA receptor GluR1 and GluR2 subunits. TERT-tg mice also exhibit increases in vesicular glutamate transporter (vGluT) 1 levels in the prefrontal cortex [86]. Furthermore, research has indicated that glutamatergic modulators may aid in the treatment of ASD in humans [83,87] and animal models [85,88,89], supporting the notion that the glutamatergic system plays a role in ASD and ASD-like phenotypes.

Male *Crmp4*-KO pups exhibit significantly greater mRNA and protein expressions of AMPA receptor subunits GluR1 and GluR2 than their WT counterparts [61]. Adult *Crmp4*-KO mice also exhibit sex- and region-dependent differences in levels of *GluR1, GluR2, vGluT1, vGluT2, GABAAα1, GABAAγ2, GABAB receptor 1*, and vesicular GABA transporter expressions. However, no significant differences in the expression of other genes (e.g., serotonin transporter mRNA in the raphe nucleus and dopamine D2 receptors (D2Rs) in the cortex) are observed between *Crmp4*-KO and WT mice of either sex [8]. These data support the notion that *Crmp4* deficiency induces alterations in glutamatergic- and some GABAergic-associated genes, which may be associated with the pathogenesis of certain autism-like features in *Crmp4*-KO mice.

Many studies have implicated altered excitatory (glutamatergic)/inhibitory (GABAergic) balance in the pathogenesis of ASD [90–93]. However, altered gene expressions in *Crmp4*-KO mice do not necessarily mean the excitatory/inhibitory balance. Future physiological investigations of *Crmp4*-KO mice may help to reveal the functional meaning of alterations in glutamatergic and GABAergic gene expressions, and whether such alterations are associated with autism-like phenotypes.

8. Sex-Specific Phenotypes Observed in *Crmp4*-KO Mice and Other Animal Models of ASD

ASD is more prevalent among boys than girls, and there are substantial sex-based differences in ASD phenotypes [94–97]. For example, male-biased differences have been observed in patients with ASD exhibiting mutations in genes that encode the synaptic cell adhesion protein neuroligin (*NLGN*), including *NLGN 3*, and *NLGN4X* [98,99]. Sex-based differences in autistic-like phenotypes have also been reported in animal models of ASD generated by exposure to chemicals or genetic manipulation [8,67,86,100–103]. For example, Schneider et al. [102] demonstrated that prenatal exposure to valproic acid (VPA), which is well known to induce autism-like phenotypes in rats or mice [104], induces some male-specific alterations in behavior and immunological function. Kim et al. [86,101] further revealed that rats exposed to VPA in utero exhibit male-specific alterations in social interactions, hyperactive behavior, and impaired postsynaptic development. Konopko et al. [103] reported sex-based differences in the induction of some exons of the brain-derived neurotrophic factor (*Bdnf*) gene in the brains of fetal mice exposed to VPA during the prenatal period, indicating that female sex may confer neuroprotection against ASD-like phenotypes.

Some animal models of ASD developed by deleting genes found to be mutated or deficient in human patients with ASD exhibit sex-based differences in autism-like phenotypes. For example, UVs in response to brief separation from the mother are more prominent in female *Nlgn4*-KO pups than in their male counterparts [105]. In addition, adult *Shank2* −/− mice exhibit limited male-biased differences in the call rate and duration of UVs [100]. Tsutiya et al. [8] identified a rare *Crmp4* mutation in male patients with ASD. Furthermore, *Crmp4*-KO mice exhibit male-biased alterations in social behavior, sensory perception, and gene expression, as described in the preceding sections (Sections 3–6). Iwakura et al. [106] further revealed that CRMP4 is among the candidate proteins involved in the sexual differentiation of the anteroventral periventricular nucleus (AVPV) in the preoptic area of the hypothalamus. The AVPV, which is known to regulate ovulatory cycles, is larger in females than in males. This difference is due to the effects of testosterone (T) secreted from the testes of perinatal males [107]. In our previous study, which involved proteomics analysis followed by real-time PCR analysis, we observed that CRMP4 and *Crmp4* mRNA expression in the AVPV is sex-dependent during the critical period of sexual differentiation. In addition, prenatal testosterone propionate

(TP) treatment increased the expression of *Crmp4* mRNA during the critical period in females [106]. Moreover, the number of dopaminergic neurons in the nucleus was influenced by *Crmp4* deletion in females, suggesting that CRMP4 plays a sex-dependent role in the regulation of dopaminergic neuronal death or survival in this region [106]. However, the relationship between decreases in the number of dopaminergic neurons in the AVPV and ASD-like phenotypes in *Crmp4*-KO females remains uncertain.

Ferri et al. [108] argued that the male predominance of ASD may be associated with interactions between risk genes, which may not be sex-specific themselves, and sex-specific hormonal or immune-related pathways. Although several candidate hormones have been proposed, it has been suggested that androgens are associated with such differences because it is well known that natural secretion of androgens from the testes during the prenatal period contributes to the increased risk of ASD in males (i.e., prenatal sex steroid theory) [109–114]. Accumulating evidence has demonstrated the important role of prenatal androgens in many aspects of neural network formation through their effects on developing neurons and glia–neuron interactions [115,116]. In these studies, it is reported that prostaglandin and gonadal steroids including T and estradiol converted from T by aromatase influence synaptogenesis via their effects on developing glial cells, astrocytes and microglia. In an intensive post mortem study, Werling et al. [117] observed increased expression of astrocyte and microglia marker genes in the brains of male patients with ASD, suggesting that interactions between glial cells and neurons may be involved in sex-based differences in ASD phenotypes. Although the mechanisms underlying the pathogenesis of ASD and the target cells of androgens and/or estrogens converted from androgens remain unclear, perinatal androgen exposure may contribute to the sexually dimorphic pathophysiology of ASD. According to the prenatal sex steroid theory of autism, loss of the suppressive role of CRMP4 in *Crmp4*-KO mice in neuronal development may exaggerate the promotive effect of prenatal sex steroids, androgens and/or estrogens converted from androgens secreted from the testes, on neuronal network development, thereby resulting in male-biased ASD-like phenotypes.

9. Conclusions

CRMPs are known to regulate various aspect of neural development, playing key roles in neurodevelopmental disorders. As summarized in Figure 2, a previous whole-exosome sequencing study identified a single mutation of the *Crmp4* gene in a patient with ASD. Neurons from *Crmp4*-KO mice or neurons transfected with the mutation observed in the patient with ASD exhibit alterations in dendritic branching and/or extension (Figure 1). In addition, axonal elongation and cell viability are affected in *Crmp4*-KO mice, and in *Crmp4*-KD or -OE cells. *Crmp4*-KO mice also exhibit alterations in the expression of multiple genes contributing to glutamatergic and GABAergic neurotransmission, and most of these differences are sex- and region-specific. Single odorant stimulation induces hyperactivity (i.e., an increase in the number of c-Fos-positive cells) in the OB of *Crmp4*-KO pups. Furthermore, male *Crmp4*-KO mice exhibit more severe social and sensory deficits than females. Since most of their ASD-like phenotypes are sexually dimorphic, *Crmp4*-KO mice may represent a powerful model for investigating the pathogenesis of ASD and the prenatal sex steroid theory of autism in addition to *Crmp4*-KO mice possibly providing an animal model for investigating some other developmental disorders including ADHD and learning disabilities associated with sensory processing issues.

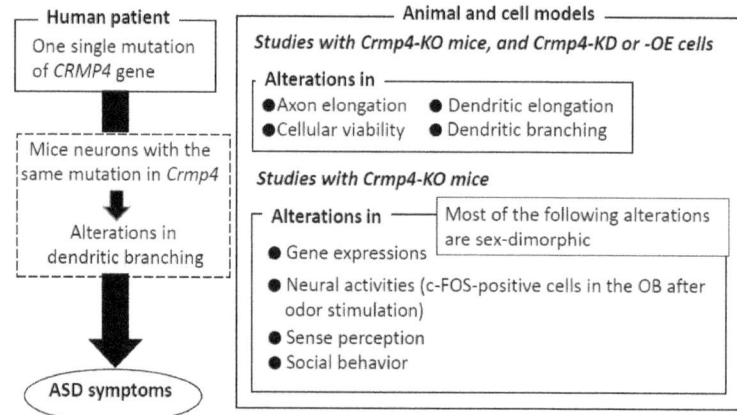

Figure 2. Summary of features associated with deficiency, overexpression, and mutation of *Crmp4*. *Crmp4*: collapsing response mediator protein; *Crmp4*-KO: *Crmp4*-knock out; *Crmp4*-KD: *Crmp4*-knockdown, *Crmp4*-OE: *Crmp4*-overexpression; OB: olfactory bulb; ASD: autism spectrum disorder.

Funding: This work was supported by Grants-in-Aid for Scientific Research (KAKENHI) from the Japan Society for the Promotion of Science (JSPS; Grant Numbers 16K07034), and partially supported by Research Center for Biomedical Engineering in Toyo University.

Acknowledgments: The author expresses sincere thanks to Y. Goshima, M. Nishihara, N. Yamashita, T. Iwakura, A. Tsutiya, Y. Nakano, A. Kitsu, K. Sato, M. Sakou, H. Watanabe, A. Kawahara, T. Kawachi, and S. Noma for their cooperation.

Conflicts of Interest: The author declares no conflict of interest.

Abbreviations

ADHD	attention-deficit/hyperactivity disorder
AMPA	α-amino-3-hydroxyl-5-methyl-4-isoxazole-propionate
ASD	autism spectrum disorder
AVPV	anteroventral periventricular nucleus
CRMP	collapsin response mediator protein
DRP	dihydropyrimidase; DPYSL3, dihydropyrimidase-like 3
EA	ethyl acetate
EPL	external plexiform layer
FMR1	fragile X mental retardation 1 gene
GCL	granule cell layer
GL	glomerular layer
GluR1	glutamate receptor 1
GluT1	glutamate transporter 1
KO	knockout
MAI	myelin-associated inhibitor
MCL	mitral cell layer
NMDA	N-methyl-D-aspartate
OB	olfactory bulb
RT	room temperature
TERT-tg mice	telomerase reverse transcriptase-overexpressing transgenic mice
TOAD-64	turned on after division 64
TUC-4	<u>T</u>OAD-64/<u>U</u>lip-1/<u>C</u>RMP4
Ulip-1	Ulip-1
UV	ultrasonic vocalization
vGluT1	vesicular glutamate transporter 1
WT	wild type

References

1. Charrier, E.; Reibel, S.; Rogemond, V.; Aguera, M.; Thomasset, N.; Honnorat, J. Collapsin response mediator proteins (CRMPs): Involvement in nervous system development and adult neurodegenerative disorders. *Mol. Neurol.* **2003**, *28*, 51–64. [CrossRef]
2. Schmidt, E.F.; Strittmatter, S.M. The CRMP family of proteins and their role in Sema3A signaling. *Adv. Exp. Med. Biol.* **2007**, *600*, 1–11. [PubMed]
3. Quach, T.T.; Honnorat, J.; Kolattukudy, P.E.; Khanna, R.; Duchemin, A.M. CRMPs: Critical molecules for neurite morphogenesis and neuropsychiatric diseases. *Mol. Psychiatry.* **2015**, *20*, 1037–1045. [CrossRef] [PubMed]
4. Hensley, K.; Venkova, K.; Christov, A.; Gunning, W.; Park, J. Collapsin response mediator protein-2: An emerging pathologic feature and therapeutic target for neurodisease indications. *Mol. Neurobiol.* **2011**, *43*, 180–191. [CrossRef] [PubMed]
5. Yamashita, N.; Takahashi, A.; Takao, K.; Yamamoto, T.; Kolattukudy, P.; Miyakawa, T.; Goshima, Y. Mice lacking collapsin response mediator protein 1 manifest hyperactivity, impaired learning and memory, and impaired prepulse inhibition. *Front. Behav. Neurosci.* **2013**, *7*, 216. [CrossRef]
6. Lee, H.; Joo, J.; Nah, S.S.; Kim, J.W.; Kim, H.K.; Kwon, J.T.; Lee, H.Y.; Kim, Y.O.; Kim, H.J. Changes in Dpysl2 expression are associated with prenatally stressed rat offspring and susceptibility to schizophrenia in humans. *Int. J. Mol. Med.* **2015**, *35*, 1574–1586. [CrossRef]
7. Pham, X.; Song, G.; Lao, S.; Goff, L.; Zhu, H.; Valle, D.; Avramopoulos, D. The DPYSL2 gene connects mTOR and schizophrenia. *Transl. Psychiatry* **2016**, *6*, e933. [CrossRef]
8. Tsutiya, A.; Nakano, Y.; Hansen-Kiss, E.; Kelly, B.; Nishihara, M.; Goshima, Y.; Corsmeier, D.; White, P.; Herman, G.E.; Ohtani-Kaneko, R. Human CRMP4 mutation and disrupted Crmp4 expression in mice are associated with ASD characteristics and sexual dimorphism. *Sci. Rep.* **2017**, *7*, 16812. [CrossRef]
9. Uchida, Y.; Ohshima, T.; Sasaki, Y.; Suzuki, H.; Yanai, S.; Yamashita, N.; Nakamura, F.; Takei, K.; Ihara, Y.; Mikoshiba, K.; et al. Semaphorin3A signalling is mediated via sequential Cdk5 and GSK3beta phosphorylation of CRMP2: Implication of common phosphorylating mechanism underlying axon guidance and Alzheimer's disease. *Genes Cells* **2005**, *10*, 165–179. [CrossRef]
10. Toba, J.; Nikkuni, M.; Ishizeki, M.; Yoshii, A.; Watamura, N.; Inoue, T.; Ohshima, T. PPARγ agonist pioglitazone improves cerebellar dysfunction at pre-Aβ deposition stage in APPswe/PS1dE9 Alzheimer's disease model mice. *Biochem. Biophys. Res. Commun.* **2016**, *473*, 1039–1044. [CrossRef]
11. Kim, A.E.; Kang, P.; Bucelli, R.C.; Ferguson, C.J.; Schmidt, R.E.; Varadhachary, A.S.; Day, G.S. Autoimmune encephalitis with multiple autoantibodies: A diagnostic and therapeutic challenge. *Neurologist* **2018**, *23*, 55–59. [CrossRef]
12. Fujisawa, H.; Ohtani-Kaneko, R.; Naiki, M.; Okada, T.; Masuko, K.; Yudoh, K.; Suematsu, N.; Okamoto, K.; Nishioka, K.; Kato, T. Involvement of post-translational modification of neuronal plasticity-related proteins in hyperalgesia revealed by a proteomic analysis. *Proteomics* **2008**, *8*, 1706–1719. [CrossRef]
13. Piekarz, A.D.; Due, M.R.; Khanna, M.; Wang, B.; Ripsch, M.S.; Wang, R.; Meroueh, S.O.; Vasko, M.R.; White, F.A.; Khanna, R. CRMP-2 peptide mediated decrease of high and low voltage-activated calcium channels, attenuation of nociceptor excitability, and anti-nociception in a model of AIDS therapy-induced painful peripheral neuropathy. *Mol. Pain* **2012**, *8*, 54. [CrossRef]
14. Harada, S.; Matsuura, W.; Takano, M.; Tokuyama, S. Proteomic profiling in the spinal cord and sciatic nerve in a global cerebral ischemia-induced mechanical allodynia mouse model. *Biol. Pharm. Bull.* **2016**, *39*, 230–238. [CrossRef]
15. Lawal, M.F.; Olotu, F.A.; Agoni, C.; Soliman, M.E. Exploring the C-Terminal Tail Dynamics: Structural and Molecular Perspectives into the Therapeutic Activities of Novel CRMP-2 Inhibitors, Naringenin and Naringenin-7-O-glucuronide, in the Treatment of Alzheimer's Disease. *Chem. Biodivers.* **2018**, *15*, e1800437. [CrossRef]
16. Kolodkin, A.L.; Matthes, D.J.; O'Connor, T.P.; Patel, N.H.; Admon, A.; Bentley, D.; Goodman, C.S. Fasciclin IV: Sequence, expression, and function during growth cone guidance in the grasshopper embryo. *Neuron* **1992**, *9*, 831–845. [CrossRef]
17. Luo, Y.; Raible, D.; Raper, J.A. Collapsin: A protein in brain that induces the collapse and paralysis of neuronal growth cones. *Cell* **1993**, *75*, 217–227. [CrossRef]

18. Raper, J.A. Semaphorins and their receptors in vertebrates and invertebrates. *Curr. Opin. Neurobiol.* **2000**, *10*, 88–94. [CrossRef]
19. Fenstermaker, V.; Chen, Y.; Ghosh, A.; Yuste, R. Regulation of dendritic length and branching by semaphorin 3A. *J. Neurobiol.* **2004**, *58*, 403–412. [CrossRef]
20. Pascual, M.; Pozas, E.; Soriano, E. Role of class 3 semaphorins in the development and maturation of the septohippocampal pathway. *Hippocampus* **2005**, *15*, 184–202. [CrossRef]
21. Yoshida, Y. Semaphorin signaling in vertebrate neural circuit assembly. *Front. Mol. Neurosci.* **2012**, *5*, 71. [CrossRef] [PubMed]
22. Goshima, Y.; Nakamura, F.; Strittmatter, P.; Strittmatter, S.M. Collapsin-induced growth cone collapse mediated by an intracellular protein related to UNC-33. *Nature* **1995**, *376*, 509–514. [CrossRef] [PubMed]
23. Minturn, J.E.; Fryer, H.J.; Geschwind, D.H.; Hockfield, S. TOAD-64, a gene expressed early in neuronal differentiation in the rat, is related to unc-33, a C. elegans gene involved in axon outgrowth. *J. Neurosci.* **1995**, *15*, 6757–6766. [CrossRef]
24. Minturn, J.E.; Geschwind, D.H.; Fryer, H.J.; Hockfield, S. Early postmitotic neurons transiently express TOAD-64, a neural specific protein. *J. Comp. Neurol.* **1995**, *355*, 369–379. [CrossRef] [PubMed]
25. Byk, T.; Dobransky, T.; Cifuentes-Diaz, C.; Sobel, A. Identification and molecular characterization of Unc-33-like phosphoprotein (Ulip), a putative mammalian homolog of the axonal guidance-associated unc-33 gene product. *J. Neurosci.* **1996**, *16*, 688–701. [CrossRef] [PubMed]
26. Hamajima, N.; Matsuda, K.; Sakata, S.; Tamaki, N.; Sasaki, M.; Nonaka, M. A novel gene family defined by human dihydropyrimidinase and three related proteins with differential tissue distribution. *Gene* **1996**, *180*, 157–163. [CrossRef]
27. Yamashita, N.; Uchida, Y.; Ohshima, T.; Hirai, S.; Nakamura, F.; Taniguchi, M.; Mikoshiba, K.; Honnorat, J.; Kolattukudy, P.; Thomasset, N.; et al. Collapsin response mediator protein 1 mediates reelin signaling in cortical neuronal migration. *J. Neurosci.* **2006**, *26*, 13357–13362. [CrossRef]
28. Alabed, Y.Z.; Poolm, M.; Tone, S.O.; Sutherland, C.; Fournier, A.E. GSK3 beta regulates myelin-dependent axon outgrowth inhibition through CRMP4. *J. Neurosci.* **2010**, *30*, 5635–5643. [CrossRef] [PubMed]
29. Charrier, E.; Mosinger, B.; Meissirel, C.; Aguera, M.; Rogemond, V.; Reibel, S.; Salin, P.; Chounlamountri, N.; Perrot, V.; Belin, M.F.; et al. Transient alterations in granule cell proliferation, apoptosis and migration in postnatal developing cerebellum of CRMP1−/− mice. *Genes Cells* **2006**, *11*, 1337–1352. [CrossRef]
30. Yamashita, N.; Morita, A.; Uchida, Y.; Nakamura, F.; Usui, H.; Ohshima, T.; Taniguchi, M.; Honnorat, J.; Thomasset, N.; Takei, K.; et al. Regulation of spine development by semaphorin3A through cyclin-dependent kinase 5 phosphorylation of collapsin response mediator protein 1. *J. Neurosci.* **2007**, *27*, 12546–12554. [CrossRef]
31. Su, K.Y.; Chien, W.L.; Fu, W.M.; Yu, I.S.; Huang, H.P.; Huang, P.H.; Lin, S.R.; Shih, J.Y.; Lin, Y.L.; Hsueh, Y.P.; et al. Mice deficient in collapsin response mediator protein-1 exhibit impaired long-term potentiation and impaired spatial learning and memory. *J. Neurosci.* **2007**, *27*, 2513–2524. [CrossRef]
32. Yamashita, N.; Goshima, Y. Collapsin response mediator proteins regulate neuronal development and plasticity by switching their phosphorylation status. *Mol. Neurobiol.* **2012**, *45*, 234–246. [CrossRef]
33. Arimura, N.; Inagaki, N.; Chihara, K.; Ménager, C.; Nakamura, N.; Amano, M.; Iwamatsu, A.; Goshima, Y.; Kaibuchi, K. Phosphorylation of collapsin response mediator protein-2 by Rho-kinase. Evidence for two separate signaling pathways for growth cone collapse. *J. Biol. Chem.* **2000**, *275*, 23973–23980. [CrossRef]
34. Arimura, N.; Ménager, C.; Kawano, Y.; Yoshimura, T.; Kawabata, S.; Hattori, A.; Fukata, Y.; Amano, M.; Goshima, Y.; Inagaki, M.; et al. Phosphorylation by Rho kinase regulates CRMP-2 activity in growth cones. *Mol. Cell Biol.* **2005**, *25*, 9973–9984. [CrossRef]
35. Yoshimura, T.; Kawano, Y.; Arimura, N.; Kawabata, S.; Kikuchi, A.; Kaibuchi, K. GSK-3beta regulates phosphorylation of CRMP-2 and neuronal polarity. *Cell* **2005**, *120*, 137–149. [CrossRef]
36. Cole, A.R.; Causeret, F.; Yadirgi, G.; Hastie, C.J.; McLauchlan, H.; McManus, E.J.; Hernández, F.; Eickholt, B.J.; Nikolic, M.; Sutherland, C. Distinct priming kinases contribute to differential regulation of collapsin response mediator proteins by glycogen synthase kinase-3 in vivo. *J. Biol. Chem.* **2006**, *281*, 16591–16598. [CrossRef]
37. Alabed, Y.Z.; Pool, M.; Ong Tone, S.; Fournier, A.E. Identification of CRMP4 as a convergent regulator of axon outgrowth inhibition. *J. Neurosci.* **2007**, *27*, 1702–1711. [CrossRef]

38. Tanaka, H.; Morimura, R.; Ohshima, T. Dpysl2 (CRMP2) and Dpysl3 (CRMP4) phosphorylation by Cdk5 and DYRK2 is required for proper positioning of Rohon-Beard neurons and neural crest cells during neurulation in zebrafish. *Dev. Biol.* **2012**, *370*, 223–236. [CrossRef]
39. Morimura, R.; Nozawa, K.; Tanaka, H.; Ohshima, T. Phosphorylation of Dpysl2 (CRMP2) and Dpysl3 (CRMP4) is required for positioning of caudal primary motor neurons in the zebrafish spinal cord. *Dev. Neurobiol.* **2013**, *73*, 911–920. [CrossRef]
40. Kowara, R.; Chen, Q.; Milliken, M.; Chakravarthy, B. Calpain-mediated truncation of dihydropyrimidinase-like 3 protein (DPYSL3) in response to NMDA and H_2O_2 toxicity. *J. Neurochem.* **2005**, *95*, 466–474. [CrossRef]
41. Kowara, R.; Moraleja, K.L.; Chakravarthy, B. Involvement of nitric oxide synthase and ROS-mediated activation of L-type voltage-gated Ca2+ channels in NMDA-induced DPYSL3 degradation. *Brain Res.* **2006**, *1119*, 40–49. [CrossRef]
42. Kowara, R.; Moraleja, K.L.; Chakravarthy, B. PLA(2) signaling is involved in calpain-mediated degradation of synaptic dihydropyrimidinase-like 3 protein in response to NMDA excitotoxicity. *Neurosci. Lett.* **2008**, *430*, 197–202. [CrossRef]
43. Liu, W.; Zhou, X.W.; Liu, S.; Hu, K.; Wang, C.; He, Q.; Li, M. Calpain-truncated CRMP-3 and -4 contribute to potassium deprivation-induced apoptosis of cerebellar granule neurons. *Proteomics* **2009**, *9*, 3712–3728. [CrossRef]
44. Quinn, C.C.; Chen, E.; Kinjo, T.G.; Kelly, G.; Bell, A.W.; Elliott, R.C.; McPherson, P.S.; Hockfield, S. TUC-4b, a novel TUC family variant, regulates neurite outgrowth and associates with vesicles in the growth cone. *J. Neurosci.* **2003**, *23*, 2815–2823. [CrossRef]
45. Yuasa-Kawada, J.; Suzuki, R.; Kano, F.; Ohkawara, T.; Murata, M.; Noda, M. Axonal morphogenesis controlled by antagonistic roles of two CRMP subtypes in microtubule organization. *Eur. J. Neurosci.* **2003**, *17*, 2329–2343. [CrossRef]
46. Tan, M.; Cha, C.; Ye, Y.; Zhang, J.; Li, S.; Wu, F.; Gong, S.; Guo, G. CRMP4 and CRMP2 interact to coordinate cytoskeleton dynamics, regulating growth cone development and axon elongation. *Neural. Plast.* **2015**, 947423. [CrossRef]
47. Seki, T. Expression patterns of immature neuronal markers PSA-NCAM, CRMP-4 and NeuroD in the hippocampus of young adult and aged rodents. *J. Neurosci. Res.* **2002**, *70*, 327–334. [CrossRef]
48. Cnops, L.; Hu, T.T.; Burnat, K.; Van der Gucht, E.; Arckens, L. Age-dependent alterations in CRMP2 and CRMP4 protein expression profiles in cat visual cortex. *Brain Res.* **2006**, *1088*, 109–119. [CrossRef]
49. Tsutiya, A.; Ohtani-Kaneko, R. Postnatal alteration of collapsin response mediator protein 4 mRNA expression in the mouse brain. *J Anat.* **2012**, *221*, 341–351. [CrossRef]
50. Koide, T.; Aleksic, B.; Ito, Y.; Usui, H.; Yoshimi, A.; Inada, T.; Suzuki, M.; Hashimoto, R.; Takeda, M.; Iwata, N.; et al. A two-stage case-control association study of the dihydropyrimidinase-like 2 gene (DPYSL2) with schizophrenia in Japanese subjects. *J. Hum. Genet.* **2010**, *55*, 469–472. [CrossRef]
51. Bader, V.; Tomppo, L.; Trossbach, S.V.; Bradshaw, N.J.; Prikulis, I.; Leliveld, S.R.; Lin, C.Y.; Ishizuka, K.; Sawa, A.; Ramos, A.; et al. Proteomic, genomic and translational approaches identify CRMP1 for a role in schizophrenia and its underlying traits. *Hum. Mol. Genet.* **2012**, *21*, 4406–4418. [CrossRef]
52. Martins-de-Souza, D.; Cassoli, J.S.; Nascimento, J.M.; Hensley, K.; Guest, P.C.; Pinzon-Velasco, A.M.; Turck, C.W. The protein interactome of collapsin response mediator protein-2 (CRMP2/DPYSL2) reveals novel partner proteins in brain tissue. *Proteomics Clin. Appl.* **2015**, *9*, 817–831. [CrossRef]
53. Liu, Y.; Pham, X.; Zhang, L.; Chen, P.L.; Burzynski, G.; McGaughey, D.M.; He, S.; McGrath, J.A.; Wolyniec, P.; Fallin, M.D.; et al. Functional variants in DPYSL2 sequence increase risk of schizophrenia and suggest a link to mTOR signaling. *G3* **2014**, *5*, 61–72. [CrossRef]
54. Nakamura, H.; Yamashita, N.; Kimura, A.; Kimura, Y.; Hirano, H.; Makihara, H.; Kawamoto, Y.; Jitsuki-Takahashi, A.; Yonezaki, K.; Takase, K.; et al. Comprehensive behavioral study and proteomic analyses of CRMP2-deficient mice. *Genes Cells* **2016**, *21*, 1059–1079. [CrossRef]
55. Nakamura, H.; Takahashi-Jitsuki, A.; Makihara, H.; Asano, T.; Kimura, Y.; Nakabayashi, J.; Yamashita, N.; Kawamoto, Y.; Nakamura, F.; Ohshima, T.; et al. Proteome and behavioral alterations in phosphorylation-deficient mutant Collapsin Response Mediator Protein2 knock-in mice. *Neurochem. Int.* **2018**, *119*, 207–217. [CrossRef]

56. Zhang, H.; Kang, E.; Wang, Y.; Yang, C.; Yu, H.; Wang, Q.; Chen, Z.; Zhang, C.; Christian, K.M.; Song, H.; et al. Brain-specific Crmp2 deletion leads to neuronal development deficits and behavioural impairments in mice. *Nat. Commun.* **2016**, *1*, 7. [CrossRef]
57. Miller, B.H.; Zeier, Z.; Xi, L.; Lanz, T.A.; Deng, S.; Strathmann, J.; Willoughby, D.; Kenny, P.J.; Elsworth, J.D.; Lawrence, M.S.; et al. MicroRNA-132 dysregulation in schizophrenia has implications for both neurodevelopment and adult brain function. *Proc. Natl. Acad. Sci. USA* **2012**, *109*, 3125–3130. [CrossRef]
58. Iossifov, I.; O'Roak, B.J.; Sanders, S.J.; Ronemus, M.; Krumm, N.; Levy, D.; Stessman, H.A.; Witherspoon, K.T.; Vives, L.; Patterson, K.E.; et al. The contribution of de novo coding mutations to autism spectrum disorder. *Nature* **2014**, *515*, 216–221. [CrossRef]
59. Tsutiya, A.; Watanabe, H.; Nakano, Y.; Nishihara, M.; Goshima, Y.; Ohtani-Kaneko, R. Deletion of collapsin response mediator protein 4 results in abnormal layer thickness and elongation of mitral cell apical dendrites in the neonatal olfactory bulb. *J. Anat.* **2016**, *228*, 792–804. [CrossRef]
60. *Diagnostic and Statistical Manual of Mental Disorders*, 5th ed (DSM-V); American Psychiatric Association: Philadelphia, PA, USA, 2013.
61. Tsutiya, A.; Nishihara, M.; Goshima, Y.; Ohtani-Kaneko, R. Mouse pups lacking collapsin response mediator protein 4 manifest impaired olfactory function and hyperactivity in the olfactory bulb. *Eur. J. Neurosci.* **2015**, *42*, 2335–2345. [CrossRef]
62. Takarae, Y.; Sablich, S.R.; White, S.P.; Sweeney, J.A. Neurophysiological hyperresponsivity to sensory input in autism spectrum disorders. *J. Neurodev. Disord.* **2016**, *8*, 29. [CrossRef]
63. Takarae, Y.; Sweeney, J. Neural Hyperexcitability in Autism Spectrum Disorders. *Brain Sci.* **2017**, *7*, 129. [CrossRef]
64. Spencer, C.M.; Alekseyenko, O.; Hamilton, S.M.; Thomas, A.M.; Serysheva, E.; Yuva-Paylor, L.A.; Paylor, R. Modifying behavioral phenotypes in Fmr1KO mice: Genetic background differences reveal autistic-like responses. *Autism Res.* **2011**, *4*, 40–56. [CrossRef]
65. He, C.X.; Cantu, D.A.; Mantri, S.S.; Zeiger, W.A.; Goel, A.; Portera-Cailliau, C. Tactile defensiveness and impaired adaptation of neuronal activity in the Fmr1 knock-out mouse model of autism. *J. Neurosci.* **2017**, *37*, 6475–6487. [CrossRef]
66. Ethridge, L.E.; White, S.P.; Mosconi, M.W.; Wang, J.; Byerly, M.J.; Sweeney, J.A. Reduced habituation of auditory evoked potentials indicate cortical hyper-excitability in Fragile X Syndrome. *Transl. Psychiatry* **2016**, *6*, e787. [CrossRef]
67. Schmeisser, M.J.; Ey, E.; Wegener, S.; Bockmann, J.; Stempel, A.V.; Kuebler, A.; Janssen, A.L.; Udvardi, P.T.; Shiban, E.; Spilker, C.; et al. Autistic-like behaviours and hyperactivity in mice lacking ProSAP1/Shank2. *Nature* **2012**, *486*, 256–260. [CrossRef]
68. Won, H.; Lee, H.R.; Gee, H.Y.; Mah, W.; Kim, J.I.; Lee, J.; Ha, S.; Chung, C.; Jung, E.S.; Cho, Y.S.; et al. Autistic-like social behaviour in Shank2-mutant mice improved by restoring NMDA receptor function. *Nature* **2012**, *486*, 261–265. [CrossRef]
69. Ko, H.G.; Oh, S.B.; Zhuo, M.; Kaang, B.K. Reduced acute nociception and chronic pain in Shank2−/− mice. *Mol. Pain* **2016**, *4*, 12. [CrossRef]
70. Scattoni, M.L.; Crawley, J.; Ricceri, L. Ultrasonic vocalizations: A tool for behavioural phenotyping of mouse models of neurodevelopmental disorders. *Neurosci. Biobehav. Rev.* **2009**, *33*, 508–515. [CrossRef]
71. Van der Gucht, E.; Clerens, S.; Cromphout, K.; Vandesande, F.; Arckens, L. Differential expression of c-fos in subtypes of GABAergic cells following sensory stimulation in the cat primary visual cortex. *Eur. J. Neurosci.* **2002**, *16*, 1620–1626. [CrossRef]
72. Sullivan, S.L.; Ressler, K.J.; Buck, L.B. Spatial patterning and information coding in the olfactory system. *Curr. Opin. Genet. Dev.* **1995**, *5*, 516–523. [CrossRef]
73. Mombaerts, P.; Wang, F.; Dulac, C.; Chao, S.K.; Nemes, A.; Mendelsohn, M.; Edmondson, J.; Axel, R. Visualizing an olfactory sensory map. *Cell* **1996**, *87*, 675–686. [CrossRef]
74. Salcedo, E.; Zhang, C.; Kronberg, E.; Restrepo, D. Analysis of training-induced changes in ethyl acetate odor maps using a new computational tool to map the glomerular layer of the olfactory bulb. *Chem. Senses.* **2005**, *30*, 615–626. [CrossRef]

75. Pathania, M.; Davenport, E.C.; Muir, J.; Sheehan, D.F.; López-Doménech, G.; Kittler, J.T. The autism and schizophrenia associated gene CYFIP1 is critical for the maintenance of dendritic complexity and the stabilization of mature spines. *Transl. Psychiatry.* **2014**, *4*, e374. [CrossRef]
76. Nagaoka, A.; Takehara, H.; Hayashi-Takagi, A.; Noguchi, J.; Ishii, K.; Shirai, F.; Yagishita, S.; Akagi, T.; Ichiki, T.; Kasai, H. Abnormal intrinsic dynamics of dendritic spines in a fragile X syndrome mouse model in vivo. *Sci. Rep.* **2016**, *6*, 26651. [CrossRef]
77. Cheng, N.; Alshammari, F.; Hughes, E.; Khanbabaei, M.; Rho, J.M. Dendritic overgrowth and elevated ERK signaling during neonatal development in a mouse model of autism. *PLoS ONE* **2017**, *12*, e0179409. [CrossRef]
78. Montani, C.; Ramon-Brossier, M.; Ponzoni, L.; Gritti, L.; Cwetsch, A.W.; Braida, D.; Saillour, Y.; Terragni, B.; Mantegazza, M.; Sala, M.; et al. The X-linked intellectual disability protein IL1RAPL1 regulates dendrite complexity. *J. Neurosci.* **2017**, *37*, 6606–6627. [CrossRef]
79. Niisato, E.; Nagai, J.; Yamashita, N.; Abe, T.; Kiyonari, H.; Goshima, Y.; Ohshima, T. CRMP4 suppresses apical dendrite bifurcation of CA1 pyramidal neurons in the mouse hippocampus. *Dev. Neurobiol.* **2012**, *72*, 1447–1457. [CrossRef]
80. Niisato, E.; Nagai, J.; Yamashita, N.; Nakamura, F.; Goshima, Y.; Ohshima, T. Phosphorylation of CRMP2 is involved in proper bifurcation of the apical dendrite of hippocampal CA1 pyramidal neurons. *Dev. Neurobiol.* **2013**, *73*, 142–151. [CrossRef]
81. Cha, C.; Zhang, J.; Ji, Z.; Tan, M.; Li, S.; Wu, F.; Chen, K.; Gong, S.; Guo, G.; Lin, H. CRMP4 regulates dendritic growth and maturation via the interaction with actin cytoskeleton in cultured hippocampal neurons. *Brain Res. Bull.* **2016**, *124*, 286–294. [CrossRef]
82. Takaya, R.; Nagai, J.; Piao, W.; Niisato, E.; Nakabayashi, T.; Yamazaki, Y.; Nakamura, F.; Yamashita, N.; Kolattukudy, P.; Goshima, Y.; et al. CRMP1 and CRMP4 are required for proper orientation of dendrites of cerebral pyramidal neurons in the developing mouse brain. *Brain Res.* **2017**, *1655*, 161–167. [CrossRef]
83. Eissa, N.; Al-Houqani, M.; Sadeq, A.; Ojha, S.K.; Sasse, A.; Sadek, B. Current enlightenment about etiology and pharmacological treatment of autism spectrum disorder. *Front. Neurosci.* **2018**, *12*, 304. [CrossRef]
84. Horder, J.; Petrinovic, M.M.; Mendez, M.A.; Bruns, A.; Takumi, T.; Spooren, W.; Barker, G.J.; Künnecke, B.; Murphy, D.G. Glutamate and GABA in autism spectrum disorder-a translational magnetic resonance spectroscopy study in man and rodent models. *Transl. Psychiatry* **2018**, *8*, 106. [CrossRef]
85. Carlson, C.G. Glutamate receptor dysfunction and drug targets across models of autism spectrum disorders. *Pharmacol. Biochem. Behav.* **2012**, *100*, 850–854. [CrossRef]
86. Kim, K.C.; Cho, K.S.; Yang, S.M.; Gonzales, E.L.; Valencia, S.; Eun, P.H.; Choi, C.S.; Mabunga, D.F.; Kim, J.W.; Noh, J.K.; et al. Sex differences in autism-like behavioral phenotypes and postsynaptic receptors expression in the prefrontal cortex of TERT transgenic mice. *Biomol. Ther.* **2017**, *25*, 374–382. [CrossRef]
87. Fung, L.K.; Hardan, A.Y. Developing medications targeting glutamatergic dysfunction in autism: Progress to date. *CNS Drugs* **2015**, *29*, 453–463. [CrossRef]
88. Silverman, J.L.; Tolu, S.S.; Barkan, C.L.; Crawley, J.N. Repetitive self-grooming behavior in the BTBR mouse model of autism is blocked by the mGluR5 antagonist MPEP. *Neuropsychopharmacology* **2010**, *35*, 976–989. [CrossRef]
89. Mehta, M.V.; Gandal, M.J.; Siegel, S.J. mGluR5-antagonist mediated reversal of elevated stereotyped, repetitive behaviors in the VPA model of autism. *PLoS ONE* **2011**, *6*, e26077. [CrossRef]
90. Gatto, C.L.; Broadie, K. Genetic controls balancing excitatory and inhibitory synaptogenesis in neurodevelopmental disorder models. *Front. Synaptic. Neurosci.* **2010**, *2*, 4. [CrossRef]
91. Rubenstein, J.L. Three hypotheses for developmental defects that may underlie some forms of autism spectrum disorder. *Curr. Opin. Neurol.* **2010**, *23*, 118–123. [CrossRef]
92. Jamain, S.; Betancur, C.; Quach, H.; Philippe, A.; Fellous, M.; Giros, B.; Gillberg, C.; Leboyer, M.; Bourgeron, T. Linkage and association of the glutamate receptor 6 gene with autism. *Mol. Psychiatry* **2002**, *7*, 302–310. [CrossRef]
93. Naaijen, J.; Bralten, J.; Poelmans, G.; Glennon, J.C.; Franke, B.; Buitelaar, J.K. Glutamatergic and GABAergic gene sets in attention-deficit/hyperactivity disorder: Association to overlapping traits in ADHD and autism. *Transl. Psychiatry.* **2017**, *7*, e999. [CrossRef]
94. Werling, D.M.; Geschwind, D.H. Sex differences in autism spectrum disorders. *Curr. Opin. Neurol.* **2013**, *26*, 146–153. [CrossRef]

95. Werling, D.M.; Geschwind, D.H. Recurrence rates provide evidence for sex-differential, familial genetic liability for autism spectrum disorders in multiplex families and twins. *Mol. Autism.* **2015**, *6*, 27. [CrossRef]
96. Rubenstein, E.; Wiggins, L.D.; Lee, L.C. A review of the differences in developmental, psychiatric, and medical endophenotypes between males and females with autism spectrum disorder. *J. Dev. Phys. Disabil.* **2015**, *27*, 119–139. [CrossRef]
97. Chen, C.; Van Horn, J.D. GENDAAR Research Consortium. Developmental neurogenetics and multimodal neuroimaging of sex differences in autism. *Brain Imaging Behav.* **2017**, *11*, 38–61. [CrossRef]
98. Yu, J.; He, X.; Yao, D.; Li, Z.; Li, H.; Zhao, Z. A sex-specific association of common variants of neuroligin genes (NLGN3 and NLGN4X) with autism spectrum disorders in a Chinese Han cohort. *Behav. Brain Funct.* **2011**, *7*, 13. [CrossRef]
99. Landini, M.; Merelli, I.; Raggi, M.E.; Galluccio, N.; Ciceri, F.; Bonfanti, A.; Camposeo, S.; Massagli, A.; Villa, L.; Salvi, E.; et al. Association Analysis of Noncoding Variants in Neuroligins 3 and 4X Genes with Autism Spectrum Disorder in an Italian Cohort. *Int. J. Mol. Sci.* **2016**, *17*, 1765. [CrossRef]
100. Ey, E.; Torquet, N.; Le Sourd, A.M.; Leblond, C.S.; Boeckers, T.M.; Faure, P.; Bourgeron, T. The Autism ProSAP1/Shank2 mouse model displays quantitative and structural abnormalities in ultrasonic vocalisations. *Behav. Brain Res.* **2013**, *256*, 677–689. [CrossRef]
101. Kim, K.C.; Kim, P.; Go, H.S.; Choi, C.S.; Park, J.H.; Kim, H.J.; Jeon, S.J.; Dela Pena, I.C.; Han, S.H.; Cheong, J.H.; et al. Male-specific alteration in excitatory post-synaptic development and social interaction in pre-natal valproic acid exposure model of autism spectrum disorder. *J. Neurochem.* **2013**, *124*, 832–843. [CrossRef]
102. Schneider, T.; Roman, A.; Basta-Kaim, A.; Kubera, M.; Budziszewska, B.; Schneider, K.; Przewłockia, R. Gender-specific behavioral and immunological alterations in an animal model of autism induced by prenatal exposure to valproic acid. *Psychoneuroendocrinology* **2008**, *33*, 728–740. [CrossRef]
103. Konopko, M.A.; Densmore, A.L.; Krueger, B.K. Sexually Dimorphic Epigenetic Regulation of Brain-Derived Neurotrophic Factor in Fetal Brain in the Valproic Acid Model of Autism Spectrum Disorder. *Dev. Neurosci.* **2017**, *39*, 507–518. [CrossRef]
104. Nicolini, C.; Fahnestock, M. The valproic acid-induced rodent model of autism. *Exp. Neurol.* **2018**, *299*, 217–227. [CrossRef]
105. Ju, A.; Hammerschmidt, K.; Tantra, M.; Krueger, D.; Brose, N.; Ehrenreich, H. Juvenile manifestation of ultrasound communication deficits in the neuroligin-4 null mutant mouse model of autism. *Behav. Brain Res.* **2014**, *270*, 159–164. [CrossRef]
106. Iwakura, T.; Sakoh, M.; Tsutiya, A.; Yamashita, N.; Ohtani, A.; Tsuda, M.C.; Ogawa, S.; Tsukahara, S.; Nishihara, M.; Shiga, T.; et al. Collapsin response mediator protein 4 affects the number of tyrosine hydroxylase-immunoreactive neurons in the sexually dimorphic nucleus in female mice. *Dev. Neurobiol.* **2013**, *73*, 502–517. [CrossRef]
107. Sumida, H.; Nishizuka, M.; Kano, Y.; Arai, Y. Sex differences in the anteroventral periventricular nucleus of the preoptic area and in the related effects of androgen in prenatal rats. *Neurosci. Lett.* **1993**, *151*, 41–44. [CrossRef]
108. Ferri, S.L.; Abel, T.; Brodkin, E.S. Sex differences in autism spectrum disorder: A review. *Curr. Psychiatry Rep.* **2018**, *20*, 9. [CrossRef]
109. Knickmeyer, R.C.; Baron-Cohen, S. Fetal testosterone and sex differences in typical social development and in autism. *J. Child. Neurol.* **2006**, *21*, 825–845. [CrossRef]
110. Auyeung, B.; Baron-Cohen, S.; Ashwin, E.; Knickmeyer, R.; Taylor, K.; Hackett, G. Fetal testosterone and autistic traits. *Br. J. Psychol.* **2009**, *100*, 1–22. [CrossRef]
111. Auyeung, B.; Taylor, K.; Hackett, G.; Baron-Cohen, S. Foetal testosterone and autistic traits in 18 to 24-month-old children. *Mol. Autism.* **2010**, *1*, 11. [CrossRef]
112. Auyeung, B.; Ahluwalia, J.; Thomson, L.; Taylor, K.; Hackett, G.; O'Donnell, K.J.; Baron-Cohen, S. Prenatal versus postnatal sex steroid hormone effects on autistic traits in children at 18 to 24 months of age. *Mol. Autism.* **2012**, *3*, 17. [CrossRef]
113. Baron-Cohen, S.; Auyeung, B.; Nørgaard-Pedersen, B.; Hougaard, D.M.; Abdallah, M.W.; Melgaard, L.; Cohen, A.S.; Chakrabarti, B.; Ruta, L.; Lombardo, M.V. Elevated fetal steroidogenic activity in autism. *Mol. Psychiatry* **2015**, *20*, 369–376. [CrossRef]
114. Cherskov, A.; Pohl, A.; Allison, C.; Zhang, H.; Payne, R.A.; Baron-Cohen, S. Polycystic ovary syndrome and autism: A test of the prenatal sex steroid theory. *Transl. Psychiatry* **2018**, *8*, 136. [CrossRef]

115. Mong, J.A.; Glaser, E.; McCarthy, M.M. Gonadal steroids promote glial differentiation and alter neuronal morphology in the developing hypothalamus in a regionally specific manner. *J. Neurosci.* **1999**, *19*, 1464–1472. [CrossRef]
116. McCarthy, M.M.; Wright, C.L. Convergence of Sex Differences and the Neuroimmune System in Autism Spectrum Disorder. *Biol. Psychiatry* **2017**, *81*, 402–410. [CrossRef]
117. Werling, D.M.; Parikshak, N.N.; Geschwind, D.H. Gene expression in human brain implicates sexually dimorphic pathways in autism spectrum disorders. *Nat. Commun.* **2016**, *7*, 10717. [CrossRef]

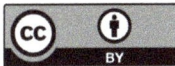 © 2019 by the author. Licensee MDPI, Basel, Switzerland. This article is an open access article distributed under the terms and conditions of the Creative Commons Attribution (CC BY) license (http://creativecommons.org/licenses/by/4.0/).

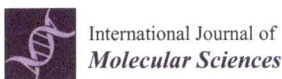

Commentary

Magnesium Supplement and the 15q11.2 BP1–BP2 Microdeletion (Burnside–Butler) Syndrome: A Potential Treatment?

Merlin G. Butler

Departments of Psychiatry & Behavioral Sciences and Pediatrics, University of Kansas Medical Center, Kansas City, KS 66160, USA; mbutler4@kumc.edu; Tel.: +1-913-588-1800

Received: 7 May 2019; Accepted: 12 June 2019; Published: 14 June 2019

Abstract: The 15q11.2 BP1–BP2 microdeletion (Burnside–Butler) syndrome is an emerging disorder that encompasses four genes (*NIPA1, NIPA2, CYFIP1,* and *TUBGCP5*). When disturbed, these four genes can lead to cognitive impairment, language and/or motor delay, psychiatric/behavioral problems (attention-deficit hyperactivity, autism, dyslexia, schizophrenia/paranoid psychosis), ataxia, seizures, poor coordination, congenital anomalies, and abnormal brain imaging. This microdeletion was reported as the most common cytogenetic finding when using ultra-high-resolution chromosomal microarrays in patients presenting for genetic services due to autism with or without additional clinical features. Additionally, those individuals with Prader–Willi or Angelman syndromes having the larger typical 15q11–q13 type I deletion which includes the 15q11.2 BP1–BP2 region containing the four genes, show higher clinical severity than those having the smaller 15q11–q13 deletion where these four genes are intact. Two of the four genes (i.e., *NIPA1* and *NIPA2*) are expressed in the brain and encode magnesium transporters. Magnesium is required in over 300 enzyme systems that are critical for multiple cellular functions, energy expenditure, protein synthesis, DNA transcription, and muscle and nerve function. Low levels of magnesium are found in those with seizures, depression, and acute or chronic brain diseases. Anecdotally, parents have administered magnesium supplements to their children with the 15q11.2 BP1–BP2 microdeletion and have observed improvement in behavior and clinical presentation. These observations require more attention from the medical community and should include controlled studies to determine if magnesium supplements could be a treatment option for this microdeletion syndrome and also for a subset of individuals with Prader–Willi and Angelman syndromes.

Keywords: 15q11.2 BP1–BP2 microdeletion (Burnside–Butler syndrome); *NIPA1*; *NIPA2*; *CYFIP1*; *TUBGCP5* genes; Prader–Willi and Angelman syndromes; magnesium transporters and supplementation; potential treatment options

1. Introduction

Clinical and behavioral differences have been reported over the past 15 years in Prader–Willi syndrome (PWS) and Angelman syndrome (AS), with the identification of specific molecular classes [1,2]. PWS and AS were the first examples of errors in genomic imprinting in humans [2–5], although they are entirely different clinical disorders. The most frequent genetic defect is a deletion of the paternal chromosome 15q11–q13 region in PWS or of the same maternal chromosome 15 region in in AS. The typical 15q11–q13 deletions are classified as either type I, involving the proximal 15q breakpoint BP1 and the distal 15q breakpoint BP3, or type II, involving the proximal 15q breakpoint BP2 and BP3 in both syndromes [2,5–9] (see Figure 1). The larger type I deletion is approximately 6.6 Mb in size and includes four genes (*TUBGCP5, CYFIFP1, NIPA,* and *NIPA2*) located in the 15q11.2 BP1–BP2 region, while the smaller type II deletion is 5.3 Mb in size and leaves the four genes intact [10]. Individuals with PWS or AS and the larger type I deletion often have increased learning, behavioral, or clinical problems compared to those with the smaller typical type II deletion [1], specifically, more frequent compulsions, self-injury episodes, and maladaptive behaviors with lower cognitive, reading, and math skills than PWS patients with type II deletions and more impaired speech and seizure activity than AS patients with the smaller deletion.

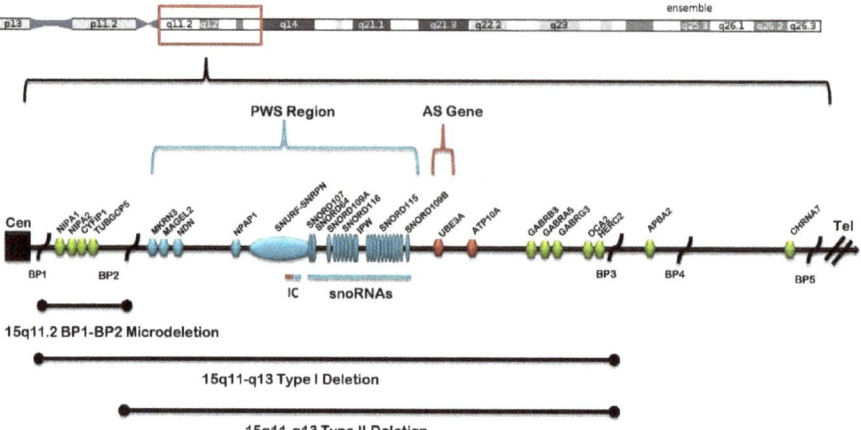

Figure 1. Chromosome 15 ideogram showing the location of genes and transcripts causing Prader–Willi syndrome (PWS) that are imprinted and paternally expressed (blue) and Angelman syndrome (AS) which are imprinted and maternally expressed (red). The location and size of the 15q11.2 BP1–BP2 microdeletion, the typical larger 15q11–q13 type I deletion involving breakpoints BP1 and BP3, and the typical smaller 15q1–q13 type II deletion involving breakpoints BP2 and BP3 are illustrated. IC: imprinting center controlling the activity of imprinted genes in the 15q11–q13 region.

2. Background and Significance

The now recognized 15q11.2 BP1–BP2 microdeletion (Burnside–Butler) syndrome involves only four genes in the region and can present with cognitive impairment, language and/or motor delay, autism, behavioral problems, poor coordination, ataxia, and congenital anomalies but not with AS or PWS. Psychiatric findings can include schizophrenia, oppositional defiant disorder, obsessive compulsive disorder, dyslexia, and structural brain defects [11–14]. Greater than two-thirds of individuals with this microdeletion present with a range of recognized clinical findings, but most individuals have not been assessed with detailed clinical, behavioral, and advanced genetic testing to identify features that may be related to the syndrome.

This emerging microdeletion syndrome encompasses the region between the proximal 15q breakpoints BP1 and BP2 including *TUBGCP5*, *CYFIP1*, *NIPA1*, and *NIPA2* genes, with an estimated prevalence from 0.6 to 1.3% based on early studies in patients presenting with unexplained behavior, cognitive, and/or psychiatric problems [11,15–19]. Later, Ho et al. [20] summarized the results of over 10,000 consecutive patients presenting with autism spectrum disorder with or without congenital anomalies or other problems using ultra-high microarray analysis and found this microdeletion to be the most common cytogenetic finding.

Cox and Butler [11] reviewed 200 individuals with the 15q11.2 BP1–BP2 microdeletion reported in the literature and grouped the findings into five categories: (1) developmental (73% of cases), speech (67%), and motor delays (42%); (2) dysmorphic ears (46%) and palatal anomalies (46%); (3) writing (60%) and reading (57%) difficulties, memory problems (60%), and verbal IQ scores ≤75 (50%); (4) general behavioral problems, unspecified (55%); and (5) abnormal brain imaging (43%). Other less frequent features observed were seizures/epilepsy (26%), autism spectrum disorder (27%), attention-deficit hyperactivity disorder (ADHD, 35%), and schizophrenia/paranoid psychosis (20%). The four genes in the 15q11.2 BP1–BP2 region are highly conserved and include *NIPA1* (non-imprinted in PWS and AS1) which causes autosomal dominant hereditary spastic paraplegia (SPG1) and postural disturbances [21,22]. An association of *NIPA1* gene repeat expansions with amyotrophic lateral sclerosis has been reported with some features in common with the 15q11.2 BP1–BP2 microdeletion syndrome [23]. This gene is known to mediate Mg^{2+} transport and is highly expressed in the brain [24]. *NIPA1* can also transport other divalent cations such as Fe^{2+}, Sr^{2+}, Ba^{2+}, Mn^{2+}, and Co^{2+} but to a lesser extent. *NIPA2* is highly selective as a magnesium transporter. Three specific *NIPA2* mutations (p.I178F, p.N244S, and p.N334_E335insD) have been reported in patients with childhood absence epilepsy [24]. Functional analysis of the mutant *NIPA2* gene variants showed decreased intracellular magnesium concentration in neurons, suggesting that lower intracellular magnesium concentrations would enhance N-methyl-D-aspartate receptor (NMDAR) currents and impact neuron excitability and brain function. Mutant proteins were not trafficked adequately to the cell membrane for normal function [24].

Magnesium transport involves the binding of fully hydrated cations to an extracellular binding loop connecting transmembrane domains and their passage through the cellular membrane without electrostatic interactions [25]. Magnesium is required for over 300 enzyme systems that are critical for multiple cellular functions, energy expenditure—including oxidative phosphorylation and glycolysis—as well as DNA transcription, protein synthesis, and muscle and nerve function. Some studies have suggested that the modern Western diet may lead to magnesium deficiency which is associated with a wide range of medical conditions including constipation, sleep disturbances, epilepsy, muscle cramps, and depression [26]. The recommended dietary allowance is 80 mg at 1–3 years of age; 130 mg at 4–8 years; 240 mg at 9–13 years, and 400 mg during adulthood. Common sources of magnesium include whole grain, spinach, almonds, peanuts, cashews, avocados, dark chocolate, and black beans.

3. Discussion

The magnesium ion fulfils several important functions in living organisms and is unique amongst the biological cations. Magnesium transporters are found in prokaryotes, but a group of newly identified transporters, including TRPM6/7, NIPA2, MagT, MMgT, and HIP14, are not found in prokaryotes. However, these mammalian magnesium transporters have no obvious amino acid similarities, indicating there are many ways to transport Mg^{2+} across membranes by using a wide variety of structural properties and physiological functions [27]. Recent studies have shown the critical role of two magnesium transporters (i.e., TRPM6 and TRPM7) that belong to the transient receptor potential (TRP) family. Transient receptor potential melastatin 7 (TRPM7) is one of these cellular receptors that mediate the entry of extracellular Mg^{2+} into cells and is required for cellular magnesium homeostasis. TRPM6 also plays a role as an epithelial magnesium transporter, and loss-of-function *TRPM6* gene mutations are found in those with a severe form of hereditary hypomagnesaemia. Both of these receptors have an atypical kinase domain that functions in the role of a transporter [28].

When disturbed, many identified Mg^{2+} transporters are also associated with congenital disorders encompassing a wide range of tissues including kidney, brain, intestine, and skin [27]. Magnesium is a potential modulator of seizure activity because of its ability to antagonize excitation of the NMDA receptors [26]. Magnesium deficiency causes NMDA-coupled calcium channels to be biased towards opening, thereby causing neuronal injury and neurological dysfunctions such as major depression [29]. Magnesium supplementation may be effective in treating depression. In addition, magnesium levels are reduced in both acute and chronic brain diseases. This has raised an interest in examining the role of magnesium in normal and injured nervous system, possibly involving the two main barrier systems. These barrier systems are the blood–brain barrier formed by brain capillary endothelial cells, which separates blood from extracellular fluid, and the blood–cerebral spinal fluid (CSF) barrier formed by choroidal epithelial cells, which separates blood from CSF. How magnesium transport takes place between the blood–brain and blood–CSF barriers is not clearly understood. It is evident that magnesium enters the brain through the blood–brain barrier and is actively transported by choroidal epithelial cells into the CSF. These epithelial cells express both *TRPM6* and *TRPM7* genes and may play a role in magnesium transport into the central nervous system [30].

Most Mg^{2+} transporter proteins transport a number of divalent cations besides Mg^{2+} across membranes, but NIPA2 is one of the few magnesium transporters that is selective for magnesium. Recent studies have shown that the absence of NIPA2 enhances neural excitability through the BK potassium channels, as evidenced from experiments in NIPA2 knockout mice versus wild-type mice using whole-cell patch-clamp recordings to measure the electrophysiological properties of neocortical somatosensory pyramidal neurons [31]. Magnesium also induces neuronal apoptosis by suppressing excitability, but the effects on brain development are unknown [32]. Information learned in these studies might lead to a better understanding of central nervous system disturbances in individuals with specific magnesium transporter gene defects. For example, *NIPA2* gene defects cause childhood epilepsy and possibly play a role in the phenotype of the 15q11.2 BP1–BP2 deletion syndrome. Patients with AS having the larger 15q11–q13 type I deletion including the four genes in the 15q11.2 BP1–BP2 region (and both *NIPA1* and *NIPA2*) are more severely affected, with increased seizure activity. Studies have shown that people with epilepsy have lower magnesium levels than individuals without epilepsy. In addition, a poor magnesium status is also recognized as a risk factor for Alzheimer's disease, but the underlying mechanism is unclear. Elevated magnesium reduces blood–brain barrier permeability and accelerates the clearance of amyloid beta peptide from the brain [33].

Recently, $MgSO_4$ and magnesium transporters were studied to determine if they have a protective effect on neurotoxicity induced in living cells. Cells that were chemically stressed and then treated with $MgSO_4$ showed improved viability and increased cellular mRNA for the protein encoded by the *NIPA1* gene located in the 15q11.2 BP1–BP2 region. These results did suggest that $MgSO_4$ may have a protective effect and that NIPA1 protein might be involved in dopaminergic neurons [34]. The *NIPA1* gene encodes a magnesium transporter protein located in early endosomes and at the cell surface of neurons. In addition, Chang et al. [35] proposed that targeting Mg^{2+} uptake mediated by NIPA1 may be an interesting option for novel therapies for conditions such as anorexia nervosa associated with 15q11.2 BP1–BP2 microduplications and other neurobehavioral disorders. A second gene in the 15q11.2 BP1–BP2 region is *NIPA2* (non-imprinted in PWS and AS2), which also encodes a protein that plays a role in magnesium transport in renal cells with mutations causing childhood absence epilepsy [36]. The *TUBGCP5* (tubulin gamma complex-associated protein 5) gene in this region is associated with ADHD and obsessive-compulsive disorder when disturbed [16]. The fourth gene is *CYFIP1* (cytoplasmic fragile X mental retardation 1 FMR1-interacting protein 1) whose protein product interacts with FMRP, the protein coded by the *FMR1* gene. Mutations of *FMR1* lead to fragile X syndrome and now recognized as the leading cause of familial intellectual disability [37].

The 15q11.2 BP1–BP2 microdeletion syndrome was found in 9% of the top 85 microarray cytogenetic results in a recent study reported by Ho et al. [20] in a large cohort of patients presenting for genetic services. However, there is a lack of detailed neuropsychiatric and behavior assessments in family members (and parents) of those with the microdeletion. More sophisticated genetic testing is now available to better characterize the relationship between the cytogenetic defect and clinical presentation, variability, and severity. Additional testing may include next-generation (exome) sequencing or targeted approaches to analyze the four genes in the 15q11.2 BP1–BP2 region and determine if there is a variant of one of the non-deleted genes in the region leading to a more severe phenotype or associated with interactive genes outside of the region but in common biological pathways.

Further research with combined behavior/psychiatric/cognitive/motor measures are needed of "affected" and "non-affected" family members with and without the microdeletion. This would allow the determination of the coding genetic status of the "normal" or "non-deleted" candidate gene alleles in families. In addition, clinical description and phenotypic findings may be incomplete, poorly characterized, or unavailable for parents and other family members having the microdeletion, without concerted efforts to undertake such testing and detailed assessments to thoroughly address these issues and examine genotype–phenotype relationships. Currently, about one-third of children inherit the microdeletion from an abnormal parent. Hence, modified genes outside of this chromosome region may also play a role but require further investigations, as suggested by examining interacting genes or pathways impacting on the phenotype and clinical presentation.

Aberrant behavior including aggression is one of the major problems that parents face with children having this microdeletion syndrome. Two of the four deleted genes in the region (i.e., *NIPA1* and *NIPA2*) encode magnesium transporter proteins and were targeted by several families exchanging information via internet communication. They administered magnesium supplements to their affected children for treatment. Their efforts were supported in the literature by Chang et al. [35] in investigations that proposed that Mg^{2+} therapy may have a positive impact. Magnesium taurate and magnesium L-threonate were used historically in anecdotal reports to improve behavior. Additionally, selenium, as an antioxidant, was also used by parents to improve mental alertness or calmness in their affected children, but magnesium with a general vitamin regime was the most effective in improving behavior, according to the parents. High iron levels reported by parents in some of their children were also lowered when magnesium taurate was introduced into the diet. Other patients showed improved behavior when administered magnesium L-threonine.

Although anecdotally, the above information from families requires more attention and investigation to address these early observations linking magnesium supplementation and improved behavior in those subjects with the 15q11.2 BP1–BP2 microdeletion. Two of the four genes in this chromosome region are involved in the transportation of magnesium and, to a lesser degree, of other cations. This information, if true, could also be applied to behavioral problems seen in PWS and AS with the larger 15q11–q13 type I deletions. Those PWS and AS patients with the larger deletion present higher clinical severity and are missing the two magnesium transporter genes in the 15q11.2 BP1–BP2 region. Controlled studies with magnesium supplementation and behavioral measures in a large cohort of subjects with the 15q11.2 BP1–BP2 microdeletion are needed to further investigate these observations.

Funding: The Smith Intellectual and Developmental Disabilities Research Center Grant (NIH U54 HD 090216), Molecular Regulation of the Cell Development and Differentiation-COBRE (5P20GM104936-10), NIH S10 High-End Instrumental Grant (NIHS10OD021743), KUMC Research Institute Clinical Pilot Research Program, University of Kansas Medical Center Grant (Y6B00030), and Prayer-Will Support PWS Organization (Family & Friends of Kyleigh Ellington) are recognized.

Acknowledgments: I thank Charlotte Iannaci and Waheeda Hossain for expert preparation of the manuscript.

Conflicts of Interest: The author declares no conflict of interest.

References

1. Butler, M.G.; Bittel, D.C.; Kibiryeva, N.; Talebizadeh, Z.; Thompson, T. Behavioral differences among subjects with Prader-Willi syndrome and type I or type II deletion and maternal disomy. *Pediatrics* **2004**, *113*, 565–573. [CrossRef] [PubMed]
2. Williams, C.A.; Driscoll, D.J.; Dagli, A.I. Clinical and genetic aspects of Angelman syndrome. *Genet. Med.* **2010**, *12*, 385–395. [CrossRef] [PubMed]
3. Nicholls, R.D.; Knoll, J.H.; Butler, M.G.; Karam, S.; Lalande, M. Genetic imprinting suggested by maternal heterodisomy in nondeletion Prader-Willi syndrome. *Nature* **1989**, *342*, 281–285. [CrossRef] [PubMed]
4. Butler, M.G. Prader-Willi syndrome: Current understanding of cause and diagnosis. *Am. J. Med. Genet.* **1990**, *35*, 319–332. [CrossRef] [PubMed]
5. Butler, M.G.; Lee, P.D.K.; Whitman, B.Y. *Management of Prader-Willi Syndrome*; Springer: New York, NY, USA, 2006.
6. Bittel, D.C.; Butler, M.G. Prader-Willi syndrome: Clinical genetics, cytogenetics and molecular biology. *Expert Rev. Mol. Med.* **2005**, *7*, 1–20. [CrossRef]

7. Cassidy, S.B.; Schwartz, S.; Miller, J.L.; Driscoll, D.J. Prader-Willi syndrome. *Genet. Med.* **2012**, *14*, 10–26. [CrossRef] [PubMed]
8. Angulo, M.A.; Butler, M.G.; Cataletto, M.E. Prader-Willi syndrome: A review of clinical, genetic, and endocrine findings. *J. Endocrinol. Invest.* **2015**, *38*, 1249–1263. [CrossRef] [PubMed]
9. Butler, M.G. Single gene and syndromic causes of obesity: Illustrative examples. *Prog. Mol. Biol. Transl. Sci.* **2016**, *140*, 1–45. [PubMed]
10. Butler, M.G.; Fischer, W.; Kibiryeva, N.; Bittel, D.C. Array comparative genomic hybridization (aCGH) analysis in Prader-Willi syndrome. *Am. J. Med. Genet. A* **2008**, *146A*, 854–860. [CrossRef]
11. Cox, D.M.; Butler, M.G. The 15q11.2 BP1-BP2 microdeletion syndrome: A review. *Int. J. Mol. Sci.* **2015**, *16*, 4068–4082. [CrossRef]
12. Butler, M.G. Clinical and genetic aspects of the 15q11.2 BP1-BP2 microdeletion disorder. *J. Intellect. Disabil. Res.* **2017**, *61*, 568–579. [CrossRef] [PubMed]
13. Ulfarsson, M.O.; Walters, G.B.; Gustafsson, O.; Steinberg, S.; Silva, A.; Doyle, O.M.; Brammer, M.; Gudbjartsson, D.F.; Arnarsdottir, S.; Jonsdottir, G.A.; et al. 15q11.2 CNV affects cognitive, structural and functional correlates of dyslexia and dyscalculia. *Transl. Psychiatry* **2017**, *7*, e1109. [CrossRef] [PubMed]
14. Davis, K.W.; Serrano, M.; Loddo, S.; Robinson, C.; Alesi, V.; Dallapiccola, B.; Novelli, A.; Butler, M.G. Parent-of-origin effects in 15q11.2 BP1-BP2 microdeletion (Burnside-Butler) syndrome. *Int. J. Mol. Sci.* **2019**, *20*, 1459. [CrossRef] [PubMed]
15. Burnside, R.D.; Pasion, R.; Mikhail, F.M.; Carroll, A.J.; Robin, N.H.; Youngs, E.L.; Gadi, I.K.; Keitges, E.; Jaswaney, V.L.; Papenhausen, P.R.; et al. Microdeletion/microduplication of proximal 15q11.2 between BP1 and BP2: A susceptibility region for neurological dysfunction including developmental and language delay. *Hum. Genet.* **2011**, *130*, 517–528. [CrossRef] [PubMed]
16. De Wolf, V.; Brison, N.; Devriendt, K.; Peeters, H. Genetic counseling for susceptibility loci and neurodevelopmental disorders: The del15q11.2 as an example. *Am. J. Med. Genet. A* **2013**, *161A*, 2846–2854. [CrossRef] [PubMed]
17. Rosenfeld, J.A.; Coe, B.P.; Eichler, E.E.; Cuckle, H.; Shaffer, L.G. Estimates of penetrance for recurrent pathogenic copy-number variations. *Genet. Med.* **2013**, *15*, 478–481. [CrossRef] [PubMed]
18. Chaste, P.; Sanders, S.J.; Mohan, K.N.; Klei, L.; Song, Y.; Murtha, M.T.; Hus, V.; Lowe, J.K.; Willsey, A.J.; Moreno-De-Luca, D.; et al. Modest impact on risk for autism spectrum disorder of rare copy number variants at 15q11.2, specifically breakpoints 1 to 2. *Autism Res.* **2014**, *7*, 355–362. [CrossRef]
19. Hashemi, B.; Bassett, A.; Chitayat, D.; Chong, K.; Feldman, M.; Flanagan, J.; Goobie, S.; Kawamura, A.; Lowther, C.; Prasad, C.; et al. Deletion of 15q11.2(BP1-BP2) region: Further evidence for lack of phenotypic specificity in a pediatric population. *Am. J. Med. Genet. A* **2015**, *67A*, 2098–2102.
20. Ho, K.S.; Wassman, E.R.; Baxter, A.L.; Hensel, C.H.; Martin, M.M.; Prasad, A.; Twede, H.; Vanzo, R.J.; Butler, M.G. Chromosomal microarray analysis of consecutive individuals with Autism Spectrum Disorders using an ultra-high resolution chromosomal microarray optimized for neurodevelopmental disorders. *Int. J. Mol. Sci.* **2016**, *17*, 2070. [CrossRef]
21. Rainier, S.; Chai, J.H.; Tokarz, D.; Nicholls, R.D.; Fink, J.K. NIPA1 gene mutations cause autosomal dominant hereditary spastic paraplegia (SPG6). *Am. J. Hum. Genet.* **2003**, *73*, 967–971. [CrossRef]
22. Chen, S.; Song, C.; Guo, H.; Xu, P.; Huang, W.; Zhou, Y.; Sun, J.; Li, C.X.; Du, Y.; Li, X.; et al. Distinct novel mutations affecting the same base in the NIPA1 gene cause autosomal dominant hereditary spastic paraplegia in two Chinese families. *Hum. Mutat.* **2005**, *25*, 135–141. [CrossRef]
23. Tazelaar, G.H.P.; Dekker, A.M.; van Vugt, J.J.F.A.; van der Spek, R.A.; Westeneng, H.J.; Kool, L.J.B.G.; Kenna, K.P.; van Rheenen, W.; Pulit, S.L.; McLaughlin, R.L.; et al. Association of NIPA1 repeat expansions with amyotrophic lateral sclerosis in a large international cohort. *Neurobiol. Aging* **2019**, *74*, 234. e9–234.e15. [CrossRef]
24. Xie, H.; Zhang, Y.; Zhang, P.; Wang, J.; Wu, Y.; Wu, X.; Netoff, T.; Jiang, Y. Functional study of NIPA2 mutations identified from the patients with childhood absence epilepsy. *PLoS ONE* **2014**, *9*, e109749. [CrossRef] [PubMed]
25. Maguire, M.E. Magnesium transporters: Properties, regulation and structure. *Front. Biosci.* **2006**, *11*, 3149–3163. [CrossRef] [PubMed]
26. Yuen, A.W.; Sander, J.W. Can magnesium supplementation reduce seizures in people with epilepsy? A hypothesis. *Epilepsy Res.* **2012**, *100*, 152–156. [CrossRef] [PubMed]

27. Quamme, G.A. Molecular identification of ancient and modern mammalian magnesium transporters. *Am. J. Physiol. Cell. Physiol.* **2010**, *298*, C407–C429. [CrossRef] [PubMed]
28. Schlingmann, K.P.; Gudermann, T. A critical role of TRPM channel-kinase for human magnesium transport. *J. Physiol.* **2005**, *566*, 301–308. [CrossRef] [PubMed]
29. Eby, G.A., 3rd; Eby, K.L. Magnesium for treatment-resistant depression: A review and hypothesis. *Med. Hypotheses* **2010**, *74*, 649–660. [CrossRef]
30. Ghabriel, M.N.; Vink, R. Magnesium transport across the blood-brain barriers. In *Magnesium in the Central Nervous System*; Vink, R., Nechifor, M., Eds.; University of Adelaide Press: Adelaide, South Australia, Australia, 2011.
31. Liu, N.N.; Xie, H.; Xiang-Wei, W.S.; Gao, K.; Wang, T.S.; Jiang, Y.W. The absence of NIPA2 enhances neural excitability through BK (big potassium) channels. *CNS Neurosci. Ther.* **2019**. [CrossRef]
32. Dribben, W.H.; Eisenman, L.N.; Mennerick, S. Magnesium induces neuronal apoptosis by suppressing excitability. Magnesium induces neuronal apoptosis by suppressing excitability. *Cell Death Dis.* **2010**. [CrossRef]
33. Zhu, D.; Su, Y.; Fu, B.; Xu, H. Magnesium Reduces Blood-Brain Barrier Permeability and Regulates Amyloid-β Transcytosis. *Mol. Neurobiol.* **2018**, *55*, 7118–7131. [CrossRef]
34. Lin, L.; Ke, Z.; Lv, M.; Lin, R.; Wu, B.; Zheng, Z. Effects of MgSO$_4$ and magnesium transporters on 6-hydroxydopamine-induced SH-SY5Y cells. *Life Sci.* **2017**, *172*, 48–54. [CrossRef] [PubMed]
35. Chang, X.; Qu, H.; Liu, Y.; Glessner, J.; Hou, C.; Wang, F.; Li, J.; Sleiman, P.; Hakonarson, H. Microduplications at the 15q11.2 BP1-BP2 locus are enriched in patients with anorexia nervosa. *J. Psychiatr. Res.* **2019**, *113*, 34–38. [CrossRef] [PubMed]
36. Goytain, A.; Hines, R.M.; El-Husseini, A.; Quamme, G.A. NIPA1 (SPG6), the basis for autosomal dominant form of hereditary spastic paraplegia, encodes a functional Mg2+ transporter. *J. Biol. Chem.* **2007**, *282*, 8060–8068. [CrossRef] [PubMed]
37. Hagerman, R.J.; Berry-Kravis, E.; Hazlett, H.C.; Bailey, D.B., Jr.; Moine, H.; Kooy, R.F.; Tassone, F.; Gantois, I.; Sonenberg, N.; Mandel, J.L.; et al. Fragile X syndrome. *Nat. Rev. Dis. Primers.* **2017**, *3*, 17065. [CrossRef] [PubMed]

 © 2019 by the author. Licensee MDPI, Basel, Switzerland. This article is an open access article distributed under the terms and conditions of the Creative Commons Attribution (CC BY) license (http://creativecommons.org/licenses/by/4.0/).

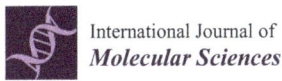

Review

IQSEC2-Associated Intellectual Disability and Autism

Nina S. Levy [1], George K. E. Umanah [2], Eli J. Rogers [1], Reem Jada [1], Orit Lache [1] and Andrew P. Levy [1,*]

1. Technion Israel Institute of Technology, 1 Efron St., Haifa, 3525422, Israel; ninal@technion.ac.il (N.S.L.); eli.rogers@rochester.edu (E.J.R.); reemjada@campus.technion.ac.il (R.J.); eorit@technion.ac.il (O.L.)
2. Department of Neurology, Johns Hopkins University, Baltimore, MD 21205, USA; gumanah1@jhmi.edu
* Correspondence: alevy@technion.ac.il; Tel.: +972-528664296

Received: 30 May 2019; Accepted: 19 June 2019; Published: 21 June 2019

Abstract: Mutations in *IQSEC2* cause intellectual disability (ID), which is often accompanied by seizures and autism. A number of studies have shown that IQSEC2 is an abundant protein in excitatory synapses and plays an important role in neuronal development as well as synaptic plasticity. Here, we review neuronal IQSEC2 signaling with emphasis on those aspects likely to be involved in autism. IQSEC2 is normally bound to N-methyl-D-aspartate (NMDA)-type glutamate receptors via post synaptic density protein 95 (PSD-95). Activation of NMDA receptors results in calcium ion influx and binding to calmodulin present on the IQSEC2 IQ domain. Calcium/calmodulin induces a conformational change in IQSEC2 leading to activation of the SEC7 catalytic domain. GTP is exchanged for GDP on ADP ribosylation factor 6 (ARF6). Activated ARF6 promotes downregulation of surface α-amino-3-hydroxy-5-methyl-4-isoxazolepropionic acid (AMPA)-type glutamate receptors through a c-jun N terminal kinase (JNK)-mediated pathway. NMDA receptors, AMPA receptors, and PSD-95 are all known to be adversely affected in autism. An *IQSEC2* transgenic mouse carrying a constitutively active mutation (A350V) shows autistic features and reduced levels of surface AMPA receptor subunit GluA2. Sec7 activity and AMPA receptor recycling are presented as two targets, which may respond to drug treatment in IQSEC2-associated ID and autism.

Keywords: intellectual disability; autism; AMPA receptors; NMDA receptors; guanine nucleotide exchange factor; synaptic plasticity

---

1. Introduction

This review will summarize our current knowledge of the molecular basis of intellectual disability (ID) in individuals with mutations in the *IQSEC2* gene and how compromised IQSEC2 function may be related to autism spectrum disorder (ASD). It is clear from clinical studies that autistic-like features are found in at least 25% of all *IQSEC2* ID cases [1–3]. This suggests a common biochemical pathway linking *IQSEC2*-associated ID and ASD. IQSEC2 is a guanine nucleotide exchange factor (GEF) that activates ADP ribosylation factor 6 (ARF6) and regulates proper membrane trafficking and synaptic structure and function in neurons. In this regard, ARF6 is important for maintaining the proper level of excitatory and inhibitory receptors essential for the normal learning process. Indeed, it is the imbalance between excitation and inhibition in synaptic transmission that has been proposed to underlie the pathophysiology of ASD. We propose a model by which IQSEC2 acts in promoting neurotransmission highlighting aspects which may be disrupted by mutations in *IQSEC2* resulting in ID and autism.

2. Clinical Connection between *IQSEC2* and ASD

Mutations in the *IQSEC2* gene associated with ID are often accompanied by autism and/or epilepsy. In the first study establishing a linkage between *IQSEC2* and non-syndromic ID [1], four distinct missense mutations in *IQSEC2* were shown to segregate with affected individuals (57 total), with each family passing along one mutation. Autism was present in two of the families and among those two families, half of the affected individuals were autistic. Since that time, numerous reports documenting *IQSEC2* mutations have been published [2,3]. A recent review summarizing 136 individuals and 70 different types of mutations showed that autism is present in 25% of affected males and 30% of affected females [3]. Although *IQSEC2* is found on the X chromosome, in females, *IQSEC2* escapes X inactivation. This may explain the relatively high prevalence of both ID and autism in heterozygous females. Due to this high level of comorbidity, it seems likely that *IQSEC2*-associated ID and autism share common biochemical abnormalities.

3. IQSEC2 Structure and Function

IQSEC2 is named for two of its conserved regions known as the IQ (aa 347–376) and the SEC7 domains (aa 746–939) (see Figure 1). IQ stands for the amino acids, isoleucine and glutamine, which make up the beginning of this approximately 30-amino-acid domain that confers calcium calmodulin binding capacity to IQSEC2. The SEC7 domain, named for the original secretory mutant SEC7 from Saccharomyces cerevisiae, is approximately 200 amino acids and is responsible for the guanine nucleotide exchange function (GEF) of IQSEC2. The substrate for IQSEC2 GEF activity is thought to be ARF6. There are six mammalian ARFs, however ARF6 is the only one found associated with the plasma membrane and has been proposed to be the primary ARF for IQSEC2 [4]. ARF binds to two forms of the guanosine nucleotide, guanosine triphosphate (GTP) and guanosine diphosphate (GDP). IQSEC2 facilitates the exchange of GDP for GTP on ARF6 resulting in its activation. Additional functional domains in IQSEC2 include an N terminal coiled coil (CC) domain (aa 23–74) thought to promote self-assembly, a pleckstrin homology (PH) domain (aa 951–1085) that binds to phosphoinositides, and two C terminal binding motifs important for cytoskeletal organization: A proline-rich motif (PRM) (aa 1424–1434) and a PDZ binding motif (aa 1484–1488) (PDZ is an initialism combining the first letters of the first three proteins found to contain this common sequence: Post synaptic density protein (PSD95), Drosophila disc large tumor suppressor (Dlg1), and zonula occludens-1 protein (zo-1)).

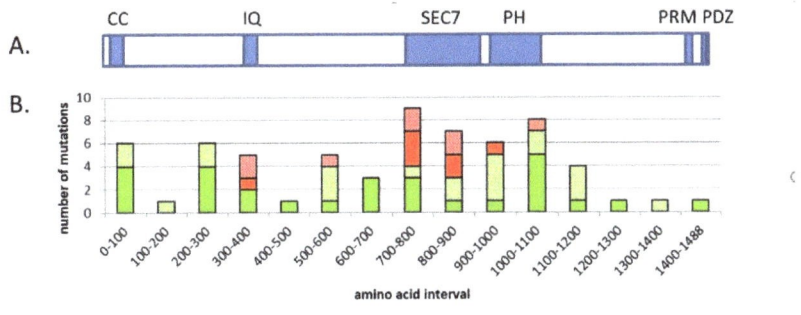

Figure 1. Schematic diagram of the conserved domains found in the human IQSEC2 protein and the distribution of mutations found in IQSEC2 cases. The top panel (A) depicts the protein encoded by the most abundant transcript for human *IQSEC2*, which contains 1488 amino acids. The known conserved domains and motifs are shown in blue. They are: CC-coiled coil, IQ–calmodulin binding site, SEC7-catalytic domain for GTP/GDP exchange on ARF, PH-pleckstrin homology domain, PRM–proline-rich motif, and PDZ-PSD-95 binding motif. The bottom panel (B) shows the distribution of mutations found in the *IQSEC2* gene (mutations were taken from Tables 2 and 3 from reference [3]) Missense mutations are shown in red; all other mutations (which include intragenic nonsense, duplication/truncation, in-frame deletions, and splicing variants) are shown in green. Hatched red bars show missense mutations associated with ASD. Hatched green bars show all other mutations associated with ASD. The positions of all mutations were arbitrarily chosen as the N terminal starting point. Mutations were considered to be associated with ASD if at least one member of the family was listed as having ASD traits or displaying autistic behavior.

Missense mutations in *IQSEC2* were concentrated in three functional domains including the IQ, SEC7, and PH domains (see Figure 1B) [3]. One missense mutation was found outside a known functional domain (R563N) and there was no ID associated with this case, only ASD traits. Other types of mutations, which mainly cause truncations or altered amino acid sequences, are scattered throughout the protein (see Figure 1 legend for details). Approximately half of all the mutations found in IQSEC2 were associated with ASD. The distribution of ASD-associated mutations across the gene was similar to non ASD mutations. This result indicates that mutations in *IQSEC2* that result in ASD cannot be attributed to any particular part of the protein. The reason that only half of the mutations in *IQSEC2* present with autism may be due to dosage effects or other variable pathology that occurs due to the stochastic nature of epileptic seizures.

An analysis of *IQSEC2* gene sequences from normal individuals has the potential to reveal mutations that do not cause ID and may be regarded as "tolerable". This type of analysis found a large discrepancy between the predicted number of missense mutations (221) and those that were observed (86) [3]. This discrepancy may be due to the fact that missense mutations in regions other than the known functional domains do cause pathology, albeit less severe than that seen in IQSEC2-associated ID. Perhaps these cases are more mild forms of ID and or ASD with no epilepsy, which is the primary reason for doing exome sequencing of IQSEC2, yet not mild enough to be included in a normal group. An example might be the R563N mutation mentioned above. A previous study of mutation intolerance showed that genes involved in early onset neurodevelopmental disorders such as the epileptic encephalopathies carry the highest level of mutational intolerance [5]. One possibility may be that genes in this class are often found in large complexes with scaffolding proteins and other proteins involved in signal transduction. The architecture and dynamics of these complexes may be so intricate that most amino acid changes would alter their proper function.

4. IQSEC2 and Spine Formation

In the brain, where IQSEC2 is predominantly expressed, it has been shown that ARF6 is important in the regulation of dendritic spine development [6]. During embryonic and neonatal growth, neuronal dendrites lengthen and become extensively branched. This process increases their surface area and allows for more connections between neurons. Maturing dendrites develop small protrusions called dendritic spines, which are the site of the majority of the excitatory synapses in the brain. Spines begin as long, thin filopodia and develop into large, mature spines with a defined spine head containing neurotransmitter receptors and a postsynaptic density (PSD). The PSD is an electron-dense region attached to the postsynaptic membrane. The PSD is in close apposition to the presynaptic membrane and ensures that receptors are in close proximity to presynaptic neurotransmitter release sites. Many proteins in the PSD are involved in the regulation of synaptic function. Key among these are postsynaptic density-95 (PSD95), NMDA receptors, AMPA receptors, calcium/calmodulin-dependent protein kinase II, and actin.

During the first few years of life, there is an intense increase in spine density, which is followed by a gradual decline in the number of spines, known as spine pruning. The elimination of spines occurs from childhood to adulthood and is the time of fine structural reorganization of the cortex. This period is associated with higher cognitive function such as learning and memory. This process is characterized by synaptic plasticity, whereby a neuron changes its synaptic strength based on previous stimuli. Synaptic strength is the average amount of current produced in the postsynaptic neuron by an action potential in the presynaptic neuron. Neurons may undergo long-term potentiation (LTP), or a sustained increase in synaptic strength. In contrast, neurons may decrease their synaptic strength for a prolonged period of time, otherwise known as long-term depression (LTD). The size of the dendritic spines and their PSDs have been observed to increase with LTP and decrease with LTD [7].

IQSEC2 has been localized to dendritic spines by immunocytochemistry of cultured rat and mouse hippocampal neurons [4,8]. The importance of IQSEC2 in spine development has been shown in studies in which knocking down IQSEC2 mRNA levels in mouse primary hippocampal cell cultures disrupted dendritic spine morphogenesis [9]. Specifically, there was an increase in the density of dendritic spines after two weeks in culture compared to controls with no change in the maturity of the spines. Overexpression of wild-type IQSEC2 in similar cultures led to a decrease in density of dendritic spines but an increase in spine maturity. IQSEC2 knockout mice gave rise to neuronal cultures that were more disorganized than their wildtype littermates. Taken together, these data suggest that the level of IQSEC2 is critical for normal spine development and maturation.

5. Proteins Implicated in ASD that Interact with IQSEC2

5.1. PSD-95

The prominence of IQSEC2 in neuronal spine formation makes it a logical candidate in affecting autism. This is because a major cellular phenotype identified in autism patients is dendritic spine aberrations. Normally, during development spine pruning occurs as part of the spinal maturation process. In brains from autistic patients, there is more rapid growth and formation during childhood and less spinal pruning and elimination during adulthood. This leads to an overabundance of spines in ASD and results in increased spine density and hyper connectivity [10,11]. Interestingly, there seems to be somewhat of an opposite effect in ID, where spines on cortical neurons from individuals with intellectual disability were described as having an immature appearance with fewer spines per dendritic branch. The dendrites of cortical neurons from ID patients have been reported to be less complex than normal subjects [11]. IQSEC2-associated ID is likely to be a very specific subclass of all ID subjects and may not be represented by the above results. Further studies on mouse models or induced pluripotent stem cells (IPSC) cells will likely clarify this issue.

One of the most abundant proteins in the PSD is PSD-95. It is a member of the membrane-associated guanylate kinase (MAGUK) family and functions as a scaffolding protein, anchoring receptor molecules in the membrane to the cytoskeleton. PSD-95 contains three PDZ domains, a common structural domain of 80–90 amino-acids that plays a key role in holding together and organizing signaling complexes at cellular membranes. There is compelling evidence that mutations in PSD-95 result in cognitive and learning deficits associated with autism and schizophrenia [10]. PSD-95 is present in the PSD in complexes as large as 1.5 MDa [12]. A subset of these complexes contains IQSEC2. In mice lacking PSD-95, IQSEC2 does not form 1.5 MDa complexes [13]. Separating and identifying the members of PSD-95/IQSEC2 super complexes will likely shed new light on the mechanism of IQSEC2 signaling.

IQSEC2 has been shown to associate with PSD-95 in the post synaptic density on excitatory synapses [8]. This binding is thought to occur via a four-amino-acid sequence STVV in the C terminus of IQSEC2. A patient with a frameshift mutation in the C terminal region of IQSEC2 quite close to the PDZ binding motif (G1468A) supports the crucial role of this domain [3]. In addition, mutations in *IQSEC2's* PDZ domain were found to disrupt glutamate receptor trafficking and neurotransmission in organotypic hippocampal cultures [14], as well as IQSEC2 localization to dendritic spines [15], as will be discussed below.

5.2. IRSp53/BAIAP2, PSD-93, SAP97, CaMKIIa

Insulin receptor substrate of 53 kDa (IRSp53), also known as brain-specific angiogenesis inhibitor 1-associated protein 2 (BAIAP2), is a multidomain scaffolding protein that is present in high levels in the PSD at excitatory synapses and regulates actin dynamics at dendritic spines [16]. IRSp53 has also been found in connection with ASD as well as other behavioral disorders. Mice that lack IRSp53 show increased NMDA receptor function and display cognitive deficits. Drug treatment that suppresses NMDA receptor activation alleviates some of these deficits. IRSp53 knockout mice display similar behaviors to *IQSEC2* A350V mutant mice [17] such as hyperactivity in open field locomotion, normal rotarod motor function, impaired Morris water maze memory, and decreased three-chamber social interaction [16].

It has been reported that the PRM region of IQSEC2 (see Figure 1) interacts with IRSp53, as evidenced by co-immunoprecipitation experiments [15]. Deletion of the 74 C-terminal amino acids of IQSEC2 prevented localization of IQSEC2 to dendritic spines versus dendritic shafts. Deletion of the last four amino acids (the PDZ binding motif) did not prevent spine localization. A separate mutation of the PRM also did not prevent spine localization, indicating a potential redundancy in this particular function by the PRM and the PDZ binding motifs. Alternatively, there may be critical sequences outside these two domains in the C terminus that are necessary for spine localization.

Other proteins that have been shown to be associated with IQSEC2 by co-immunoprecipitation are PSD93, synapse-associated protein 97 (SAP97), and calcium calmodulin kinase IIa (CaMKIIa) [4]. SAP97 and PSD-93 are members of the MAGUK family of scaffold proteins and contain PDZ domains. PSD-93, along with PSD-95 and the NMDA receptor subunit GluN2B, were found to be essential for the formation of 1.5 MDa NMDA supercomplexes [12]. As mentioned above, IQSEC2 is a member of a subset of these complexes. CaMKII is also present at very high levels in the PSD and is thought to be an important mediator of learning and memory. Aside from its phosphorylation function, CaMKII has protein docking capability. Specifically, CaMKII is a central organizer of the postsynaptic F-actin network and can autoregulate its position in the PSD while binding to other effector proteins [18] It is becoming clear that understanding IQSEC2 signal transduction will require teasing apart the biochemical composition and dynamics of the large PSD complexes.

5.3. Glutamate Receptors

IQSEC2 is as abundant as many of the NMDA and AMPA glutamate receptors in the PSD of glutamatergic synapses [19]. These two receptor types are responsible for mediating excitatory neurotransmission and neuronal plasticity, the process by which neurons acquire a long-term change in their excitability based on previous stimuli. Neuronal synaptic plasticity is critical for learning and memory. Disruption of these pathways leads to neurodevelopmental diseases, including ID and autism. A recent review summarizes the disturbances in AMPA/NMDA receptor expression and function for 31 different synaptic genes implicated in autism [20]. In two well-known mouse models of autism, it was shown that expression of AMPA receptors was disturbed [21].

The importance of IQSEC2 in glutamate receptor function was shown using organotypic rat hippocampal slices. Transfection of normal IQSEC2 resulted in decreased electrophysiological responses characteristic of AMPA receptors [22]. There was no change in NMDA receptor response. Transfection of an N terminal deletion construct (213 aa), which removes the coiled coil domain, resulted in an increased AMPA receptor response, possibly due to a dominant negative effect. Blocking of NMDA receptors reversed the effects of wild-type and N terminally deleted IQSEC2, indicating that spontaneous synaptic activity activates NMDA receptors, which, in turn, activates IQSEC2, producing a decrease in AMPA receptors. This decrease was shown to be dependent on SEC7 activity. Transfection of the IQSEC2 construct BRAG-IQ containing a mutated IQ region (rendering it unable to bind to calmodulin) resulted in a decreased AMPA receptor response that was not dependent on NMDA receptor signaling. The authors suggest that the BRAG-IQ mutant is constitutively active and does not require calcium-induced release of calmodulin to undergo an activating conformational change [22].

A second group studying synaptic transmission found that transfection of wild-type *IQSEC2* into organotypic hippocampal neurons resulted in an increase in AMPA receptor signaling that was independent of SEC7 activity but required the presence of the PDZ binding motif [14]. In addition, surface expression of GluA2 was shown to be increased by IQSEC2. The increase in AMPA signaling in this study is opposite to that discussed above [22] where a decrease in AMPA signaling was seen with wild-type IQSEC2. Differences in the age of the cell cultures used by both groups may be an important factor in resolving the discrepant results. It has been shown that during postnatal weeks 2–3, there is a switch from NMDA receptor subunit GluN2B-IQSEC2 signaling to GluN2A-IQSEC1 signaling in cortical cultures [23]. These effects were also seen in hippocampal neurons and may be responsible for the differences seen above.

Additional experiments by the second group [14] involved induction of long-term potentiation (LTP) and long-term depression (LTD) in *IQSEC2*-transfected organotypic hippocampal slices. The results showed that IQSEC2 was not involved in LTP, whereas LTD was dependent on IQSEC2 containing a functional SEC7 domain and the C terminal PDZ binding motif. In addition, immunoprecipitation experiments showed that in addition to PSD-95, IQSEC2 was found in complexes containing the NR1 and NR2A subunits of NMDA receptors. These results are in agreement with the finding that IQSEC2 plays a role in AMPA receptor removal mediated by NMDA receptor activity [22].

A recent study has been conducted using a transgenic mouse model of *IQSEC2* carrying a mutation in the IQ region (A350V) originally found in a young male subject with moderate to severe ID and ASD [24]. The mice display seizures between days 14–21 which results in an approximately 40% mortality rate among hemizygous males and 20% mortality among heterozygous females [17]. Biochemical analysis revealed that transgenic mice carrying the A350V mutation displayed decreased levels of surface AMPA receptor subunit GluA2, as assessed by FACS analysis of hippocampal cells, immunocytochemistry of hippocampal brain slices, and immunoblotting of crosslinked cell surface proteins from hippocampi [17]. This mutation was associated with a calcium-independent GEF activity as assessed by the GGA3 pull down assay in cells treated with or without ionomycin, similar to the BRAG1-IQ mutation discussed above [22].

It was further shown that wild-type IQSEC2 does bind to calcium/calmodulin as measured by binding to calmodulin sepharose, with half maximal binding occurring at 1 µM [17]. The A350V mutant protein also bound to calcium/calmodulin sepharose with similar affinity. However, when measured in HEK cells using the Lumier assay, the A350V mutant IQSEC2 bound much less efficiently to apocalmodulin when compared to wild-type IQSEC2. Discrepant results stating that calcium releases calmodulin bound to IQSEC2 [22] may have been due to different concentrations of Triton X-100 present in the lysis buffer used by the two groups.

In summary, we can suggest that the initial steps in IQSEC2 signaling are as follows (see Figure 2): IQSEC2 is normally bound to apocalmodulin in the cell under basal conditions. IQSEC2/calmodulin is found in complex with PSD-95 and NMDA receptors and likely a large number of additional proteins. When glutamate binds to the NMDA receptor, it becomes activated, allowing an influx of calcium, which binds to calmodulin present on IQSEC2 and causes a conformational change. This alteration in protein conformation activates the SEC7 domain and leads to an increase in ARF-GTP. In the case of the A350V mutant, IQSEC2 adopts a constitutively active conformation, leading to increased ARF6-GTP and a decrease in AMPA receptors. The steps leading from active ARF-GTP to changes in surface AMPA receptors are less well understood but appear to involve JNK kinase [22].

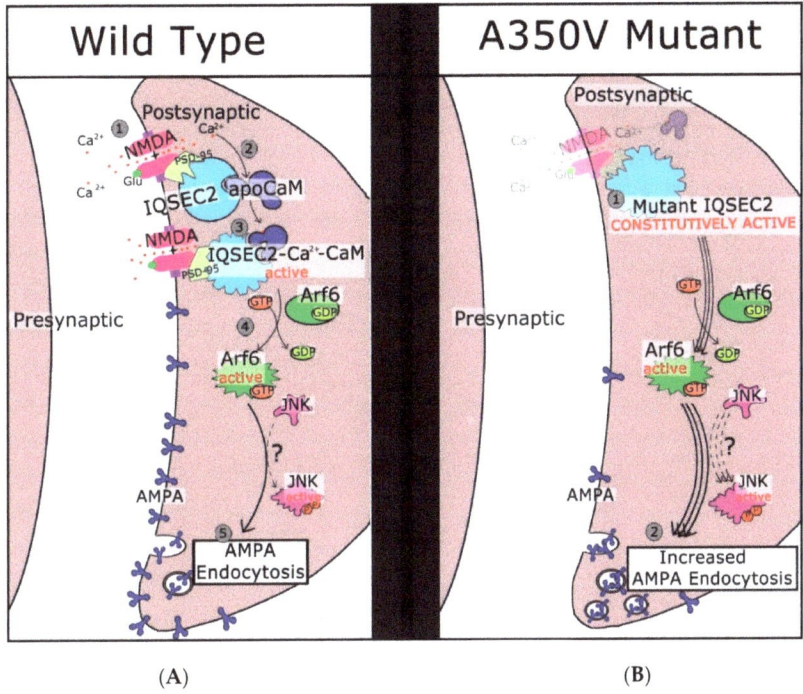

Figure 2. Signal transduction pathway in wild type and A350V mutant IQSEC2. In the left panel (**A**), binding of glutamine to the NMDA receptor (pink shape) allows calcium ion influx (step 1). Binding of calcium to calmodulin present on IQSEC2 (light blue shape) causes a conformational change (step 2) in IQSEC2 resulting in activation of the SEC7 catalytic domain (step 3). GDP is exchanged for GTP on ARF6 (green shape), resulting in active ARF6 (step 4). Additional steps including JNK activation (purple shape) lead to endocytosis of AMPA receptors (step 5). In the right panel (**B**), the A350V mutant IQSEC2 is constitutively active (step 1) leading to constant activation of ARF6 and JNK, enhanced endocytosis of AMPA receptors (step 2), and decreased surface AMPA expression. (Reproduced from reference 17.)

6. Therapeutic Treatment of IQSEC2-Associated ID and Autism

The above data suggest possible targets for drug treatment in *IQSEC2*-associated ID and autism based on the molecular pathophysiology associated with specific mutations. One potential target is the Sec7 activity of IQSEC2. A second potential target is the regulation of AMPA receptor recycling. With regards to the constitutively elevated Sec7 activity demonstrated by the A350V mutation, the objective would be to restore the normal situation wherein the Sec7 activity is normally inactive and is only induced by calcium influx through the NMDA receptor. A precise personalized medicine for this mutation would be a drug that was specific for the Sec7 domain of A350V IQSEC2 and whose activity would itself be inhibited by intracellular calcium. We are currently working on designing such a drug. For the second target, the recycling of AMPA receptors, several drugs are currently in existence [25]. Specifically, the drug parampanel inhibits recycling, while ritalin and aniracetam increase recycling. The recently described positive allosteric modulators (PAM) of AMPA receptor activity such as PF-4778574 may serve to increase AMPAR activity in the setting of an absolute decrease in AMPAR levels.

The importance of understanding the precise mechanism underlying a given mutation for personalized therapy is underscored by the apparent difference in the molecular pathophysiology of different *IQSEC2* mutations. The work of a number of investigators [14,22] proposes that many IQSEC2 mutations (specifically truncations or missense mutations in Sec7) result in a down regulation of IQSEC2 Sec7 activity and a corresponding increase in surface AMPAR. This precisely represents the opposite pathophysiology of what is seen with A350V *IQSEC2*. A similar paradigm whereby two different mutations in the same gene can oppositely regulate AMPA receptors was recently demonstrated for the thorase gene where some mutations decrease thorase activity and are associated with an increase in AMPA receptors (treatable with parampanel) while other mutations increase thorase activity and they are associated with a decrease in surface AMPA receptors, which might be treatable with AMPA receptor PAMS [26,27]. Transgenic mice carrying *IQSEC2* mutations as well as pluripotent stem cells derived from patient tissue may serve as models for testing these approaches to treat specific *IQSEC2* mutations associated with ID and autism.

Author Contributions: Conceptualization, writing, reviewing, and editing were done by N.S.L., G.K.E.U., E.J.R., R.J., O.L., and A.P.L.

Funding: This work was funded in part by the Rappaport Research Institute to APL and NIH/NINDS NS099362 to GU and by the Technion Institute-Johns Hopkins University Collaborative Research Fund 2026496 to APL.

Conflicts of Interest: Authors declare that the research was conducted in the absence of any commercial or financial relationships that could be construed as a potential conflict of interest.

Abbreviations

ID	Intellectual disability
NMDA	N-methyl-D-aspartate
PSD	Post synaptic density
GTP	Guanosine triphosphate
GDP	Guanosine diphosphate
ARF	ADP ribosylation factor
AMPA	α-Amino-3-hydroxy-5-methyl-4-isoxazolepropionic acid
GABA	Gamma-aminobutyric acid
ASD	Autism spectrum disorder
CC	Coiled coil
PH	Pleckstrin homology
PRM	Proline rich motif
PDZ	Post synaptic density protein (PSD95), Drosophila disc large tumor suppressor (Dlg1), and zonula occludens-1 protein (zo-1)
GEF	Guanine nucleotide exchange factor
MAGUK	Membrane associated guanylate kinase
IRSp53	Insulin receptor substrate of 53 kda
BAIAP2	Brain specific angiogenesis inhibitor 1-associated protein 2
SAP97	Synapse associated protein 97
CaMKIIa	Calcium calmodulin kinase iia
GGA3	Golgi associated gamma adaptin ear containing ARF binding protein 3
JNK	C-jun N terminal kinase
PAM	Positive allosteric modulators

References

1. Shoubridge, C.; Tarpey, P.S.; Abidi, F.; Ramsden, S.L.; Rujirabanjerd, S.; Murphy, J.S.; Boyle, J.; Shaw, M.; Gardner, A.; Proos, A.; et al. Mutations in the guanine nucleotide exchange factor gene IQSEC2 cause non-syndromic intellectual disability. *Nat. Genet.* **2010**, *42*, 486–488. [CrossRef] [PubMed]
2. Mignot, C.; McMahon, A.C.; Bar, C.; Campeau, P.M.; Davidson, C.; Buratti, J.; Nava, C.; Jacquemont, M.L.; Tallot, M.; Milh, M.; et al. IQSEC2-related encephalopathy in males and females: a comparative study including 37 novel patients. *Genet. Med.* **2019**, *4*, 837–849. [CrossRef] [PubMed]
3. Shoubridge, C.; Harvey, R.J.; Dudding-Byth, T. IQSEC2 mutation update and review of the female-specific phenotype spectrum including intellectual disability and epilepsy. *Hum. Mutat.* **2019**, *40*, 5–24. [CrossRef] [PubMed]
4. Sakagami, H.; Sanda, M.; Fukaya, M.; Miyazaki, T.; Sukegawa, J.; Yanagisawa, T.; Suzuki, T.; Fukunaga, K.; Watanabe, M.; Kondo, H. IQ-ArfGEF/BRAG1 is a guanine nucleotide exchange factor for Arf6 that interacts with PSD-95 at postsynaptic density of excitatory synapses. *Neurosci. Res.* **2008**, *60*, 199–212. [CrossRef] [PubMed]
5. Petrovski, S.; Wang, Q.; Erin, L.; Heinzen, E.L.; Allen, A.S.; Goldstein, D.B. Genic Intolerance to Functional Variation and the Interpretation of Personal Genomes. *PLoS Genet.* **2013**, *9*, 1–13. [CrossRef]
6. Kim, Y.; Lee, S.-E.; Park, J.; Kim, M.; Lee, B.; Hwang, D.; Chang, S. ADP-ribosylation Factor 6 (ARF6) Bidirectionally Regulates Dendritic Spine Formation Depending on Neuronal Maturation and Activity. *J. Biol. Chem.* **2015**, *290*, 7323–7335. [CrossRef]
7. Straub, C.; Sabatini, B.L. How to Grow a Synapse. *Neuron* **2014**, *82*, 256. [CrossRef]
8. Murphy, J.A.; Jensenb, O.N.; Walikonis, R.S. BRAG1, a Sec7 domain-containing protein, is a component of the postsynaptic density of excitatory synapses. *Brain Res.* **2006**, *1120*, 35–45. [CrossRef] [PubMed]
9. Hinze, S.J.; Jackson, M.R.; Lie, S.; Jolly, L.; Field, M.; Barry, S.C.; Harvey, R.J.; Shoubridge, C. Incorrect dosage of IQSEC2, a known intellectual disability and epilepsy gene, disrupts dendritic spine morphogenesis. *Transl. Psychiatry* **2017**, *7*, 1–11. [CrossRef] [PubMed]
10. Coley, A.A.; Gao, W.-J. PSD95: A synaptic protein implicated in schizophrenia or autism? *Prog. Neuro-Psychoph.* **2017**, *82*, 187–194. [CrossRef] [PubMed]
11. Forrest, M.P.; Euan Parnell, E.; Penzes, P. Dendritic structural plasticity and neuropsychiatric disease. *Nat. Rev. Neurosci.* **2018**, *19*, 215–234. [CrossRef] [PubMed]
12. Frank, R.A.; Komiyama, N.H.; Ryan, T.J.; Zhu, F.; O'Dell, T.J.; Grant, S.G. NMDA receptors are selectively partitioned into complexes and supercomplexes during synapse maturation. *Nat. Commun.* **2016**, *7*, 11264. [CrossRef] [PubMed]
13. Frank, R.A.W.; Zhu, F.; Komiyama, N.H.; Grant, S.G.N. Hierarchical organisation and genetically separable subfamilies of PSD95 postsynaptic supercomplexes. *J. Neurochem.* **2017**, *142*, 504–511. [CrossRef] [PubMed]
14. Brown, J.C.; Petersen, A.; Zhong, L.; Himelright, M.L.; Murphy, J.A.; Walikonis, R.S.; Gerges, N.Z. Bidirectional regulation of synaptic transmission by BRAG1/IQSEC2 and its requirement in long-term depression. *Nat. Commun.* **2015**, *7*, 11080. [CrossRef] [PubMed]
15. Kang, J.; Park, H.; Kim, E. IRSp53/BAIAP2 in dendritic spine development, NMDA receptor regulation, and psychiatric disorders. *Neuropharm.* **2016**, *100*, 27–39. [CrossRef] [PubMed]
16. Rogers, E.J.; Jada, R.; Schragenheim-Rozales, K.; Sah, M.; Cortes, M.; Florence, M.; Levy, N.S.; Moss, R.; Walikonis, R.S.; Palty, R.; et al. An IQSEC2 mutation associated with intellectual disability and autism results in decreased surface AMPA receptors. *Front. Mol. Neurosci.* **2019**, *12*, 43. [CrossRef]
17. Sanda, M.; Kamata, A.; Katsumata, O.; Fukunaga, K.; Watanabe, M.; Kondo, H.; Sakagami, H. The postsynaptic density protein, IQ-ArfGEF/BRAG1, can interact with IRSp53 through its proline-rich sequence. *Brain Res.* **2009**, *1251*, 7–15. [CrossRef] [PubMed]
18. Hell, J.W. CaMKII: Claiming Center Stage in Postsynaptic Function and Organization. *Neuron* **2014**, *81*, 249–265. [CrossRef]
19. Dosemeci, A.; Makusky, A.J.; Jankowska-Stephens, E.; Yang, X.; Slotta, D.J.; Markey, S.M. Composition of the Synaptic PSD-95 Complex. *Mol Cell Proteomics* **2007**, *6*, 1749–1760. [CrossRef]
20. Guang, S.; Pang, N.; Deng, X.; Yang, L.; He, F.; Wu, L.; Chen, C.; Yin, F.; Peng, J. Synaptopathology Involved in Autism Spectrum Disorder. *Front. Cell. Neurosci.* **2018**, *12*, 470. [CrossRef]

21. Kim, J.-W.; Park, K.; Kang, J.; Gonzales, E.L.T.; Kim, D.G.; Oh, H.A.; Seung, H.; Ko, M.J.; Kwon, K.J.; Kim, K.C.; et al. Pharmacological modulation of AMPA receptor rescues social impairments in animal models of autism. *Neuropsychopharmacology* **2019**, *44*, 314–323. [CrossRef] [PubMed]
22. Myers, K.R.; Wang, G.; Sheng, Y.; Conger, K.K.; Casanova, J.E.; Zhu, J.J. Arf6-BRAG1 regulates JNK-mediated synaptic removal of GluA1-containing AMPA receptors: A new mechanism for nonsyndromic X-linked mental disorder. *J. Neurosci.* **2012**, *32*, 11716–11726. [CrossRef] [PubMed]
23. Elagabani, M.N.; Brisevac, D.; Kintscher, M.; Pohle, J.; Kohr, G.; Schmitz, D.; Kornau, H.-C. Subunit-selective N-Methyl-D-aspartate (NMDA) receptor signaling through brefeldan A-resistant Arf guanine nucleotide exchange factors BRAG1 and BRAG2 during synapse maturation. *J. Biol. Chem.* **2016**, *291*, 9105–9118. [CrossRef] [PubMed]
24. Zerem, A.; Haginoya, K.; Lev, D.; Blumkin, L.; Kivity, S.; Liner, I.; Lerman-Sagie, T. The molecular and phenotypic spectrum of IQSEC2-related epilepsy. *Epilepsia* **2016**, *57*, 1858. [CrossRef] [PubMed]
25. Ahrens-Nicklas, R.C.; Umanah, G.K.; Sondheimer, N.; Deardorff, M.A.; Wilkens, A.B.; Conlin, L.K.; Santani, A.B.; Nesbitt, A.; Juulsola, J.; Ma, E.; et al. Precision therapy for a new disorder of AMPA receptor recycling due to mutations in ATAD1. *Neurol. Genet.* **2017**, *3*, e130. [CrossRef] [PubMed]
26. Piard, J.; Umanah, G.K.E.; Harms, F.L.; Abalde-Atristain, L.; Amram, D.; Chang, M.; Chen, R.; Alawi, M.; Salpietro, V.; Rees, M.I.; et al. A homozygous ATAD1 mutation impairs postsynaptic AMPA receptor trafficking and causes a lethal encephalopathy. *Brain* **2018**, *141*, 651–661. [CrossRef] [PubMed]
27. Umanah, G.K.E.; Pignatelli, M.; Yin, X.; Chen, R.; Crawford, J.; Neifert, S.; Scarffe, L.; Behensky, A.A.; Guiberson, N.; Chang, M.; et al. Thorase variants are associated with defects in glutamatergic neurotransmission that can be rescued by perampanel. *Sci. Transl. Med.* **2017**, *13*, 420. [CrossRef]

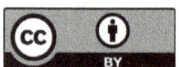

© 2019 by the authors. Licensee MDPI, Basel, Switzerland. This article is an open access article distributed under the terms and conditions of the Creative Commons Attribution (CC BY) license (http://creativecommons.org/licenses/by/4.0/).

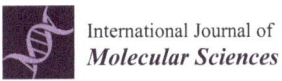

Article

High Functioning Autism with Missense Mutations in Synaptotagmin-Like Protein 4 (SYTL4) and Transmembrane Protein 187 (TMEM187) Genes: SYTL4- Protein Modeling, Protein-Protein Interaction, Expression Profiling and MicroRNA Studies

Syed K. Rafi [1,*], Alberto Fernández-Jaén [2], Sara Álvarez [3], Owen W. Nadeau [4] and Merlin G. Butler [1,*]

[1] Departments of Psychiatry & Behavioral Sciences and Pediatrics, University of Kansas Medical Center, Kansas City, KS 66160, USA
[2] Department of Pediatric Neurology, Hospital Universitario Quirón, 28223 Madrid, Spain
[3] Genomics and Medicine, NIM Genetics, 28108 Madrid, Spain
[4] Department of Biochemistry and Molecular Biology, University of Kansas Medical Center, Kansas City, KS 66160, USA
* Correspondence: rafigene@yahoo.com (S.K.R.); mbutler4@kumc.edu (M.G.B.); Tel.: +816-787-4366 (S.K.R.); +913-588-1800 (M.G.B.)

Received: 25 March 2019; Accepted: 17 June 2019; Published: 9 July 2019

Abstract: We describe a 7-year-old male with high functioning autism spectrum disorder (ASD) and maternally-inherited rare missense variant of Synaptotagmin-like protein 4 (*SYTL4*) gene (Xq22.1; c.835C>T; p.Arg279Cys) and an unknown missense variant of Transmembrane protein 187 (*TMEM187*) gene (Xq28; c.708G>T; p. Gln236His). Multiple in-silico predictions described in our study indicate a potentially damaging status for both X-linked genes. Analysis of predicted atomic threading models of the mutant and the native SYTL4 proteins suggest a potential structural change induced by the R279C variant which eliminates the stabilizing Arg279-Asp60 salt bridge in the N-terminal half of the SYTL4, affecting the functionality of the protein's critical RAB-Binding Domain. In the European (Non-Finnish) population, the allele frequency for this variant is 0.00042. The *SYTL4* gene is known to directly interact with several members of the RAB family of genes, such as, *RAB27A*, *RAB27B*, *RAB8A*, and *RAB3A* which are known autism spectrum disorder genes. The *SYTL4* gene also directly interacts with three known autism genes: *STX1A*, *SNAP25* and *STXBP1*. Through a literature-based analytical approach, we identified three of five (60%) autism-associated serum microRNAs (miRs) with high predictive power among the total of 298 mouse Sytl4 associated/predicted microRNA interactions. Five of 13 (38%) miRs were differentially expressed in serum from ASD individuals which were predicted to interact with the mouse equivalent *Sytl4* gene. *TMEM187* gene, like *SYTL4*, is a protein-coding gene that belongs to a group of genes which host microRNA genes in their introns or exons. The novel Q236H amino acid variant in the TMEM187 in our patient is near the terminal end region of the protein which is represented by multiple sequence alignments and hidden Markov models, preventing comparative structural analysis of the variant harboring region. Like *SYTL4*, the *TMEM187* gene is expressed in the brain and interacts with four known ASD genes, namely, *HCFC1*; *TMLHE*; *MECP2*; and *GPHN*. TMM187 is in linkage with *MECP2*, which is a well-known determinant of brain structure and size and is a well-known autism gene. Other members of the *TMEM* gene family, *TMEM132E* and *TMEM132D* genes are associated with bipolar and panic disorders, respectively, while *TMEM231* is a known syndromic autism gene. Together, *TMEM187* and *SYTL4* genes directly interact with recognized important ASD genes, and their mRNAs are found in extracellular vesicles in the nervous system and stimulate target cells to translate into active protein. Our evidence shows that both these genes should be considered as candidate genes for autism. Additional biological testing is warranted to further determine the pathogenicity of these gene variants in the causation of autism.

Keywords: autism candidate genes; synaptotagmin-like protein 4 (SYTL4); transmembrane protein 187 (TMEM187); SYTL4-protein structure; STRING-protein-protein interaction; expression profile; microRNA- interactions

1. Introduction

Whole exome sequencing (WES) and occasionally whole-genome sequencing (WGS) are increasingly used in clinical practice for diagnosis, medical intervention and prognosis [1–3]. High heritability estimates and family studies have supported a definite role of genetics in autism spectrum disorder (ASD). In neurodevelopmental disorders, particularly ASD and intellectual disability have diagnostic rates using WES which fluctuates in part from differences in clinical features from one study to another with rates up to 50% [4–7]. We describe a 7-year-old male with high-functioning autism spectrum disorder presenting for genetic services and whole exome sequencing following a normal microarray analysis, and variants were found in two X-linked genes: *SYTL4* and *TMEM187*.

1.1. Synaptotagmin-Like Protein 4 (SYTL4) Gene

SYTL4 gene, also known as Granuphilin/SLP4, encodes a member of the synaptotagmin-like protein family. Members of this family are characterized by an N-terminal RAB27-binding domain and C-terminal tandem C2 domains (Figures 1 and 2). The first C2 domain binds phospholipids in a calcium-independent manner, whereas the second C2 domain does not (http://omim.org/entry/300723). The encoded protein binds to specific small RAB-GTPases involved in intracellular membrane trafficking. This protein binds to RAB27 and may be involved in inhibiting dense core vesicle exocytosis. Alternate splicing results in multiple transcript variants that encode the same protein.

SYTL4 gene is relevant in neuronal system development and implicated in neurological and psychological diseases [8] (Entrez Gene ID # 94121 (Human); ID # 27359 (Mouse). This gene is highly expressed in the bed nucleus of the stria terminalis (BNTS) [9], a brain region that regulates mood, motivation for social behavior and social attachment [10]. *SYTL4* expression is down regulated in the dorsal raphe nucleus from patients with major depressive disorder [11]. In a mouse model of anxiety, significant change in Sytl4 was observed among the altered protein networks in the brain proteome [12].

Targeted Null/Knockout mutant *Sytl4* mammalian phenotypes for *Sytl4* showed abnormal behavior and neurological phenotype [13–15]. This gene interacts directly with other known autism genes. Confirmatively, gene expression knock-out *Sytl4* mutant mouse includes abnormal behavior and neurological problems [13,14]. Diseases already associated with *SYTL4* include Epileptic Encephalopathy (early Infantile) and Branchiootic syndrome (www.genecards.org/cgi-Fbin/carddisp.pl?gene=SYTL4&keywords=sytl4). A missense mutation in *SYTL4* was also recently reported in a female with autism and non-skewed X-chromosome inactivation [16].

1.2. Transmembrane Protein 187 (TEM187) Gene

The second gene in our study, *TMEM187*, is additionally known as *ITBA1/CXORF12/DXS9878E*-gene and consists of two exons which encode a multi-pass membrane protein expressed in all regions of the brain (www.genecards.org/cgi-bin/carddisp.pl?gene=TMEM187&keywords=TMEM187). This is a conserved gene that codes a 261-amino-acid protein with six transmembrane helical domains. Unlike *SYTL4*, not much is known about this gene, but it belongs to a group of genes which host microRNA genes in their introns or exons [17]. One of this gene's related phenotypes is schizophrenia (GWAS catalog for *TMEM187* gene: Gene relation via enhancers containing phenotype SNP: Enhancer ID: GH0XJ153980). The latest STRING- network of protein interactions for this gene reveals that it directly interacts with four known ASD genes, namely, *HCFC1*; *TMLHE*; *MECP2* and *GPHN*. (https://gene.sfari.org/database/human-gene/).

2. Results

2.1. Genomic Study

Whole exome sequencing performed in trios revealed maternally inherited X-linked missense variants: c.835C>T, p. Arg279Cys in the *SYTL4* gene and c.708G>T; and p. Gln236His in the *TMEM187* gene. Research findings will be discussed that relate specifically to *SYTL4* and *TMEM187* gene variants seen in our patient and as emerging candidate genes for autism.

2.2. Synaptotagmin-Like 4 (SYTL4) Gene

2.2.1. Deleterious and Damaging Nature of the SYTL4- Variant

The maternally inherited variant in Synaptotagmin-like protein 4 gene *(SYTL4)* at chromosome-X position g.99944930G>A, c.835C>T, p. Arg279Cys [NM_001174068.1] sits within exon 9 of the *SYTL4* gene located at the Xq22.1 cytoband (Figure 1). This particular *SYTL4* nucleotide variant CGC⇒TGC at position 835 (exon 9; alternating) has been predicted by large-scale genomic sequencing studies, such as the 1000 Genome project, to be deleterious (SIFT score 0.01) and possibly damaging (Polyphen score 0.79), which is further validated with a MAF score of 0.0005/2. The Exome Aggregation Consortium (ExAC) database including data from 1000 genomes further indicated that the *SYTL4* variant is also damaging.

Our patient is from Spain and according to Exome Aggregation Consortium, the allele frequency among European (Non-Finnish) population for this variant is 0.0004222. No homozygotes were found, but eight hemizygotes (male) were observed in 47372 alleles which presumably included both isoforms. There is no reported information from these individuals regarding findings related to ASD when examining clinical information-sharing resources such as Phenome Central, Gene Matcher or ClinVar.

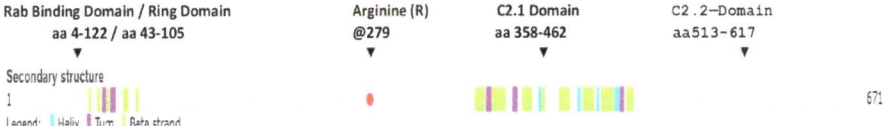

Figure 1. Graphic representation of the secondary structure of *SYTL4* gene indicating the location of Rab binding domain, ring domain, C2 domains, and the location of arginine at amino acid position 279.

2.2.2. Modeling of Native and R279C Mutant for SYTL4 Gene

There is limited high-resolution structural information about *SYTL4*. The crystal [18] and NMR [19] structure of C2(1) (residues 354-483) and ring domain (residues 43-105) cover only 29% of the protein primary structure. A structural comparison of *SYTL4* and the R279C mutant was carried out using the I-TASSER multiple threading approach [20]. The protein structure closest to both forms of SYTL4 found in the Protein Data Bank (PDB) [21] is human synaptotagmin 2 (PDB #4P42) [22,23], with TM scores (0.658 and 0.661) and RMSD values (1.15 Å and 0.96 Å), respectively, for the native and R279C form (Figure 2).

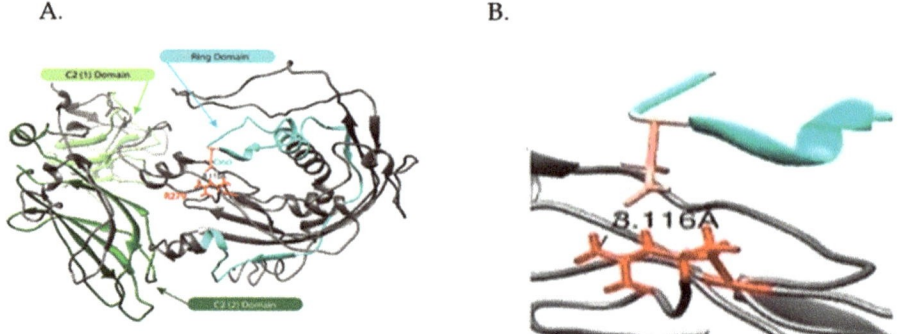

Figure 2. The native SYTL4 protein structure contains the C2 domains, ring domain, and an apparent salt bridge between arginine (R279) and aspartic acid (D60) as noted in (**A**). Arginine 279 (side chain in red) is part of a large extended loop conformation that appears to be stabilized by an apparent salt bridge formed between it and Asp60 (side chain in Salmon) in the ring domain. The distance (3.116Å) calculated between the Arg guanidinium nitrogen and Asp carboxyl oxygen is well within the threshold distance observed for salt bridges in a comprehensive survey of crystal structures as noted in (**B**).

2.2.3. Hierarchical Protein Structural Modeling Study of Both Native and R (279) C SYTL4

Both atomic models preserved the canonical C2 structures of synaptotagmins; [21–23], however, only the native SYTL4 preserved the extended structure of the ring domain (Figure 3) [18]. An overlay (Figure 3C) of two atomic models demonstrated good alignment of the C-terminal C2 domains, whereas the structures of the region comprising both the ring domain and the 279 amino acid change sites for the two SYTL4 forms differed considerably. In the native SYTL4 model, Arg 279 (side chain in red) is part of a large extended loop conformation that appears to be stabilized by an apparent salt bridge formed between it and Asp60 (side chain in Salmon) in the ring domain. The distance (3.116 Å) calculated between the Arginine guanidinium nitrogen and Asp carboxyl oxygen (magnified in Figure 3B) is well within the threshold distance observed for salt bridges in a comprehensive survey of crystal structures [24]. In the R279C model, Cys279 is in a beta sheet, with no apparent hydrogen bonding contacts observed within distance constraints for such interactions [25] (Figure 3A,B). Our modeling suggests a potential structural change induced by the R279C variant, which eliminates the stabilizing Arg279-Asp60 salt bridge and, therefore, leads to significant structural changes in the N-terminal half of the SYTL4.

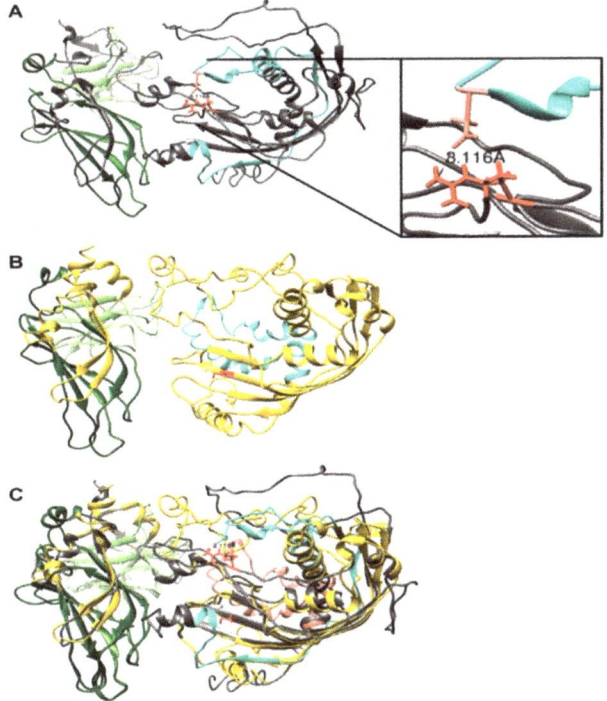

Figure 3. Effect of the R[Arg]⇒C[Cys] amino acid change at 279 on the structure of SYTL4 Proteins. Theoretical 3D structures of native and R279C SYTL4. Hierarchical protein structural modeling of both native (**A**) and R279C (**B**) SYTL4 proteins were carried out using I-TASSER. Three X-ray crystal structures of human Synaptotagmin C2 domains (Protein Data Bank ID: 2R83, 4P42 and 3HN8) among the top 10 templates used for both SYTL4 forms. Native SYTL4 (grey ribbon trace) and R279C variant (gold ribbon trace) are shown with C2(1), C2(2) and ring domains rendered as light green, dark green and cyan traces, respectively, in Panels (**A,B**). Panel (**A**): SYTL4 native protein structure indicating the C2 domains, ring domain, and an apparent salt bridge between arginine (R279) and aspartic acid (D60). Shown magnified in the native SYTL4 structure is the apparent salt bridge formed between D60 and R279. Panel (**B**): SYTL4 R279C variant (gold ribbon trace) shows significant displacement of both the 279 amino acid site (salmon ribbon trace) and ring domains of native (cyan ribbon trace). Panel (**C**): An overlay of native (**A**) and R279C (**B**) SYTL4 structures demonstrates relatively good alignment for the C terminal C2 domains and confirms the significant displacement of both the 279 amino acid site (salmon ribbon trace) and ring domains of native (cyan ribbon trace) SYTL4.

2.2.4. STRING- Protein–Protein Interaction Network Study Reveals Direct Interaction of *SYTL4* with Other Known Autism Genes

SYTL4 directly interacts with three known *ASD* genes, *STX1A*, *SNAP25* and *STXBP1* (https://gene.sfari.org/database/human-gene/). *SYTL4* also interacts with 14 other genes, namely, *FGF4*, *STX1B*, *SNAP29*, *RAB3A*, *SNAP23*, *RAB27B*, *RAB8A*, *SNAP47*, *STX4*, *STX19*, *STX3*, *STX11*, *STX2*, and *RAB27A*, whose transcriptome-wide isoform-level multiple related gene family members are known ASD genes (https://gene.sfari.org/database/human-gene/). SYTL4 also directly interacts with several members of the RAB-family of genes, such as *RAB27A*, *RAB27B*, *RAB8A*, and *RAB3A* [26] (Figure 4).

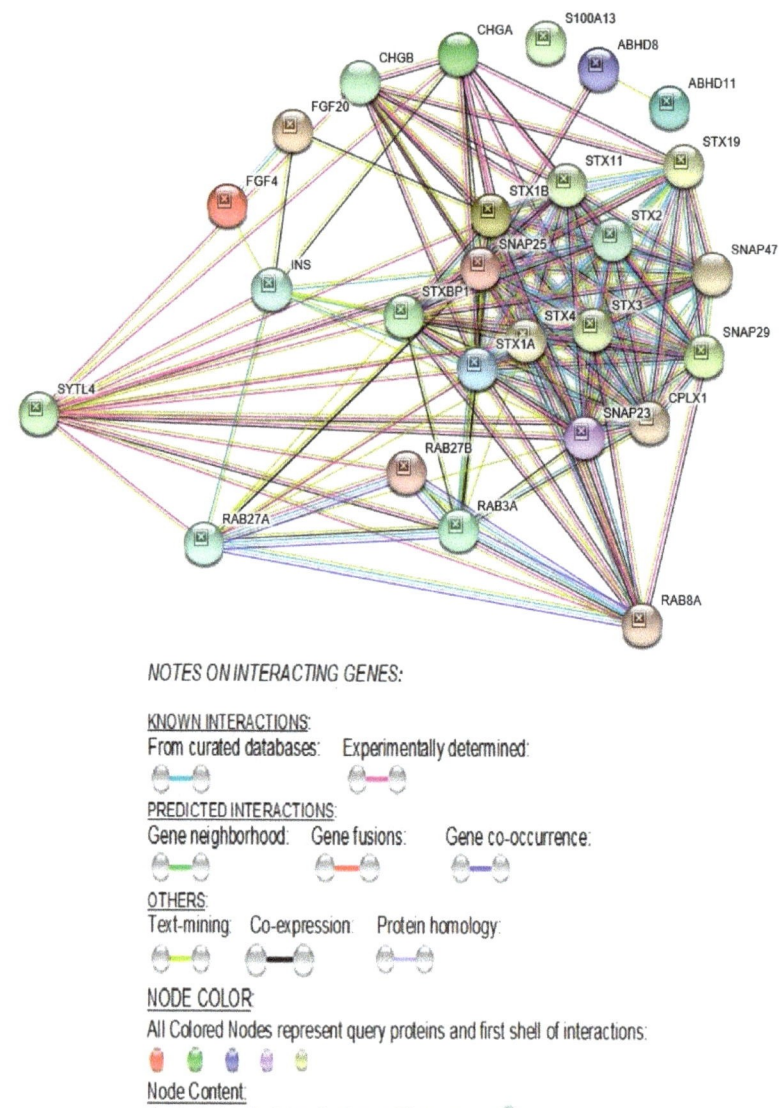

Figure 4. STRING- Protein-Protein Interaction Network of SYTL4. [https://version11.string-db.org/cgi/network.pl?taskId=f7upTuHlbV0A]. SYTL4- Interacting ASD Genes; *SYTL4*: Synaptotagmin-like protein 4; modulates exocytosis of dense-core granules and secretion of hormones in the pancreas and the pituitary. Interacts with vesicles containing negatively charged phospholipids in a Ca (2+)-independent manner; synaptotagmin-like tandem C2 proteins. STXBP1: Syntaxin-binding protein 1; may participate in the regulation of synaptic vesicle docking and fusion. Essential for neurotransmission and binds syntaxin, a component of the synaptic vesicle fusion machinery (Score: 0.746). STX1A: Syntaxin-1A; plays a role in hormone and neurotransmitter exocytosis. Potentially involved in docking of synaptic vesicles at presynaptic active zones (Score: 0.805). SNAP25: Synaptosomal-associated protein 25; t-SNARE involved in the molecular regulation of neurotransmitter release. May play an important role in the synaptic function of specific neuronal systems (Score: 0.551).

2.2.5. SYTL4- Molecular Pathways and Associated Diseases

The molecular pathways of the *SYTL4* gene includes a synaptic vesicle cycle, insulin secretion, AMPK- signaling, and SNARE interactions in vesicular transport (Table 1). Diseases associated with synaptic vesicle cycle defects include early infantile epileptic encephalopathy and defects in insulin secretion including defects in degradation of gangliosides which are abundantly expressed in the nervous system. The deficiency of certain gangliosides will affect the regenerative ability of injured hypoglossal nerves [27]. Lastly, defective SNARE interactions in vesicular transport have been implicated in CEDNIK-syndrome, which includes cerebral dysgenesis and neuropathy. All the noted pathways and their associated diseases broadly impact nervous system function which are relevant to autism (Table 1) [26].

Table 1. SYTL4 Molecular Pathways and Associated Diseases.

Pathway ID	Pathway Description	Count in Gene Set	False Discovery Rate	Functional Description
4721	Synaptic vesicle cycle	3	0.0161	Communication between neurons is mediated by the release of neurotransmitter from synaptic vesicles (SVs). At the nerve terminal, SVs cycle through repetitive episodes of exocytosis and endocytosis. SVs are filled with neurotransmitters by active transport. DISEASES: Early infantile epileptic encephalopathy; Centronuclear myopathy; Episodic ataxias; Familial or sporadic hemiplegic migraine
4911	Insulin secretion	3	0.0161	Insulin secretion is regulated by several hormones and neurotransmitters. Peptide hormones, such as glucagon-like peptide 1 (GLP-1), increase cAMP levels and thereby potentiate insulin secretion via the combined action of PKA and Epac2. Acetylcholine (Ach), a major parasympathetic neurotransmitter. DISEASES: Type II diabetes mellitus; Defects in the degradation of ganglioside.
4152	AMPK signaling pathway	3	0.0325	AMP-activated protein kinase (AMPK) is a serine threonine kinase that is highly conserved through evolution. AMPK system acts as a sensor of cellular energy status.
4130	SNARE interactions	2	0.0432	SNARE proteins (an acronym derived from "SNAP (Soluble NSF Attachment Protein) Receptor"). The primary role of SNARE proteins is to mediate vesicle fusion, that is, the fusion of vesicles with their target membrane-bound compartments. The best studied SNAREs are those that mediate docking of synaptic vesicles with the presynaptic membrane in neurons. DISEASES: Pseudohypoparathyroidism and Cerebral dysgenesis, neuropathy, ichthyosis, and palmoplantar keratoderma syndrome; CEDNIK syndrome.

2.2.6. SYTL4- Networks of Biological Processes

As presented in Table 2 [26], extensive biological processes of the *SYTL4* gene pertain to synaptic vesicle functions, including neurotransmitter secretion and regulation of signaling, RAB protein signal transduction, glutamate secretion, neuro-muscular synaptic transmission, and axonogenesis, all of which are relevant for proper neuronal function, and thus important in autism.

Table 2. SYTL4- Network: Biological Processes

Pathway ID	Pathway Description	Count in Gene Set	False Discovery Rate
GO:0048489	synaptic vesicle transport	8	1.14×10^{-9}
GO:0097479	synaptic vesicle localization	8	1.14×10^{-9}
GO:0016079	synaptic vesicle exocytosis	7	1.79×10^{-9}
GO:0016082	synaptic vesicle priming	4	1.14×10^{-7}
GO:0031629	synaptic vesicle fusion to presynaptic membrane	4	5.45×10^{-7}
GO:0007269	neurotransmitter secretion	6	3.06×10^{-6}
GO:0048167	regulation of synaptic plasticity	5	0.000171
GO:0032482	RAB protein signal transduction	4	0.000701
GO:0031630	regulation of synaptic vesicle fusion to presynaptic membrane	2	0.00156
GO:0014047	glutamate secretion	3	0.00165
GO:0007268	synaptic transmission	6	0.0115
GO:0023051	regulation of signaling	1	0.0211
GO:0050803	regulation of synapse structure or activity	4	0.0249
GO:0050804	modulation of synaptic transmission	4	0.0356
GO:0007274	neuromuscular synaptic transmission	2	0.0385
GO:0065008	regulation of biological quality	1	0.0389
GO:0007409	axonogenesis	5	0.0393

2.2.7. SYTL4- Molecular Functions

The molecular function of the *SYTL4* gene includes syntaxin binding, which is essential for neurotransmission (Table 3) [26] and directly interacts with syntaxin-binding protein 1 (STXBP1) (Figure 4). Mutations in STXBP1 are associated with infantile-epileptic encephalopathy-4 [28]. *SYTL4* molecular gene function also relates to synaptosomal-associated protein receptor (SNAPRe) activity which regulates neurotransmitter release to ensure vesicle-to-target specificity [29]. In addition, the molecular function of the *SYTL4* gene pertains to trimeric-G-protein (GDP binding protein) which plays a pivotal role in signal transduction pathways for numerous hormones and neurotransmitters [30].

Table 3. Molecular Function (GO)

Pathway ID	Pathway Description	Count in Gene Set	False Discovery Rate	Functional Description and Associated Diseases
GO:0019905; GO:0017075	Syntaxin binding	6	5.46×10^{-7}	Syntaxin binding is essential for neurotransmission: syntaxin is a component of the synaptic vesicle fusion machinery. Mutations in Syntaxin binding protein 1 (STXBP1) have been associated with infantile-epileptic encephalopathy-4 [28].
GO:0005484	SNAP receptor activity	4	0.000161	SNAPRE activity also regulates neurotransmitter release to ensure vesicle-to-target specificity (SNAP receptors implicated in vesicle targeting and fusion [29].
GO:0019003	GDP binding	3	0.019	The trimeric-G-protein (GTP binding proteins) play a pivotal role in the signal transduction pathways for numerous hormones and neurotransmitters [30].

2.2.8. Missense Mutation Causing R (279) C Amino Acid Change Affects the Structures of Canonical *SYTL4* Gene as Well as Its Shorter Isoform

The amino acid change found in our study, R(arg)279C(cys) in exon 9 (Figure 1), is integral for the full length 'canonical' sequence of the SYTL4 protein with 671 amino acids. It is also part of the shorter isoform containing 349 amino acids shown in Figure 5. The R>C amino acid variation at residue 279 has been classified by the Human Genome Variation Society (HGVS) as a missense variant (variation ID # rs141441277) and determined to be least common with a Minor Allele Frequency (MAF) of 0.000529801. It is further predicted as "possible damaging" with a PolyPhen score of 0.79, while SIFT predicts the effect of this amino acid change on protein function as "deleterious" (https://gnomad.broadinstitute.org/variant/X-99944930-G-A; Variant Effect Predictor (VEP) program: https://useast.ensembl.org/info/docs/tools/vep/index.html.

```
1    MSELLDLSFL SEEEKDLILS VLQRDEEVRK ADEKRIRRLK NELLEIKRKG
51   AKRGSQHYSD [60] RTCARCQESL GRLSPKTNTC RGCNHLVCRD CRIQESNGTW
101  RCKVCAKEIE LKKATGDWFY DQKVNRFAYR TGSEIIRMSL RHKPAVSKRE
151  TVGQSLLHQT QMGDIWPGRK IIQERQKEPS VLFEVPKLKS GKSALEAESE
201  SLDSFTADSD STSRRDSLDK SGLFPEWKKM SAPKSQVERE TQPGGQNVVF
251  VDEGEMIFKK NTRKILRPSE YTKSVIDLR[279]⇒CP EDVVHESGSL DRSKSVPGL
301  NVDMEEEEEE EDIDHLVKLH RQKLARSSMQ SGSSMSTIGS MMSIYSEAGD
351  FGNIFVTGRI AFSLKYEQQT QSLVVHVKEC HQLAYADEAK KRSNPYVKTY
401  LLPDKSRQGK RKTSIKRDTI NPLYDETLRY EIPESLLAQR TLQFSVWHHG
451  RFGRNTFLGE AEIQMDSWKL DKKLDHCLPL HGKISAESPT GLPSHKGELV
501  VSLKYIPASK TPVGGDRKKS KGGEGGELQV WIKEAKNLTA AKAGGTSDSF
551  VKGYLLPMRN KASKRKTPVM KKTLNPHYNH TFVYNGVRLE DLQHMCLELT
601  VWDREPLASN DFLGGVRLGV GTGISNGEVV DWMDSTGEEV SLWQKMRQYP
651  GSWAEGTLQL RSSMAKQKLG L
658-671: VSSIRSVVTGMLGY (in Isoform 2)
```

Figure 5. SYTL4 amino acids sequence data for the "canonical" form and its truncated isoform 2, both encompassing the alternating exon 9 with the missense mutation resulting in R[Arg]⇒C[Cys] at 279: Amino acid sequences that are highlighted in blue are the first 335 amino acids which are common to both the full length 'canonical' sequence of the SYTL4 protein and its truncated isoform 2, both containing the alternating exon 9 Glu(E) 270–Met(M) 304, highlighted in yellow with the R[Arg]⇒C[Cys] at 279. The location of native arginine residue (at 279) in-between two Serine(S) amino acid residues at 274 and 289 positions (which have been shown to undergo post-translational phosphorylation) is underlined. The RAB-Binding Domain (comprised of amino acids 4 through 122) is also indicated with underline, within which lies D[Asp] at position 60 and takes part in the apparent salt bridge formation with R[Arg] at 279 in the native protein configuration. The presence of mutant C[Cys] at 279 leads to the formation of an extended beta-pleated sheet therein instead (as seen in Figure 3A,B).

2.2.9. Autism Predictive Human Serum MicroRNAs with Predicted Interaction with Mouse *Sytl4* Gene

Among the total of 298 mouse Sytl4 associated/predicted miRs, three of the five miRs (60%), namely, miR181b-5p, miR320a, and miR130a-3p- are with good ASD predictive power in serum, as identified in Table 4. Apart from the five-serum miRNAs with good ASD predictive power, miR106b-5p and miR328- were up and down regulated (respectively) in the serum ASD study. Both miRs have been reported as showing altered expression among schizophrenics [31–34]. Interestingly, these two miRs have been predicted to interact with mouse *Sytl4* gene (Table 4). In addition, four other miRs (miR98, miR103, miR132, and miR320) have been found to be dysregulated in the superior temporal gyrus of ASD [35] and predicted to interact with mouse *Sytl4* gene. Furthermore, miR106b, miR181b-5p, miR320, and miR328 are differentially expressed in the ASD cerebellar cortex [35,36] and predicted to interact with mouse *Sytl4* gene (Table 4).

Table 4. Showing the Five Autism Predictive Human Serum MicroRNAs with Predicted Interaction with Mouse *Sytl4* Gene.

Sytl4-miR=ASD-miR	Mouse Sytl4- miRs: Predicted Interactions with ASD & Schizophrenia- Associated miRs	Validation	Reference
miR93	Sytl4	predicted	MGI:1351606c
miR93	ASD	Dysregulated in superior temporal gyrus of ASD	Stomova, et al., 2015 [37]
miR103-1; miR103-2	Sytl4	Predicted	MGI:1351606c
miR103	ASD	Dysregulated in superior temporal gyrus of ASD	Stomova, et al., 2015 [37]
miR106b	Sytl4	Predicted	MGI:1351606c
miR106b-5p (miR106b) *	ASD	Upregulated in ASD-serum; differentially expressed in ASD cerebellar cortex	Vasu, et al., 2014 [34] and Abu-Elneel K, et al., 2008 [35]
miR106b	Schizophrenia	Altered expression (serum/cortical)	Vasu, et al., 2014 [34] and Shi, et al., 2012 [33], Beveridge and Cairns, 2012 [32].
miR130a	Sytl4	Predicted	MGI:1351606c
miR130a-3p (miR130a) **	ASD	Good predictive power for ASD-serum	Vasu, et al., 2014 [34]
miR-130a	Schizophrenia	Altered expression (serum/cortical)	Vasu, et al., 2014 [34]; Shi, et al., 2012 [33], Beveridge and Cairns, 2012 [32]
miR132	Sytl4	Predicted	MGI:1351606c
miR132	ASD	Dysregulated in superior temporal gyrus of ASD	Stomova, et al., 2015 [37]
miR181b-1 (miR181b) ***	Sytl4	Predicted	MGI:1351606c
miR181b-2	Sytl4	Predicted	MGI:1351606c
miR181b-5p (miR181b/b1) ***	ASD	Good predictive power for ASD in serum; differentially expressed in ASD cerebellar cortex	Vasu, et al. 2014 [34]. Abu-Elneel K, et al. 2008 [35]. Ghahramani Seno et al., 2011 [36].
miR181b	Schizophrenia	Altered expression (serum/cortical)	Vasu, et al., 2014 [34]; Shi, et al., 2012 [33], Beveridge and Cairns, 2012 [32].
miR320	Sytl4	Predicted	MGI:1351606c
miR320a (miR320) ****	ASD	Good predictive power for ASD in serum	Vasu, et al., 2014 [34]
miR320	ASD	Dysregulated in superior temporal gyrus of ASD	Stomova, et al., 2015 [37]
miR320	ASD	Differentially expressed in ASD cerebellar cortex	Abu-Elneel K, et al. 2008 [35]
miR328	Sytl4	Predicted	MGI:1351606c
miR328	ASD	Down regulated in serum; differentially expressed in ASD cerebellar cortex	Vasu, et al., 2014 [34] and Abu-Elneel K, et al., 2008 [35]
miR328	Schizophrenia	Altered expression (serum/cortical)	Vasu, et al., 2014 [34] and Shi, et al., 2012 [33]; Beveridge and Cairns, 2012 [32]

* http://www.mirbase.org/cgi-bin/mirna_entry.pl?acc=MI0000407; ** http://www.mirbase.org/cgi-bin/mirna_entry.pl?acc=MI0000156; *** http://www.mirbase.org/cgi-bin/mature.pl?mature_acc=MIMAT0000673; **** http://www.mirbase.org/cgi-bin/mirna_entry.pl?acc=MI0000542; C. http://www.informatics.jax.org/interaction/explorer?markerIDs=MGI:1351606.

2.3. Transmembrane Protein 187 (TEM187) Gene

2.3.1. Structure of *TMEM187* Gene, Expression and Location of the Novel Variant

TMEM187 gene consists of two exons and encodes a multi-pass membrane protein (Figure 6).

The maternally inherited *TMEM187* missense variant lies beyond the last transmembrane helix region at the near terminal end of the *Pfam* domain 8-245aa represented by multiple sequence alignments and hidden Markov models (https://pfam.xfam.org/family/tmem187; TMEM187 (PF15100)). The *TMEM187* gene has three transcripts (splice variants) and 35 orthologs.

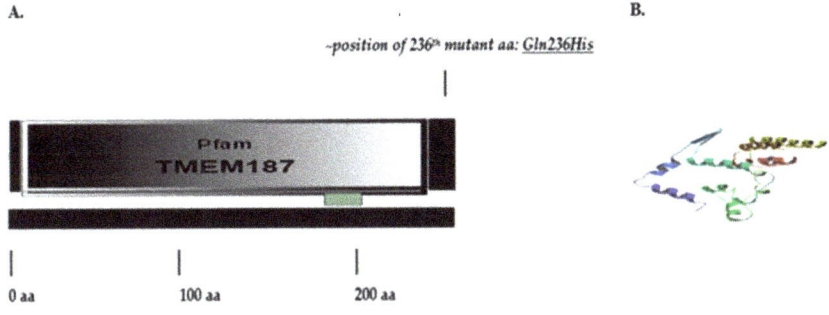

Green bar represents the Last (6th) transmembrane helix region: 185-207 aa.

Figure 6. (**A**). Graphic representation of TMEM187 protein indicating the location of Q236H amino acid variation beyond the last (6th) transmembrane helical domain (191-210aa), at the near terminal end of the *Pfam* domain (8-245aa) (https://pfam.xfam.org/family/tmem187; TMEM187 (PF15100)). (**B**). Theoretical partial 3D protein structure of the encoded multi-pass transmembrane protein targeting the 15-200aa region (https://modbase.compbio.ucsf.edu/), excluding the Q236H amino acid variant near the terminal end region of the protein which is represented by multiple sequence alignments and hidden Markov models preventing comparative structural analysis of the variant harboring region.

2.3.2. Deleterious and Damaging Nature of the Novel *TMEM187* Gene Variant

Unlike the *SYTL4* gene variant, the *TMEM187* missense gene variant (c.708G>T; p. Gln236His) is neither found in the Exome Aggregation Consortium (ExAC) database (which includes the 1000 genome data) or in the *Ensemble.org* data base. The nature of this novel Glutamine(Q)236 to Histidine(H) variation in TMEM187 is considered deleterious as determined by the PROVEAN (Protein Variation Effect Analyzer v1.1) score of = −4.474 with prediction cutoff of −2.5; SIFT score as deleterious (0.05); and PolyPhen-2 score as probably damaging (0.432). (http://gnomad.broadinstitute.org/variant/X-153248221-G-T). PROVEAN prediction generated score of −4.47 is termed as deleterious (scores <−2.5 considered deleterious), while the SIFT score of 0.05 approaches 0.0 which is the most damaging score.

2.3.3. TMEM187 Gene Is Expressed in the Brain

The *TMEM187* gene is ubiquitously expressed in all systems including all parts of the brain (www.uniprot.org/uniprot/Q14656; www.genecards.org/).

2.3.4. Latest STRING- Gene Interaction Network Study Reveals Direct Protein–Protein Interactions of TMEM187 with Several Other Known Autism Genes

Analysis of its STRING- network of interactions (Figure 7) reveals that it directly interacts with four known ASD genes, namely *HCFC1, TMLHE, MECP2,* and *GPHN* (https://gene.sfari.org/database/human-gene/). Moreover, three other directly interacting genes, namely *UBL4A, RBM25,* and *AKAP4,* though not known ASD genes, do show other transcriptome-wide isoform-level family member genes known as ASD genes: *UBL7, RBM27, RBM8A, RBMS3,* and *AKAP9* (https://gene.sfari.org/database/human-gene/).

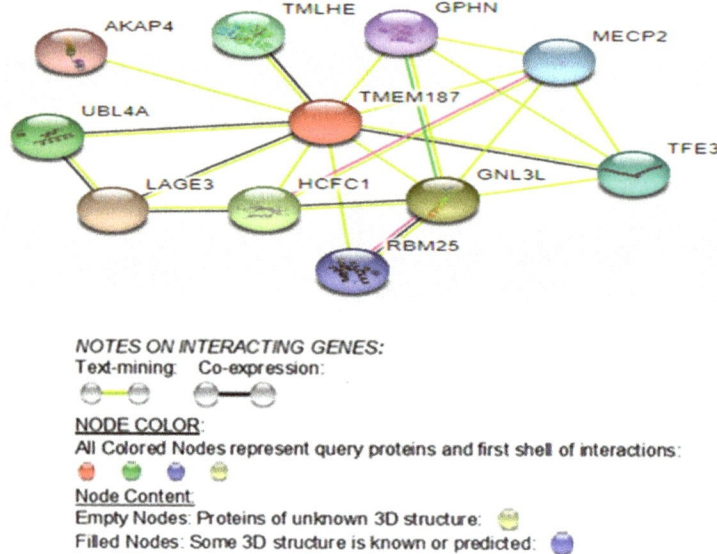

Figure 7. STRING-Protein–Protein Interactions of TMEM187. (https://string-db.org/network/9606.ENSP00000358999). TMEM187- Interacting ASD Genes: HCFC1: *Host cell factor 1*: Involved in control of the cell cycle; Coactivator for EGR2 and GABP2 (Score: 0.747); TMLHE: Trimethyllysine dioxygenase, mitochondrial: Converts trimethyllysine (TML) into Hydroxytrimethyllysine (HTML). (Score: 0.657); MECP2: Methyl-CpG-binding protein 2: Chromosomal protein that binds to methylated DNA; Mediates transcriptional repression through interaction with histone deacetylase and the corepressor SIN3A (Score: 0.555); GPHN: Gephyrin: Microtubule-associated protein involved in membrane protein-cytoskeleton interactions (Score: 0.531).

3. Discussion

Our research findings will be discussed related specifically to both the *SYTL4* and *TMEM187* gene variants seen in our patient and evidence for the two gene variants playing a role in the causation of high-functioning autism spectrum disorder.

3.1. Synaptotagmin-Like 4 (SYTL4) Gene

As an emerging candidate gene for autism with analyzed protein modeling, protein interactome networks, expression profiling and microRNA interactions will follow.

3.1.1. Protein Structure Altering Rare Variants Have Been Observed to Be More Frequent in Individuals with Autism

Though common variants are a large driving factors in autism spectrum disorder, the effect size of individual common variants is estimated to be small [38,39]. Therefore, the search for rare variants exhibiting a much larger individual effect is ongoing. Protein structure-altering rare variants have been observed more frequently in ASD cases, and ASD risks are increased when two rare variants may deleteriously affect both copies for an autosomal protein, or a single copy of an X-chromosomal protein among ASD males [40]. Rare hemizygous mutations on the X-chromosome are found to be more enriched in male ASD patients compared to controls. Furthermore, if rare hemizygous mutations on the X-chromosome in males alter gene expression known to be present in the brain, then the overall odds-ratio for ASD will be increased [41].

3.1.2. Deleterious and Damaging Nature of the *SYTL4* Gene Variant

It is important to note that this particular SYTL4 nucleotide variant CGC⇒TGC resulting in p. Arg279Cys (Figure 1) has been predicted through large-scale genomic sequencing studies, such as the 1000 Genome project, and has been judged to be deleterious (SIFT score 0.01) and possibly damaging (Polyphen score 0.79) with a MAF score of 0.0005/2.

It should also be noted that ExAC database which includes the 1000 genomes data, also calls this SYTL4 variant damaging and deleterious based on Polyphen and SIFT, respectively. Our patient being from Spain, according to ExAC, among the European (Non-Finnish) population, the allele frequency for this variant is 0.0004222 without any homozygotes and with eight hemizygotes (male) for 47,372 alleles, which presumably includes both isoforms. There is no information available as to any of these eight hemizygotes, or any other hemizygote being reported as exhibiting ASD in any of the clinical information-sharing resources such as Phenome Central, Gene Matcher and ClinVar.

3.1.3. Randomness of X Chromosome Inactivation Could Render the Mother Asymptomatic

It is important to note that our male heterozygous carrier of the R (279) C variant is expected to be fully penetrant for the mutant allele. The proband's mother is a heterozygous carrier of the R (279) C variant and due to randomness of X chromosome inactivation may render her as asymptomatic given that the X-linked *SYTL4* gene is not over expressed among females, indicating that it does not escape inactivation [42]. The proband's mother is expected to express equally her normal SYTL4 allele along with the mutant allele.

3.1.4. Our Modeling Results Show Large Conformational Changes Proximal to the R (279) C Amino Acid Variation

It is possible that the structure and function of both the canonical and the truncated isoform of SYTL4 protein will be affected, particularly considering their interactions at membrane surfaces. Our modeling results show large conformational changes proximal to the R (279) C amino acid variation within exon 9. The flanking regions contain two known phosphorylatable serines (YTKS (@274) VIDLR (@279) P EDVVHESGS (@289) L) as shown in Figure 5.

3.1.5. Missense Mutations Change the Size or Properties of Amino Acids Preventing the Function of Proteins

A study (reported by our co-authors: SKR, MGB) in whole exome sequencing in females with autism, a non-synonymous missense mutation (X: 99941091; C>G; p.H448D) of the SYTL4 gene was observed in a female with autism and random X-chromosome inactivation (46–54%). This patient additionally harbored four other autosomal missense gene mutations [16]. Missense mutations are of importance in understanding the structure or function of a protein since they usually occur in amino acid residues of structural or functional significance by changing the size or properties of the amino acid there by preventing the function of that protein [43,44]. The effect of such a mutation is additionally dependent on the sequence and structure context of the alteration [45]. Proteins fold according to minimum free energy [46]. Only correctly folded proteins can deliver the functional properties of a protein, and even minor changes in the size or properties of an amino acid side chain can alter or prevent the function of the protein [47]. On the other hand, even large deletions or insertions may be tolerated in numerous positions within a protein [48].

Protein function and interactions require both stability and specificity. Since most disease-causing mutations produce structural effects, the importance of a specific gene location and protein production is emphasized [47]. Structural information is needed to fully understand the effects and consequences of mutations, whether disease-causing or used purposefully to modify the properties of a protein. Three-dimensional structures and computer models have been used to elucidate disease mechanisms from specific amino acid substitutions [49,50]. For example, in a study of 4236 mutations from

436 genes, mutations at arginine and glycine residues are collectively responsible for about 30% of genetic diseases [43].

3.1.6. SYTL4 Amino Acid Change R (279) C in Exon 9: RAB-Binding Domain

The amino acid change in our study patient, *SYTL4* R(279)C in exon 9 (Figures 1, 3 and 5), has been determined to severely affect the critical functioning of this gene's encoded RAB protein binding region at its N-terminal [51,52], which is perhaps analogous to the effect of a significant change in Sytl4 gene expression observed among the altered protein networks in the mouse brain proteome in a mouse model of anxiety [12]. The SYTL4 RAB-Binding Domain within which lies D[Asp], at 60 takes part in the apparent salt bridge formation with R[Arg] at 279 only in the native protein configuration with the presence of mutant C[Cys] at 279 leading to the formation of an extended beta-pleated sheet (see Figure 3A,B).

3.1.7. Effect of the R[Arg]⇒C[Cys] Amino Acid Change at 279 on the functionality of the RAB-Binding Domain

Our analysis of the mutant and native SYTL4 protein structure models shows that in the native protein, arginine (R279) forms an apparent salt bridge with aspartic acid (D60) (Figures 2 and 3A). This arginine is part of a large extended loop conformation that appears to be stabilized by the apparent salt bridge formed between it and Asp60 within the RAB-Binding Domain [aa 4-122] and the Ring Domain [aa 43-105] (Figures 2 and 3A).

In our R (279) C mutant protein structure model (Figure 3B), cysteine (C279) is located amidst a beta sheet with no apparent hydrogen bonding contacts observed within distance constraints for such interactions. Our modeling suggests a potential structural change induced by the R (279) C variation eliminating the stabilizing Arg279-Asp60 salt bridge and leads to significant structural changes in the N-terminal half of SYTL4 (Figure 3B,C). This change could very well affect the functionality of the RAB-Binding Domain, not only for the canonical-full-length SYTL4 protein (isoform-1), but also for the truncated SYTL4 protein: isoform-2 (Figure 5).

3.1.8. Potentially Deleterious R (279) C Amino Acid Change "Likely" To Affect Its Neighboring Active Phosphorylation Sites

Given our modeling and profiling results, large conformational changes were seen proximal to the R279C amino acid variation within exon 9. Flanking regions do contain two known phosphorylatable serines (YTKS (@274) VIDLR (@279) P EDVVHESGS (@289) L) (Figure 5). The structure and function of both canonical and truncated isoforms of the SYTL4 protein may be affected, particularly considering their interactions at membrane surfaces.

3.1.9. Role of Arginine (R279) in SYTL4 Protein Structure and Function

The missense mutation identified in our study causes a change in the amino acid at 279 from R [Arginine] to C [Cysteine] (Figures 1 and 2B). Arginine is a large polar amino acid with sidechains that prefers to reside in an aqueous environment and is found more commonly on the surface of a protein. SYTL4 is a protein that anchors to the cell membrane and is exposed to both sides of the membrane by aqueous environments of the luminal and cytoplasmic sides. The C2 domain of SYTL4 protein facilitates binding of this protein to cell membranes and is often found in the active centers of proteins that bind phosphorylated substrates [53,54].

The arginine (R279) residue is in-fact located in between two Serine(S) residues at 274 and 289- positions (YTKS (@274) VIDLR (@279) PEDVVHESGS (@289) L) (Figure 5) and is shown to undergo post-translational phosphorylation [55–57]. Arginine is capable of "salt bridging" by forming non-bonded and hydrogen-bonded paired electrostatic interactions between acidic carboxyl groups and basic amino groups in single or adjacent protein chains [58]. One important role of "salt bridging" is connecting protein subunits or joining two secondary structures to form quaternary structures where they can connect as many as five secondary structure units [58].

3.1.10. Arginine Disfavors Cysteine for Substitution

Given the above contrasting basic differences between arginine and cysteine in their properties and their role in protein structure and function, arginine disfavors cysteine for substitution, particularly in extracellular and membrane proteins, such as SYTL4. Since such substitution can be devastating to protein stability and function given the loss of arginine's ability to create stabilizing hydrogen bonds, the substituted cysteine residue's ability to alter the native three-dimensional conformation of the protein molecule is important [44]. Thus, the potential for a structural and functional change induced by the SYTL4 R279C amino acid change is consistent with the noted physiochemical differences between arginine and cysteine [44].

3.1.11. Dysfunction of Evolutionarily Conserved RAB-Binding GTPases Play a Role in Autism and Neuronal Disorders

Among the transcriptome-wide RAB family of genes, *RAB2A, RAB11FIP5, RAB19, RAB39B,* and *RAB43* are also known ASD genes [59–61] (https://gene.sfari.org/database/human-gene/) and SYTL4 protein interacts with several other members of the RAB family of proteins including RAB3A, RAB8A, RAB27A, and RAB27B (Figure 4). Therefore, the defect in the RAB protein-binding region in the N-terminal half of the SYTL4 protein is due to the R (279) C amino acid variant and may be a causal factor for the high-functioning autism in our patient.

In addition, the *SYTL4* gene directly interacts with Syntax Binding Protein 1 (STXBP1). Both SYTL4 and STXBP1 are known to interact with RAB3A. STXBP1 interaction with RAB3A promotes RAB3A dissociation from the vesicle membrane (https://www.uniprot.org/uniprot/P61764). SYTL4 protein additionally interacts with several other members of the RAB family of proteins, including RAB3A, RAB8A, RAB27A, and RAB27B. Further, RAB-binding domain of SYTL4 serves as a preferred effector binding site for the GTP-bound form of the RAB27A protein that regulates the exocytosis of secretary granules [62–64]. RAB27A binds to the N-terminus SLP homology domains 1 and 2 of SYTL4 protein and the C-terminal domain (Figures 1 and 2A). It appears to play a role in the localization of RAB27A to specific sites in a cell [51,52,65]. Upregulation of RAB27A protein in basal forebrain neurons has been associated with mild cognitive impairment and Alzheimer's disease [52].

Further, specific evolutionarily conserved RAB-binding GTPases function as regulators of membrane trafficking and binding and act as binary molecular switches turned on by binding GTP and off by hydrolyzing GTP to GDP [66]. Their dysfunction through mutations has also been shown to play a crucial role in causing diverse patho-physiologies including X-linked mental retardation associated with autism, epilepsy and macrocephaly. This suggests a major role for specific RAB-binding effector proteins, such as SYTL4 and interacting RAB-activating GTPases (RAB GTPases) in the maintenance of normal neuronal function [51,59–61,64–66].

3.1.12. Significance of Defect in RAB- Protein Binding Region of N-Terminal Half of SYTL4 Protein due to R (279) C Amino Acid Variant

The potentially deleterious R (279) C amino acid change could critically affect the RAB-binding domain of SYTL4 proteins. Our analysis of the mutant and native SYTL4 protein structure models shows that in the native protein, arginine (R279) forms an apparent salt bridge with aspartic acid (D60). This arginine is part of a large extended loop conformation that appears to be stabilized by the apparent salt bridge formed between it and Asp60 within the RAB-Binding Domain [aa 4-122] and the Ring Domain [aa 43-105].

In our R279C mutant model, cysteine (C279) is located amidst a beta sheet with no apparent hydrogen bonding contacts observed within distance constraints for such interactions. Our modeling thus suggests a potential structural change induced by the R279C variation which eliminates the stabilizing Arg279-Asp60 salt bridge and leads to significant structural changes in the N-terminal half of SYTL4 (Figure 3B). This could very well affect the functionality of the RAB-Binding Domain, not only for the canonical-full-length SYTL4 protein (isoform-1), but also for the truncated SYTL4 protein: isoform-2.

3.1.13. SYTL4-Protein-Protein Interactions with RAB27A and with Other RAB-Family of Genes

As seen in Figure 4, the SYTL4 protein directly interacts with several members of the RAB (Ras-Associated proteins in Brain) family of proteins, RAB3A, RAB8A, RAB27A, and RAB27B. Further, RAB- binding domain of the SYTL4 protein serves as a preferred effector binding site for the GTP-bound form of RAB27A protein that regulates the exocytosis of secretory granules [62–64]. Among the RAB-family of genes, *RAB2A*, *RAB11FIP5*, *RAB19*, *RAB39B*, and *RAB43* are known ASD genes [59–61] (https://gene.sfari.org/database/human-gene/).

3.1.14. Upregulation of RAB27A Protein Associated with Mild Cognitive Impairment and Alzheimer Disease

RAB27A binds to the N-terminus SLP homology domains 1 and 2 of the SYTL4 protein, and the C-terminal domain seems to play a role in the localization of RAB27A to specific sites in a cell [51,52,65]. It important to note that upregulation of the RAB27A protein in basal forebrain neurons has been associated with mild cognitive impairment and Alzheimer disease [52].

3.1.15. Dysfunction of Conserved RAB-Binding GTPases Play a Role in X-Linked Mental Retardation with Autism

As indicated earlier, specific evolutionarily conserved RAB-binding GTPases do function as regulators of membrane trafficking and binding by acting as binary molecular switches that are turned on by binding GTP and off by hydrolyzing GTP to GDP. Their dysfunction through mutations has been shown to play a crucial role in causing diverse patho-physiologies including X-linked mental retardation associated with autism, epilepsy, and macrocephaly, suggesting a major role for specific RAB-binding effector proteins, such as the SYTL4, and interacting RAB-activating GTPases (RAB-GTPases) in the maintenance of normal neuronal function [51,52,59–61,66,67].

3.1.16. *SYTL4* Gene Is Relevant to Neuronal System Function and Disorders

The *SYTL4* gene is relevant for neuronal system development, function and behavior, and is implicated in neurological and psychological diseases (Entrez Gene ID # 94121 (Human); ID # 27359 (Mouse). The *SYTL4* gene expression is down regulated in the dorsal raphe nucleus of patients with major depressive disorders [11]. In addition, in a mouse model of anxiety, significant changes in *Sytl4* were observed among the altered protein networks in the brain proteome [12].

3.1.17. SYTL4 Protein Is Abundantly Expressed in the Bed Nucleus of Stria Terminalis and Is Upregulated in Male Brain

The bed nucleus of stria terminalis (BNST) is a heterogeneous complex limbic forebrain structure, which plays an important role in controlling autonomic, neuroendocrine, and behavioral responses, and is thought to serve as a key relay connecting limbic forebrain structures to hypothalamic and brainstem regions associated with autonomic and neuroendocrine functions [10,14]. Its control of physiological and behavioral activity is mediated by local action of numerous neurotransmitters [68]. Therefore, one could argue that the abundantly-expressed SYTL4 mutant protein in the bed nucleus of stria terminalis could potentially affect normal behavioral responses resulting in an autistic phenotype, given that *Sytl4* is upregulated in the brain of male mice, specifically in the posteromedial area of the medial BNST [9].

Furthermore, in mouse brain, the expression of Sytl4 protein is sexually dimorphic due to the sex hormone (estrogen and testosterone)-specific control of this gene and the developmental influence of sex hormone can lead to enduring effects on brain and behavior [9,69]. Mice with targeted disruptions of the *Sytl4* gene exhibit specific deficits in sex-specific behavior and deficits. *Sytl4* is required for patterning male sexual behavior [9]. Given the increased risk estimates of ASD among males [70,71], the overall odds-ratio for ASD increases if the rare hemizygous mutation on the X-chromosome pertains to gene expression that is known to express in the brain [41].

3.1.18. Targeted Knockout Mutant Mammalian Phenotypes for *Sytl4* Includes Abnormal Behavior and Abnormal Neurological Phenotype

The amino acid changes of SYTL4 R279C in exon 9 in our patient have been determined to severely affect the RAB protein-binding region at its N-terminal [51,52], which may be analogous to the partial or full effect of targeted Null/Knockout mutant *Sytl4* mammalian phenotypes. Gomi et al. [16] found that a targeted (Null/Knockout) mutation for Granuphilin (*Sytl4*) in XY-male mouse with 129P2/OlaHsd- genetic background replaced exons 3–5: targeted mutation 1, Tetsuro Izumi (tm1Tiz): Grn−/Y (*Sytl4* tm1Tiz/Y) particularly affected its endocrine and nervous systems with abnormal corticotroph morphology and hypersecretion of adrenocorticotropin [16,72]. Importantly, the same mammalian-targeted *Sytl4* knock-outs in 129P2/OlaHsd*C3H/He (*Sytl4*tm1Tiz/*Sytl4*tm1Tiz) and in 129P2/OlaHsd (*Sytl4*tm1Tiz/Y) have been associated with abnormal behavior and neurological phenotypes encompassing alertness, behavioral response to light, circadian rhythm, cognition, consumption behavior, emotion/affect behavior, grooming behavior, impulsive behavior, motor capabilities/coordination/movement, sensory capabilities/reflexes/nociception, sheltering behavior, sleep behavior, vocalization, and social interaction [13,14].

3.1.19. Targeted *Sytl4* Knock Out Mouse Model Studies Affirm That Defective SYTL4 Protein Function is Likely to Effectuate Neurological and Phenotypic Defects

A wide range of functions of the SYTL4 protein is noted for various cellular components, such as intracellular protein transport and positive regulation of protein secretion involving nucleoplasm, cytoplasm, endosome, centrosome, and plasma membrane which govern diverse molecular functions. These include protein and phospholipid binding, zinc and metal ion binding, clathrin binding, and neurexin protein binding. One could postulate that the observed low birth weight and height, as well as the down-slanting palpebral fissures, mild hypertelorism, thin upper lip, and pointed chin seen in our patient could relate to the abnormal SYTL4 protein. These phenotypic abnormalities are perhaps not observable in the Tetsuro Izumi (tm1Tiz) and Grn−/Y (*Sytl4* tm1Tiz/Y) mice models [16,72], however, decreased body weight has been reported in targeted *Sytl4* knock-out (*Sytl4*tm1Tiz/*Sytl4*tm1Tiz) mice with 129P2/OlaHsd*C3H/He genetic background. Thus, targeted *Sytl4* knock out mouse model studies affirm that defective SYTL4 protein function may effectuate neurological and phenotypic defects.

3.1.20. SYTL4 Protein Directly Interacts with Proteins Known to Cause Autism

Our protein–protein interactions study of the *SYTL4* gene shows that the SYTL4 protein directly interacts with three other proteins which are known to cause autism, namely, STX1A, SNAP25 and STXBP1 (Figure 4; https://gene.sfari.org/database/human-gene/). In addition, the SYTL4 protein directly interacts with FGF4, STX1B, SNAP29, SNAP23, SNAP47, RAB3A, RAB27A, RAB27B, RAB8A, STX4, STX19, STX3, STX11, and STX2 whose numerous transcriptome-wide isoforms are known as autism genes (https://gene.sfari.org/database/human-gene/).

3.1.21. *SYTL4* Gene Sequence Shows Similarity to a Known Autism Gene: *SYT1*

Moreover, the *SYTL4* gene sequence alignment shows similarity to the *SYT1* gene which is a known autism gene (https://gene.sfari.org/database/human-gene/). Yet another larger Synaptotagmin gene family member, *SYT17*, is also a known ASD gene (https://gene.sfari.org/database/human-gene/).

3.1.22. *SYTL4* Gene Sequence Alignment Shows Similarity to *SYT1*(Synaptotagmin 1) Gene Which is a Known ASD Gene

Although the *SYTL4* gene is presented here as a candidate gene, its transcriptome-wide isoform-level related gene family members, such as *SYT1*, *SYT17*, and *SYT3* are known ASD genes (https://gene.sfari.org/database/human-gene/). Moreover, the *SYTL4* gene sequence alignment shows similarity to the *SYT1* gene [70]. Synaptotagmins are integral membrane proteins of synaptic vesicles thought to serve as Ca (2+) sensors in the process of vesicular trafficking and exocytosis. Calcium binding to synaptotagmin-1 participates in triggering neurotransmitter release at the synapse [70].

3.1.23. Direct Protein-Protein STRING Interactions of the *SYTL4* Gene with Other ASD Genes

More significantly, the SYTL4 protein directly interacts with three known ASD proteins, STX1A, STXBP1 and SNAP25 (Figure 4) (https://gene.sfari.org/database/human-gene/). STX1A (Syntaxin 1A (brain)) encodes a protein involved in the regulation of serotonergic and GABAergic systems and its expression is altered in autism [70]. Rare single gene mutations in *STX1A* have been implicated in ASD. This gene is located at 7q11.23. Common *STX1A* variants are nominally associated with high-functioning autism and Asperger syndrome (https://gene.sfari.org/database/human-gene/). This protein governs the release and uptake of extracellular vesicles in the nervous system and glial cells facilitating transcellular communication [73] and serves as a key molecule in ion channel regulation and synaptic exocytosis (https://gene.sfari.org/database/human-gene/).

The *SYTL4* gene also directly interacts with Syntax binding protein 1 (STXBP1). A frameshift mutation in the *STXBP1* gene has been implicated in a study of quartet families with autism spectrum disorder [74–76] and is a known autism gene (https://gene.sfari.org/database/human-gene/). *SYTL4* recruits and binds *STXBP1* to promote exocytosis [26] (http://www.genecards.org/cgi-bin/carddisp.pl?gene=STXBP1&keywords=STXBP]. It is important to note that like *STXBP1*, *SYTL4* is also associated with early onset epileptic encephalopathy and both these genes are expressed in every part of the brain [http://www.genecards.org/). *SYTL4* as well as *STXBP1* are known to be expressed in the frontal cortex and brain and are essential for protein–protein interactions at synapses and the neurotransmitter release cycle in human neurons (http://www.genecards.org/). STXBP1 is overexpressed in the frontal cortex and even heterozygous mutations cause early onset epileptic encephalopathy, specifically through presynaptic impairment and autism [74–76]. Like STXBP1, SYTL4 is also associated with early onset epileptic encephalopathy and is expressed in brain regions (http://www.genecards.org/). Polymorphisms in the *SNAP25* (Synaptosomal-associated protein, 25 kDa) gene are associated with ADHD. *SNAP25+/−* mice also exhibit hyperactivity and cognitive and social impairment [77]. In addition to the SYTL4 protein's direct interactions with three known ASD proteins, STX1A, STXBP1 and SNAP25, it interacts with 14 other genes, namely, *FGF4, STX1B, SNAP29, RAB3A, SNAP23, RAB27B, RAB8A, SNAP47, STX4, STX19, STX3, STX11, STX2*, and *RAB27A*, whose numerous transcriptome-wide isoform-level multiple gene family members are known ASD genes (https://gene.sfari.org/database/human-gene/).

3.1.24. *SYTL4*- Molecular Pathways, Biological Processes and Molecular Functions

Significant *SYTL4* gene-involved molecular pathways are the synaptic vesicle cycle, insulin secretion, AMPK-signaling pathway, and SNARE interactions (Table 1). The synaptic vesicle cycle pertains to synaptic vesicles that are filled with neurotransmitters by active transport, and the diseases that are associated with defects in this cycle are early infantile epileptic encephalopathy; centronuclear myopathy; episodic ataxias; and familial or sporadic hemiplegic migraine. Insulin secretion is regulated by several hormones and neurotransmitters, and the diseases associated with this pathway are defects in the degradation of ganglioside and type II diabetes mellitus. AMPK signaling acts as a sensor of cellular energy status while SNARE interactions mediate the docking of synaptic vesicles with the presynaptic membrane in neurons. Diseases associated with defective SNARE interactions are pseudohypoparathyroidism and cerebral dysgenesis, neuropathy, ichthyosis, and palmoplantar keratoderma or CEDNIK syndrome (Table 1).

The *SYTL4* gene's extensive biological processes (Table 2) pertain to RAB-protein signal transduction along with synaptic vesicle functions, neurotransmitter secretion, regulation of signaling, glutamate secretion, neuro-muscular synaptic transmission, and axonogenesis, which are all relevant for proper neuronal function, and thus also relevant to autism. The *SYTL4* gene's molecular functions (Table 3), biological processes (Table 2) and molecular pathways (Table 1) are indicative of its significant role in neuronal function that is meaningful in the causation of high-functioning autism in our proband. Moreover, in recent studies, disturbed *SYTL4* gene function has been associated with neuropsychiatric disorders, such as autism, schizophrenia and depression as well as the immune system. It is also considered a major modulator of central nervous system function [11,12].

3.1.25. Synaptic Dysfunction in Neurodevelopmental Disorders Is Associated with Autism and Intellectual Disabilities

The SYTL4 modulates exocytosis of dense-core granules and secretion of hormones in the pancreas and the pituitary. It interacts with vesicles containing negatively charged phospholipids in a Ca (2+)-independent manner (http://www.genecards.org/). The significant SYTL4 molecular pathways are the synaptic vesicle cycle, insulin secretion, AMPK-signaling pathway, and SNARE interactions (Table 1). Like *SYTL4*, *SYT1*, *STX1A*, *STXBP1* and *SNAP25* genes play an important role in the extravesicular synaptic function of neuronal systems and neurotransmission (https://gene.sfari.org/database/human-gene/; www.genecards.org/). Thus, these proteins are generally involved in the functioning of the synaptic vesicles' (or neurotransmitter vesicles) cycle to facilitate synaptic vesicle exocytosis by which a synaptic vesicle fuses with the plasma membrane of the pre-synaptic axon terminal and releases its contents in the synaptic cleft, which is essential for propagating nerve impulses between neurons and are constantly created by the cells to facilitate transcellular communication [73].

It should be noted that the *SYTL4* mRNAs are found in extracellular vesicles and stimulate target cells to translate into active protein [78]. The *SNAP25* gene encodes t-SNARE which is involved in the molecular regulation of neurotransmitter release that associates with proteins in vesicle docking and membrane fusion. It may play an important role in the synaptic function of specific neuronal systems [77] (https://gene.sfari.org/database/human-gene/). Similarly, STXBP1 protein is essential for neurotransmission and binds to syntaxin, a component of the synaptic vesicle fusion machinery (https://www.uniprot.org/uniprot/P61764).

Genes that regulate presynaptic processes ultimately affect neurotransmitter release when disturbed [79,80]. Synaptic dysfunction in neurodevelopmental disorders is associated with autism and intellectual disabilities [81–84] as noted by Baker et al. [80] who reported the first case of a rare missense variant (I368T) in the Synaptotagmin1 (*SYT1*) gene causing a human neurodevelopmental disorder. It has a dominant negative effect involving both synaptic vesicle exocytosis and endocytosis [80].

Significant molecular pathways, functions and biological processes (Tables 1–3) of the *SYTL4* gene include synaptic vesicle cycle and fusion, exocytosis and neurotransmitter secretion, akin to the molecular functions of its directly interacting known ASD genes: *STXBP1* and *SNAP25*. Therefore, deficiency in the functioning of the SYTL4 protein due to the R (279) C amino acid change affects the canonical structures of the *SYTL4* gene as well as its shorter isoform affecting synaptic vesicle cycle and fusion, exocytosis, and neurotransmitter secretion likely to cause autism and intellectual disabilities.

3.1.26. ASD-Predictive MicroRNAs among Mouse *Sytl4*- Interacting MicroRNAs

Our analysis of 298 validated/predicted microRNA interactions with mouse *Sytl4* gene [34,85–88] has identified three of five autism-associated serum miRs (60%), namely, miR181b-5p, miR320a, and miR130a-3p, which have good predictive power in serum [34]. Among these three miRs, miR320 has the greatest ASD predictive power reported in serum as well as in the superior temporal gyrus and cerebellar cortex of ASD individuals [34,35,37]. In addition, 5 of 13 (38%) miRs that were differentially expressed in ASD serum samples were predicted to be interacting with mouse *Sytl4* gene [34]. Three of these five miRs, namely, miR130a-3p, miR181b-5p, and miR328 are predicted to be associated with the mouse *Sytl4* gene. They have been shown to be differentially expressed in schizophrenics [31,32].

3.1.27. Dysregulation of miR-320—Most Predictive for ASD in Serum and Brain Tissues

Recently, miR-320, along with miR-197 in human follicular fluid were found to be associated with embryonic development potential [89]. Knocking down miR-320 in mouse oocytes negatively affects embryonic developmental potentially by inhibiting the expression of the Wnt-signaling pathway and therefore miRNAs in human follicular fluid might reflect an effect on embryo quality [89]. Furthermore, autopsy tissue sections showed concordantly dysregulated miR-320a and voltage-dependent anion channel 1 levels in HIV-1 patients suffering from mild cognitive impairment [90]. One could consider dysregulation of miR-320 as the most predictive for ASD in serum and brain tissues, since it was also found to be dysregulated in the superior temporal gyrus of ASD specimens [37]. Additionally, miR-320 and miR-197 are differentially expressed in the ASD cerebellar cortex [35,36]. Given the fact that miR-320 has been predicted to interact with mouse *Sytl4* gene, it gives credence to the *SYTL4* gene as a plausible new gene ASD.

3.1.28. *SYTL4* Interacting miR181b-1- Being Predictive of ASD

The micro RNA second in line to miR320 is miR181b-1 as the most predictive for ASD. It not only showed good predictive power for ASD in serum [34] but is also differentially expressed in the ASD cerebellar cortex [35,36]. Unlike miR-320, miR181b-1 has additionally been found to show altered expression in the cortical regions in schizophrenia [32–34], supporting the contention that ASD and schizophrenia share common neurobiological features [32–34]. In a recent study, significant down-regulation of miRNA-181b expression in schizophrenics predicted improvement of negative symptoms to treatment, and thus miRNA-181b is predicted to serve as a potential plasma-molecular marker for antipsychotic responses [91].

3.1.29. SYTL4 Interacting miR130a-Being Predictive of ASD

Another potentially important micro RNA is miR130a (miR130a-3p) for prediction of ASD but is lacking corroboration from any ASD brain tissue studies (unlike miR320 and miR181b-1, above). However, like miRNA-181b, miR130a also showed altered expression (serum/cortical) in schizophrenia, again supporting the contention that ASD and schizophrenia share common neurobiological features [32–34].

3.1.30. *SYTL4*-Interacting miR106b and miR328 Dysregulated in ASD Cerebellar Cortex and Altered among Schizophrenics

Other SYTL4-associated miRs, miR106b (106b-3p) and miR328, have shown up and down regulation, respectively, in ASD serum and are differentially expressed in the ASD cerebellar cortex [34,35]. In addition, both miRs have also been shown to be altered among schizophrenics [32–34].

3.1.31. *SYTL* Interacting miR63, miR103, 5nd miR132 Are Dysregulated in Superior Temporal Gyrus of ASD

Other predicted *SYTL4*-interacting miRs, such as, miR93, miR103 (miR103-1 and miR103-2), and miR132, have been found to be dysregulated in superior temporal gyrus of ASD [37]. Thus, a total of eight microRNAs which are predicted to be associated with mouse *Sytl4* are found to be altered in ASD serum and/or brain, thereby, augmenting our contention that the *SYTL4* gene is a plausible new ASD candidate gene. Fifty percent (4/8) of the ASD-associated miRs (miRs106, miRs130a, miRs181b, and miRs328) that are predicated to interact with the mouse *Sytl4* gene are also known to be associated with schizophrenia, supporting the contention that ASD and schizophrenia share common neurobiological features [34,92,93] (Table 4).

Fifty percent (4/8) of the ASD-associated mirRs (mirRs93, mirRs103, mirRs132, mirRs320) that are predicted to interact with mouse Sytl4 have also been determined to be dysregulated in superior temporal gyrus of ASD [37]. Yet again, 50% (4/8) of the ASD-associated mirRs (mirRs106b, mirRs181b-5p, mirRs320, mirRs328) predicted to interact with the mouse *Sytl4* have also been determined to be differentially expressed in the ASD cerebellar cortex [35]. Over expression of miR142-5p, miR142-3p, miR451a, miR144-3p, and miR21-5p has been reported in ASD brain tissue along with hypomethylation of the promoter region of the miR142 gene in the same samples, suggesting dysregulation of these microRNAs [94]. However, the mouse *Sytl4* gene has not been predicted to interact with any of the miRs that were found to be over expressed by Mor et al. [94]. Furthermore, these five miRs are not represented among the 13 differentially expressed miRs in ASD serum [34] (Table 4). Other studies have also not reported any of the five miRs to be over expressed by Mor et al., [94] based on specific regions of ASD brains, such as the superior temporal gyrus [37] and cerebellar cortex [35].

3.2. Transmembrane Protein 187 (TMEM187) Gene

TMEM187 is an emerging candidate gene for autism with a discussion undertaken on protein interactome networks, expression profiling and microRNA interaction studies.

3.2.1. TMEM187 Gene Belongs to a Group of Genes Which Host MicroRNA Genes in Their Introns or Exons

At the outset, it should be noted that unlike the *SYTL4* gene, not much is known about the *TMEM187* gene, and there is limited information available regarding its biological processes, molecular pathways and functions or microRNA interactions. The *TMEM187* gene, like *SYTL4*, is a protein-coding gene, but belongs to a group of genes which host microRNA genes in their introns or exons [17]. However, we introduce the *TMEM187* gene as an emerging candidate gene for autism with our mutation analysis of its novel missense variant c.708G>T; p. Gln236His, its STRING-protein interactome network and its expression profiling.

3.2.2. Novel *TMEM187* Missense Variant c.708G>T: Glutamine(Q)236 Histidine(H)

Unlike the *SYTL4* gene variant, *TMEM187* Glutamine(Q)236 Histidine(H) variant in our patient is not found in the Exome Aggregation Consortium (ExAC) database. It is also not found in the listed 261 previous variants currently listed at ensembl.org.

3.2.3. Deleterious and Damaging Nature of the Novel *TMEM187*- Variant

Our extensive analyses of this novel variant, as detailed in the Results section, was often determined to be deleterious or damaging. Glutamine, which is a polar amino acid, was changed to histidine and this alters the protein [43,44].

3.2.4. TMEM187 Protein Is Expressed in Brain

Like *SYTL4*, the *TMEM187* gene is ubiquitously expressed in all systems including all parts of the brain (www.uniprot.org/uniprot/Q14656; www.genecards.org/).

3.2.5. STRING–Gene Interaction Network Study Reveals Direct Protein–Protein Interactions of the TMEM187 Gene with Several Other Known Autism Genes

Although the novel X-linked *TMEM187* missense gene variant c.708G>T; p.Gln236His found in our high-functioning autism patient is not known as an ASD gene, but analysis of the latest STRING network interactions reveal direct interactions with four known ASD genes, namely *HCFC1*, *TMLHE*, *MECP2*, and *GPHN* (https://gene.sfari.org/database/human-gene/) (Figure 7).

3.2.6. Significance of *TMEM187* Protein-Protein Interacting Autism Genes

HCFC1 is a syndromic ASD gene that interacts with *TMEM187*, while *TMLHE*, *MECP2* and *GPHN* are rare single gene autism genes (https://gene.sfari.org/database/human-gene/). *HCFC1* is involved in control of the cell cycle with mutations in this X-linked (Xq28) gene associated with intellectual disability [26]. The two genes (*TMEM187* and *HCFC1*) lie just 2kb apart [95]. Over expression of *HCFC1* due to a variant is linked to intellectual disability [26]. A rare mutation in *TMLHE* has been identified with autism (https://gene.sfari.org/database/human-gene/).

The *TMEM187* gene is in linkage with the *MECP2* gene which is a well-known determinant of brain structure, and amino acid variations in the MECP2 protein cause micro-encephalopathy and are also associated with several neurodevelopmental disorders that affect both brain morphology and cognition [96]. Mutations in this gene underlie Rett syndrome, a well-known autism disorder (https://gene.sfari.org/database/human-gene/). Rare single gene mutations in the *GPHN* gene are associated with ASD and this gene encodes a neuronal assembly protein that anchors inhibitors of neurotransmitter receptors to postsynaptic cytoskeleton (https://gene.sfari.org/database/human-gene/).

3.2.7. Significance of Other Protein-Protein Interactions of TMEM187

The TMEM187 protein interacts directly with *UBL4A*, *RBM25*, and *AKAP4* (Figure 7). Though these genes are not known ASD genes, their other transcriptome-wide isoform-level family member genes are known ASD genes: *UBL7*, *RBM27*, *RBM8A*, *RBMS3* and *AKAP9* (https://gene.sfari.org/database/human-gene/).

Additionally, the TMEM187 protein directly interacts with the LAGE3 (L Antigen Family Member 3) protein (Figure 7), however, *LAGE3* is not a known ASD gene. It is associated with Galloway-Mowat syndrome 2, an X-linked early-onset nephrotic syndrome associated with microcephaly, central nervous system abnormalities, developmental delay, and a propensity for seizures. Brain anomalies include gyration defects such as lissencephaly, pachygyria, polymicrogyria, and cerebellar hypoplasia. Most patients show facial dysmorphism characterized by a small, narrow forehead, large/floppy ears, deep-set eyes, hypertelorism, and micrognathia (www.uniprot.org/uniprot/Q14657).

3.2.8. Other TMEM Proteins Gene Family Members Are Known Autism, Bipolar and Panic Disorder Genes

Other transmembrane proteins gene family members, such as *TMEM231*, are known syndromic autism genes (https://gene.sfari.org/database/human-gene/). This gene is associated with two neurological syndromes: Joubert syndrome-20 [MIM:614970] and Meckel syndrome 11 (https://gene.sfari.org/database/human-gene/; MIM:615397). Additionally, two other members (TMEM132E and TMEM132D) are known to be associated with bipolar and panic disorders [97,98].

3.2.9. X-chromosome Harbors Disproportionately Higher Number of *TMEM187*-Interacting Autism and Nervous System Disorder Genes: Implications for Boys vs Girls Ratio

Except for *GPHN* gene located on chromosome 14, all the other genes (*TMEM187*, *HCFC1*, *TMLHE*, *MECP2*, *LAGE3* and *SYTL4*) are located exclusively on the long arm of the X-chromosome. The *LAGE3* gene, whose family of genes are clustered together at Xq28, is like that of *TMEM187*, *HCFC1*, *TMLHE*, and *MECP2*. SYTL4 is also located on the X-chromosome at q22.1, proximal to the centromere. This augments the assertion that X-chromosome harbors a disproportionately higher number of ASD and nervous system disorder genes [99], and consequently, disproportionately affects more boys than girls, given that the overall odds-ratio for ASD is increased if the rare hemizygous mutation is on the X-chromosome and X-linked genes expressed in the brain [41] as is the case in all six of these X-linked genes (www.genecards.org).

4. Materials and Methods

4.1. Clinical Report

The 7-year-old male proband was the only child born to healthy young non-consanguineous parents. There was no family history of genetic disorders, malformations, epilepsy, autism, or intellectual disability. Our proband was the product of a 38-week pregnancy to a primigravida mother via an uncomplicated C-section due to a transverse presentation. The Apgar scores were 9 and 9 at 1 and 5 min, respectively. The birth weight was 3600 gm (55th percentile), length was 52 cm (85th percentile), and head circumference was 35 cm (55th percentile).

The proband was evaluated in the Department of Pediatric Neurology, Hospital Universitario Quirón, Madrid, Spain at the age of 4.5 years due to longstanding impairment in social and communicative functioning. Although an early intervention program was established in the first months of life for motor, cognitive, speech development, and social behavior, the proband exhibited mild psychomotor delay during his first years of life. He walked unsupported at 11 months but had significant problems with walking, squatting or dressing at 4.5 years of age. First bi-syllabic babbling occurred at 18 months; at the age of 3 years, he only spoke words without making sentences. His social development was markedly affected; he showed atypical behaviors, refused playing with other children, had a limited amount of interests, and eye contact was minimal.

His weight was 19 kg (65th percentile) and height was 109 cm (65th percentile). He had down-slanting palpebral fissures, mild hypertelorism, thin upper lip, and a pointed chin. Conventional genetic studies (karyotype and array comparative genomic hybridization) showed no abnormalities. The neurological exam was normal. He had impaired social interaction during the examination and lacked eye contact, had peculiar language (echolalias, verbosity, and abnormal pitch), stereotyped mannerisms, and restricted patterns of interest. Brain MRI and sleep video-EEG tests displayed normal results. Cognitive assessment using the Wechsler Preschool and Primary Test of Intelligence-III (WPPSI-III) revealed a verbal and non-verbal IQ at above-average level without significant discrepancies. The Behavior Assessment System for Children (BASC) completed by his parents and preschool teachers revealed significant problems in "social skills," "adaptability" and "atypicality" domains.

At the age of 6 years, his neurological examination remained normal, but he had an unusually high-pitched voice with stereotyped phrases and echolalia. He tended to perseverate on repetitive interests and activities (chronology of history, borders of countries). His eye contact was inconsistent and poorly integrated with other communicative efforts. He reacted aversely to sensory stimuli (e.g., loud noise, flavors). Autism Spectrum Screening Questionnaire (ASSQ), the Autism Diagnostic Interview-Revised (ADI-R), and the Autism Diagnostic Observation Scale (ADOS, Module 3) were administered. His total score on the ASSQ was 31 and 29 according to the evaluation by the teachers and parents (high-functioning autism cut-off = 22 and 19, respectively). His ADI-R algorithm scores were 15 on the social domain (autism cut-off = 10), 11 on the communication domain for verbal children (autism cut-off = 8), and 5 on the repetitive behavior's domain (autism cut-off = 3). His total score on the ADOS communication and social algorithm items were 6 and 9 (autism cut-off = 3 and 6, respectively). The clinical and neuropsychological evaluations were consistent with high-functioning autism. The patients allowed for us to undertake research investigations. The study was approved by the local ethics committees on January 7, 2016 and was conducted in accordance with the ethical principles of the Declaration of Helsinki and Good Clinical Practice standards. Informed consent was obtained from parents, with the child giving assent.

4.2. Genomic Investigations

Exome sequencing was performed using genomic DNA isolated (MagnaPure, Roche Applied Science, Manheim, Germany) from whole blood from the proband and parents. Libraries were prepared using the Ion AmpliSeq™ Exome Kit (Life Technologies, Carlsbad, California, USA) and quantified by qPCR. The enriched libraries were prepared using Ion Chef™ and sequenced on PI™ Chip in the

Ion Proton™ System (Life Technologies) to provide >90% of amplicons covered with at least 20X. Signal processing, base calling, alignment and variant calling were performed on a Proton™ Torrent Server using the Torrent Suite™ Software (v4.4 Life Technologies, Carlsbad, CA, USA). Variants were annotated using Ion Reporter™ Software with the human genome reference assemble GRCh37 (hg19) and pedigree analysis performed using the Genetic Disease Screen (GDS) trio workflow.

Candidate variants were visualized using IGV (Integrative Genomics Viewer, Cambridge, MA, USA) and evaluated based on stringent assessments at both the gene and variant levels, taking into consideration both the patient's phenotype and the inheritance pattern. Variants in the *SYTL4* and *TMEM187* genes were recognized as probable pathogenic and confirmed by Sanger sequencing. However, due to the lack of cooperation from other family members, additional testing was not available.

4.3. Modeling of Native and R279C Variant for SYTL4 Gene

The theoretical atomic models of native and R279C *SYTL4* were constructed using I-TASSER [20,100,101]. With human SYTL4 sequence (UniProtKB Accession # = Q96C24) as query, multiple sequence-template alignments were initially generated by the meta-threading program LOMETS [20,102,103], followed by generation of the predicted atomic structures. Native SYTL4 matched well with several moderately high-scoring templates corresponding to synaptotagmin family members, with an estimated TM score of 0.5 ± 0.15 and RMSD of 12.2 ± 4.4 Å. The R279C variant also matched to synaptotagmin family member templates, with slightly lower scores, yielding a TM score and RMSD of 0.45 ± 0.15 and 13.5 ± 4.0 Å, respectively.

Both structures were close to the threshold (TM score >0.5) for correct topology. Molecular graphics and analyses were performed with the UCSF Chimera package. Chimera is developed by the Resource for Biocomputing, Visualization, and Informatics at the University of California, San Francisco (supported by NIGMS P41-GM103311) [85].

4.4. MicroRNAs

MicroRNAs (miRNAs / miRs) play a key role in the transcriptional networks of the developing human brain, as regulators of gene expression. Autism spectrum disorder (ASD), being a complex neurodevelopmental disorder, is characterized by multiple deficits in communication, social interaction and behavior [34]. Vasu et al. [34] examined the serum expression profiles of 125 neurologically relevant miRNAs expression profiles in 55 individuals with ASD. These neurologically relevant miRNAs represented pathways involved in axon guidance, TGF-beta signaling, MAPK signaling, adherents' junction, regulation of actin cytoskeleton, oxidative phosphorylation, hedgehog signaling, focal adhesion, mTOR signaling, and Wnt signaling [34].

Vasu et al. [34] found that only 13 miRNAs (out of the selected 125 miRs; ~10%) were differentially expressed among the 55 ASD individuals compared to the controls in their serum. Of these 13, miR151a-3p, miR181b-5p, miR320a, miR328, miR433, miR489, miR572, and miR663a were downregulated (61.5%), while miR101-3p, miR106b-5p, miR130a-3p, miR195-5p, and miR19b-3p were upregulated (38.5%) [34]. Furthermore, of these 13 miRs, only five miRs (38.5%), namely, miR181b-5p, miR320a, miR572, miR130a-3p and miR19b-3p had high values for sensitivity, specificity and area under the curve, thereby showing good predictive power for distinguishing individuals with ASD [34]. Therefore, it was decided to screen for the presence of these five miRNAs with good ASD predictive power, namely, miR181b-5p, miR320a, miR572, miR130a-3p and miR19b-3p as well as the other five miRs that were also differentially expressed among the 55 ASD individuals among the 298 validated/predicted microRNA interactions of mouse *Sytl4* gene [86–88,104]. Additionally, we screened for the presence of other significantly ASD-associated miRs from brain-specific micro RNA expression studies by others [35–37].

5. Conclusions

1. *TMEM187* as well as *SYTL4* genes are: X-linked and both located on the long arm of the X-chromosome at Xq28 and Xq22.1, respectively;

2. Both *Q236H TMEM187* and *R279C SYTL4* gene variants have been predicted to be damaging or deleterious by SIFT, PolyPhen2, MutationTaster, Provean, and LRT variant calling programs;

3. Both *TMEM187* and *SYTL4* mRNAs are found in extracellular vesicles and stimulate target cells to translate into active protein [17], and the release and uptake of extracellular vesicles in the nervous system and glial cells provides novel mechanisms of transcellular communication [73];

4. Together, *TMEM187* and *SYTL4* genes directly interact with seven known ASD genes: four and three ASD genes, respectively (Figures 4 and 7; https://gene.sfari.org/database/human-gene/);

5. Another transmembrane protein gene family member, *TMEM231*, is a known syndromic autism gene: *TMEM231* gene is associated with two neurological syndromes: Joubert syndrome-20 [MIM:614970] and Meckel syndrome 11 (https://gene.sfari.org/database/human-gene/; MIM:615397);

6. The SYTl4-RAB-binding protein RAB27A is specifically associated with mild cognitive impairment and Alzheimer disease [52];

7. RAB-binding GTPases play a crucial role in causing diverse patho-physiologies including X-linked mental retardation (intellectual disability) associated with autism, epilepsy, and macrocephaly, suggesting a major role for specific RAB-binding effector proteins, such as SYTL4, and interacting RAB-activating GTPases (RAB GTPases) in the maintenance of normal neuronal function [51,59–61,64–66];

8. Two other members of the transmembrane protein gene family, *TMEM132E* and *TMEM132D*, are known to be associated with bipolar and panic disorders, respectively [97,98];

9. One of the *TMEM187* genes' related phenotypes is schizophrenia (GWAS catalog for TMEM187 gene: Gene relation via enhancers containing phenotype SNP: Enhancer ID: GH0XJ153980; https://genecards.weizmann.ac.il/geneloc-bin/display_map.pl?chr_nr=0X&range_type=gh_id&gh_id=GH0XJ153941#GH0XJ153941). Similarly, our extensive ASD predictive mouse Sytl4-interacting microRNAs study reveals that 50% of the ASD-associated miRs are known to be associated with schizophrenia (Table 4);

10. A recent large study of gene expression patterns from postmortem brain tissues found transcriptome-wide isoform-level dysregulation in ASD, schizophrenia, bipolar disorder, panic disorder, and other related neurological disorders [105], supporting our above findings in *SYTL4* and *TMEM187* gene variants that ASD and schizophrenia share common neurobiological features [34,92,93];

11. Both *SYTL4* and the *TMM187* genes are ubiquitously expressed, including in the brain [9,10,14] (www.GeneCards.Org; www.Uniprot.Org). The overall odds-ratio for ASD is increased if rare hemizygous mutations on the X-chromosome in male patients are found as these genes have known expression in the brain [41].

Given the above analytical analyses, there is evidence to support that the missense mutations seen in both the *TMEM187* and *SYTL4* genes, either synergistically or individually, are causal mutations for the high-functioning autism seen in our patient. Consequently, both genes are proposed as novel autism candidate genes.

It is probable that both gene variants synergistically are causative of the high-functioning autism seen in our patient. Oligogenic heterozygosity or involvement of more than one gene observed in patients, suggests a new potential mechanism in the pathogenesis of autism spectrum disorders [106], further supporting the suggestion that the multifactorial model of ASD risk or monogenic may be too simplistic even for the most penetrant causes of ASD [107]. Pathogenicity of mutations individually or synergistically would require biological assays, such as in-vivo models, for study. Meanwhile, publications of similar findings by others in the study of autism involving either of these two gene variants would lend credence to our findings and assertions.

Author Contributions: The manuscript was conceived and entirely drafted by S.K.R., including the title, figures, tables, microRNA study, interpretation, discussion, conclusion, materials and methods, and references. M.G.B. reviewed, contributed and edited the entire manuscript. The clinical studies were conducted by A.F.-J., Neuro-pediatrician at the Department of Pediatric Neurology, Hospital Universitario Quirón, Madrid, Spain. The clinical case report was by A.F.-J. The genomic studies were conducted by S.Á., at the Genomics and Medicine, NIM Genetics, Madrid, Spain. The theoretical 3D structural modeling of native SYTL4 as well as the analysis of predicted atomic threading models of the mutant and native SYTL4 proteins, and the interpretation thereof was by O.W.N., at the Department of Biochemistry & Molecular Biology, University of Kansas Medical Center. Kansas City, USA. S.K.R. was granted permissions to reproduce in this manuscript the following: (1) the gene interaction STRING networks (by M.S., Head of GeneCards Development, Weizmann Institute of Science, Israel (www.GeneCards.Org & STRING Consortium)) and (2) the SYTL4 protein secondary structure graphics by E.G., SIB Swiss Institute of Bioinformatics, Geneva, Switzerland (UniProtKB/Swiss-Prot; WWW.Uniprot.Org; Q96C24).

Funding: Owen W. Nadeau acknowledges the research funding support for this project from NIH grant # DK32953. Merlin G. Butler acknowledges National Institute of Child Health and Human Development (NICHD) grant HD02528.

Acknowledgments: Waheeda Hossain in the Departments of Psychiatry & Behavioral Sciences, University of Kansas Medical Center (Kansas City, KS., 66160 USA) reviewed and edited the manuscript. Charlotte Iannachi in the Departments of Psychiatry & Behavioral Sciences, University of Kansas Medical Center rendered valuable help with the manuscript processing. Mark Grubb (Kansas City, MO. 64171 USA) and Azhar Mohammed (Falls Church, VA. 22044 USA) assisted in the production of figures. We acknowledge the seminal contribution of the proband's family to this study.

Conflicts of Interest: The authors declare no conflict of interest.

References

1. Shashi, V.; McConkie-Rosell, A.; Rosell, B.; Schoch, K.; Vellore, K.; McDonald, M.; Jiang, Y.H.; Xie, P.; Need, A.; Goldstein, D.B. The utility of the traditional medical genetic diagnostic evaluation in the context of next-generation sequencing for undiagnosed genetic disorders. *Genet. Med.* **2014**, *16*, 176–182. [CrossRef] [PubMed]
2. LePichon, J.B.; Saunders, C.; Soden, S.E. The future of next-generation sequencing in neurology. *JAMA Neurol.* **2015**, *72*, 971–972. [CrossRef] [PubMed]
3. Xue, Y.; Ankala, A.; Wilcox, W.R.; Hegde, M.R. Solving the molecular diagnostic testing conundrum for Mendelian disorders in the era of next-generation sequencing: Single-gene, gene panel, or exome/genome sequencing. *Genet. Med.* **2015**, *17*, 444–451. [CrossRef] [PubMed]
4. O'Roak, B.J.; Deriziotis, P.; Lee, C.; Vives, L.; Schwartz, J.J.; Girirajan, S.; Karakoc, E.; Mackenzie, A.P.; Ng, S.B.; Baker, C.; et al. Exome sequencing in sporadic autism spectrum disorders identifies severe de novo mutations. *Nat. Genet.* **2011**, *43*, 585–589. [CrossRef] [PubMed]
5. Dixon-Salazar, T.J.; Silhavy, J.L.; Udpa, N.; Schroth, J.; Bielas, S.; Schaffer, A.E.; Olvera, J.; Bafna, V.; Zaki, M.S.; Abdel-Salam, G.H.; et al. Exome sequencing can improve diagnosis and alter patient management. *Sci. Transl. Med.* **2012**, *4*, 138ra78. [CrossRef] [PubMed]
6. Sanders, S.J.; Murtha, M.T.; Gupta, A.R.; Murdoch, J.D.; Raubeson, M.J.; Willsey, A.J.; Ercan-Sencicek, A.G.; DiLullo, N.M.; Parikshak, N.N.; Stein, J.L.; et al. De novo mutations revealed by whole-exome sequencing are strongly associated with autism. *Nature* **2012**, *485*, 237–241. [CrossRef]
7. Yu, T.W.; Chahrour, M.H.; Coulter, M.E.; Jiralerspong, S.; Okamura-Ikeda, K.; Ataman, B.; Schmitz-Abe, K.; Harmin, D.A.; Adli, M.; Malik, A.N.; et al. Using whole-exome sequencing to identify inherited causes of autism. *Neuron* **2013**, *77*, 259–273. [CrossRef]
8. Vasieva, O.; Cetiner, S.; Savage, A.; Schumann, G.G.; Bubb, J.V.; Quinn, J.P. Primate specific retrotransposons, SVAs, in the evolution of networks that alter brain function in Neurons and Cognition. *arXiv* **2016**, arXiv:1602.07642v2.
9. Xu, X.; Coats, J.K.; Yang, C.F.; Wang, A.; Ahmed, O.M.; Alvarado, M.; Izumi, T.; Shah, N.M. Modular genetic control of sexually dimorphic behaviors. *Cell* **2012**, *48*, 596–607. [CrossRef]
10. Lebow, M.; Chen, A. Overshadowed by the amygdala: The bed nucleus of the stria terminalis emerges as key to psychiatric disorders. *Mol. Psychiatry* **2016**, *21*, 450–463. [CrossRef]
11. Kerman, I.A.; Bernard, R.; Bunney, W.E.; Jones, E.G.; Schatzberg, A.F.; Myers, R.M.; Barchas, J.D.; Akil, H.; Watson, S.J.; Thompson, R.C. Evidence for transcriptional factor dysregulation in the dorsal raphe nucleus of patients with major depressive disorder. *Front. Neurosci.* **2012**, *6*, 135. [CrossRef] [PubMed]
12. Szego, E.M.; Janáky, T.; Szabó, Z.; Csorba, A.; Kompagne, H.; Müller, G.; Lévay, G.; Simor, A.; Juhász, G.; Kékesi, K.A. A mouse model of anxiety molecularly characterized by altered protein networks in the brain proteome. *Eur. Neuropsychopharmacol.* **2010**, *20*, 96–111. [CrossRef] [PubMed]
13. Wang, H.; Ishizaki, R.; Xu, J.; Kasai, K.; Kobayashi, E.; Gomi, H.; Izumi, T. The Rab27a effector exophilin7 promotes fusion of secretory granules that have not been docked to the plasma membrane. *Mol. Biol. Cell* **2013**, *24*, 319–330. [CrossRef] [PubMed]

14. Xu, X. Modular genetic control of innate behaviors. *Bioessays* **2013**, *35*, 421–424. [CrossRef]
15. Butler, M.G.; Rafi, S.K.; Hossain, W.; Stephan, D.A.; Manzardo, A.M. Whole exome sequencing in females with autism implicates novel and candidate genes. *Int. J. Mol. Sci.* **2015**, *16*, 1312–1335. [CrossRef] [PubMed]
16. Gomi, H.; Mori, K.; Itohara, S.; Izumi, T. Rab27b is expressed in a wide range of exocytic cells and involved in the delivery of secretory granules near the plasma membrane. *Mol. Biol. Cell* **2007**, *18*, 4377–4386. [CrossRef] [PubMed]
17. Boivin, V.; Deschamps-Francoeur, G.; Scott, M.S. Protein coding genes as hosts for noncoding RNA expression. *Semin. Cell Dev. Biol.* **2018**, *75*, 3–12. [CrossRef] [PubMed]
18. Bonanno, J.B.; Rutter, M.; Bain, K.T.; Miller, S.; Romero, R.; Wasserman, S.; Sauder, J.M.; Burley, S.K.; Almo, S.C. *Protein Data Bank in Europe (PDBe) ID: 3fdw: Crystal Structure of a C2 Domain from Human Synaptotagmin-Like Protein 4*; New York SGX Research Center for Structural Genomics (NYSGXRC): New York, NY, USA, 2008.
19. Miyamoto, K.; Sato, M.; Koshiba, S.; Inoue, M.; Kigawa, T.; Yokoyama, S. Protein Data Bank (PDB) ID: 2CSZ: Solution Structure of the RING Domain of the Synaptotagmin-Like Protein 4. RIKEN Structural Genomics/Proteomics Initiative (RSGI), 2005. Available online: https://www.ncbi.nlm.nih.gov/Structure/pdb/2CSZ (accessed on 8 July 2018).
20. Zhang, Y. I-TASSER server for protein 3D structure prediction. *BMC Bioinform.* **2008**, *9*, 40. [CrossRef] [PubMed]
21. Berman, H.M.; Westbrook, J.; Feng, Z.; Gilliland, G.; Bhat, T.N.; Weissig, H.; Shindyalov, I.N.; Bourne, P.E. The protein data bank. *Nucleic Acids Res.* **2000**, *28*, 235–242. [CrossRef] [PubMed]
22. Fuson, K.L.; Montes, M.; Robert, J.J.; Sutton, R.B. Structure of human synaptotagmin 1 C2AB in the absence of Ca2+ reveals a novel domain association. *Biochemistry* **2007**, *46*, 13041–13048. [CrossRef]
23. Schauder, C.M.; Wu, X.; Saheki, Y.; Narayanaswamy, P.; Torta, F.; Wenk, M.R.; De Camilli, P.; Reinisch, K.M. Structure of a lipid-bound extended synaptotagmin indicates a role in lipid transfer. *Nature* **2014**, *510*, 552–555. [CrossRef] [PubMed]
24. Donald, J.E.; Kulp, D.W.; DeGrado, W.F. Salt bridges: Geometrically specific, designable interactions. *Proteins* **2011**, *79*, 898–915. [CrossRef]
25. Gregoret, L.M.; Rade, S.D.; Fletterick, R.J.; Cohen, F.E. Hydrogen bonds involving sulfur atoms in proteins. *Proteins* **1991**, *9*, 99–107. [CrossRef] [PubMed]
26. Szklarczyk, D.; Franceschini, A.; Wyder, S.; Forslund, K.; Heller, D.; Huerta-Cepas, J.; Simonovic, M.; Roth, A.; Santos, A.; Tsafou, K.P.; et al. STRING v10: Protein-protein interaction networks, integrated over the tree of life. *Nucleic Acids Res.* **2015**, *43*, D447–D452. [CrossRef] [PubMed]
27. Okada, M.; Itoh, M.; Haraguchi, M.; Okajima, T.; Inoue, M.; Oishi, H.; Matsuda, Y.; Iwamoto, T.; Kawano, T.; Fukumoto, S.; et al. b-series Ganglioside deficiency exhibits no definite changes in the neurogenesis and the sensitivity to Fas-mediated apoptosis but impairs regeneration of the lesioned hypoglossal nerve. *J. Biol. Chem.* **2002**, *277*, 1633–1636. [CrossRef] [PubMed]
28. Stamberger, H.; Nikanorova, M.; Willemsen, M.H.; Accorsi, P.; Angriman, M.; Baier, H.; Benkel-Herrenbrueck, I.; Benoit, V.; Budetta, M.; Caliebe, A.; et al. STXBP1 Encephalopathy: A neurodevelopmental disorder including epilepsy. *Neurology* **2016**, *86*, 954–962. [CrossRef]
29. Söllner, T.; Bennett, M.K.; Whiteheart, S.W.; Scheller, R.H.; Rothman, J.E. A protein assembly-disassembly pathway in vitro that may correspond to sequential steps of synaptic vesicle docking, activation, and fusion. *Cell* **1993**, *75*, 409–430. [CrossRef]
30. Neves, S.R.; Ram, P.T.; Iyengar, R. G protein pathways. *Science* **2002**, *296*, 1636–1639. [CrossRef]
31. Rapoport, J.; Chavez, A.; Greenstein, D.; Addington, A.; Gogtay, N. Autism spectrum disorders and childhood-onset schizophrenia: Clinical and biological contributions to a relation revisited. *J. Am. Acad. Child Adolesc. Psychiatry* **2009**, *48*, 10–18. [CrossRef]
32. Beveridge, N.J.; Cairns, M.J. MicroRNA dysregulation in schizophrenia. *Neurobiol. Dis.* **2012**, *46*, 263–271. [CrossRef]
33. Shi, W.; Du, J.; Qi, Y.; Liang, G.; Wang, T.; Li, S.; Xie, S.; Zeshan, B.; Xiao, Z. Aberrant expression of serum miRNAs in schizophrenia. *J. Psychiatr. Res.* **2012**, *46*, 198–204. [CrossRef] [PubMed]
34. Vasu, M.; Anitha, A.; Thanseem, I.; Suzuki, K.; Yamada, K.; Takahashi, T.; Wakuda, T.; Iwata, K.; Tsujii, M.; Sugiyama, T.; et al. Serum microRNA profiles in children with autism. *Mol. Autism* **2014**, *5*, 40. [CrossRef] [PubMed]

35. Abu-Elneel, K.; Liu, T.; Gazzaniga, F.S.; Nishimura, Y.; Wall, D.P.; Geschwind, D.H.; Lao, K.; Kosik, K.S. Heterogeneous dysregulation of microRNAs across the autism spectrum. *Neurogenetics* **2008**, *9*, 153–161. [CrossRef] [PubMed]
36. Ghahramani Seno, M.M.; Hu, P.; Gwadry, F.G.; Pinto, D.; Marshall, C.R.; Casallo, G.; Scherer, S.W. Gene and miRNA expression profiles in autism spectrum disorders. *Brain Res.* **2011**, *1380*, 85–97. [CrossRef] [PubMed]
37. Stamova, B.; Ander, B.P.; Barger, N.; Sharp, F.R.; Schumann, C.M. Specific regional and age-related small noncoding RNA expression patterns within superior temporal gyrus of typical human brains are less distinct in autism brains. *J. Child Neurol.* **2015**, *30*, 1930–1946. [CrossRef] [PubMed]
38. Anney, R.; Klei, L.; Pinto, D.; Almeida, J.; Bacchelli, E.; Baird, G.; Bolshakova, N.; Bölte, S.; Bolton, P.F.; Bourgeron, T.; et al. Individual common variants exert weak effects on the risk for autism spectrum disorders. *Hum. Mol. Genet.* **2012**, *21*, 4781–4792. [CrossRef] [PubMed]
39. Klei, L.; Sanders, S.J.; Murtha, M.T.; Hus, V.; Lowe, J.K.; Willsey, A.J.; Moreno-De-Luca, D.; Yu, T.W.; Fombonne, E.; Geschwind, D.; et al. Common genetic variants, acting additively, are a major source of risk for autism. *Mol. Autism* **2012**, *3*, 9. [CrossRef]
40. Stein, J.L.; Parikshak, N.N.; Geschwind, D.H. Rare inherited variation in autism: Beginning to see the forest. *Neuron* **2013**, *77*, 209–211. [CrossRef]
41. Crestani, C.C.; Alves, F.H.; Gomes, F.V.; Resstel, L.B.; Correa, F.M.; Herman, J.P. Mechanisms in the bed nucleus of the stria terminalis involved in control of autonomic and neuroendocrine functions: A review. *Curr. Neuropharmacol.* **2013**, *11*, 141–159. [CrossRef]
42. Lopes, A.M.; Burgoyne, P.S.; Ojarikre, A.; Bauer, J.; Sargent, C.A.; Amorim, A.; Affara, N.A. Transcriptional changes in response to X chromosome dosage in the mouse: Implications for X inactivation and the molecular basis of Turner Syndrome. *BMC Genom.* **2010**, *11*, 82. [CrossRef]
43. Vitkup, D.; Sander, C.; Church, G.M. The amino-acid mutational spectrum of human genetic disease. *Genome Biol.* **2003**, *4*, R72. [CrossRef] [PubMed]
44. Betts, M.J.; Russell, R.B. Amino acid properties and consequences of substitutions. In *Bioinformatics for Geneticists*; Barnes, M.R., Gray, I.C., Eds.; John Wiley & Sons: New York, NY, USA, 2003.
45. Khan, S.; Vihinen, M. Spectrum of disease-causing mutations in protein secondary structures. *BMC Struct. Biol.* **2007**, *7*, 56. [CrossRef] [PubMed]
46. Poussu, E.; Vihinen, M.; Paulin, L.; Savilahti, H. Probing the alpha-complementing domain of E. coli beta-galactosidase with use of an insertional pentapeptide mutagenesis strategy based on Mu in vitro DNA transposition. *Proteins* **2004**, *54*, 681–692. [CrossRef]
47. Vihinen, M.; Vetri, D.; Maniar, H.S.; Ochs, H.D.; Zhu, Q.; Vorechovský, I.; Webster, A.D.; Notarangelo, L.D.; Nilsson, L.; Sowadski, J.M.; et al. Structural basis for chromosome X-linked agammaglobulinemia: A tyrosine kinase disease. *Proc. Natl. Acad. Sci. USA* **1994**, *91*, 12803–12807. [CrossRef] [PubMed]
48. Yue, P.; Li, Z.; Moult, J. Loss of protein structure stability as a major causative factor in monogenic disease. *J. Mol. Biol.* **2005**, *353*, 459–473. [CrossRef] [PubMed]
49. Rong, S.B.; Vihinen, M. Structural basis of Wiskott-Aldrich syndrome causing mutations in the WH1 domain. *J. Mol. Med. (Berl.)* **2000**, *78*, 530–537. [CrossRef] [PubMed]
50. Lappalainen, I.; Vihinen, M. Structural basis of ICF-causing mutations in the methyltransferase domain of DNMT3B. *Protein Eng.* **2002**, *15*, 1005–1014. [CrossRef] [PubMed]
51. Strom, M.; Hume, A.N.; Tarafder, A.K.; Barkagianni, E.; Seabra, M.C. A family of Rab27-binding proteins. Melanophilin links Rab27a and myosin Va function in melanosome transport. *J. Biol. Chem.* **2002**, *277*, 25423–25430. [CrossRef] [PubMed]
52. Mufson, E.J.; Counts, S.E.; Ginsberg, S.D. Gene expression profiles of cholinergic nucleus basalis neurons in Alzheimer's disease. *Neurochem. Res.* **2002**, *27*, 1035–1048. [CrossRef] [PubMed]
53. Zhang, D.; Aravind, L. Identification of novel families and classification of the C2 domain superfamily elucidate the origin and evolution of membrane targeting activities in eukaryotes. *Gene* **2010**, *469*, 18–30. [CrossRef] [PubMed]
54. Lyakhova, T.A.; Knight, J.D. The C2 domains of granuphilin are high-affinity sensors for plasma membrane lipids. *Chem. Phys. Lipids* **2014**, *182*, 29–37. [CrossRef] [PubMed]
55. Dephoure, N.; Zhou, C.; Villén, J.; Beausoleil, S.; Bakalarski, C.E.; Elledge, S.J.; Gygi, S.P. A quantitative atlas of mitotic phosphorylation. *Proc. Natl. Acad. Sci. USA* **2008**, *105*, 10762–10767. [CrossRef] [PubMed]

56. Bian, Y.; Song, C.; Cheng, K.; Dong, M.; Wang, F.; Huang, J.; Sun, D.; Wang, L.; Ye, M.; Zou, H. An enzyme assisted RP-RPLC approach for in-depth analysis of human liver phosphoproteome. *J. Proteom.* **2014**, *96*, 253–262. [CrossRef] [PubMed]
57. Sharma, K.; D'Souza, R.C.; Tyanova, S.; Schaab, C.; Wiśniewski, J.R.; Cox, J.; Mann, M. Ultradeep human phosphoproteome reveals a distinct regulatory nature of Tyr and Ser/Thr-based signaling. *Cell Rep.* **2014**, *8*, 1583–1594. [CrossRef] [PubMed]
58. Musafia, B.; Buchner, V.; Arad, D. Complex salt bridges in proteins: Statistical analysis of structure and function. *J. Mol. Biol.* **1995**, *254*, 761–770. [CrossRef] [PubMed]
59. Mitra, S.; Cheng, K.W.; Mills, G.B. Rab GTPases implicated in inherited and acquired disorders. *Semin. Cell Dev. Biol.* **2010**, *22*, 57–68. [CrossRef] [PubMed]
60. Zhen, Y.; Stenmark, H. Cellular functions of Rab GTPases at a glance. *J. Cell Sci.* **2015**, *128*, 3171–3176. [CrossRef] [PubMed]
61. Zerial, M.; McBride, H. Rab proteins as membrane organizers. *Nat. Rev. Mol. Cell Biol.* **2001**, *2*, 107–117. [CrossRef] [PubMed]
62. Fukuda, M.; Kanno, E. Analysis of the role of Rab27 effector Slp4-a/Granuphilin-a in dense-core vesicle exocytosis. *Methods Enzymol.* **2005**, *403*, 445–457.
63. Izumi, T.; Gomi, H.; Torii, S. Functional analysis of Rab27a effector granuphilin in insulin exocytosis. *Methods Enzymol.* **2005**, *403*, 216–229.
64. Chavas, L.M.; Ihara, K.; Kawasaki, M.; Torii, S.; Uejima, T.; Kato, R.; Izumi, T.; Wakatsuki, S. Elucidation of Rab27 recruitment by its effectors: Structure of Rab27a bound to Exophilin4/Slp2-a. *Structure* **2008**, *16*, 1468–1477. [CrossRef] [PubMed]
65. Krzewski, K.; Cullinane, A.R. Evidence for defective Rab GTPase-dependent cargo traffic in immune disorders. *Exp. Cell Res.* **2013**, *319*, 2360–2367. [CrossRef] [PubMed]
66. Giannandrea, M.; Bianchi, V.; Mignogna, M.L.; Sirri, A.; Carrabino, S.; D'Elia, E.; Vecellio, M.; Russo, S.; Cogliati, F.; Larizza, L.; et al. Mutations in the small GTPase gene RAB39B are responsible for X-linked mental retardation associated with autism, epilepsy, and macrocephaly. *Am. J. Hum. Genet.* **2010**, *86*, 185–195. [CrossRef] [PubMed]
67. Goitre, L.; Trapani, E.; Trabalzini, L.; Retta, S.F. The Ras superfamily of small GTPases: The unlocked secrets. *Methods Mol. Biol.* **2014**, *1120*, 1–18. [PubMed]
68. Yang, C.F.; Shah, N.M. Representing sex in the brain, one module at a time. *Neuron* **2014**, *8*, 261–278. [CrossRef] [PubMed]
69. Palmer, N.; Beam, A.; Agniel, D.; Eran, A.; Manrai, A.; Spettell, C.; Steinberg, G.; Mandl, K.; Fox, K.; Nelson, S.F.; et al. Association of Sex with Recurrence of Autism Spectrum Disorder among Siblings. *JAMA Pediatr.* **2017**, *171*, 1107–1112. [CrossRef] [PubMed]
70. Durdiakova, J.; Warrier, V.; Banerjee-Basu, S.; Baron-Cohen, S.; Chakrabarti, B. STX1A and Asperger syndrome: A replication study. *Mol. Autism* **2014**, *5*, 14. [CrossRef] [PubMed]
71. Halladay, A.K.; Bishop, S.; Constantino, J.M.; Daniels, A.M.; Koenig, K.; Palmer, K.; Messinger, D.; Pelphrey, K.; Sanders, S.J.; Singer, A.T.; et al. Sex and gender differences in autism spectrum disorder: Summarizing evidence gaps and identifying emerging areas of priority. *Mol. Autism* **2015**, *6*, 36. [CrossRef] [PubMed]
72. Gomi, H.; Mizutani, S.; Kasai, K.; Itohara, S.; Izumi, T. Granuphilin molecularly docks insulin granules to the fusion machinery. *J. Cell Biol.* **2005**, *171*, 99–109. [CrossRef] [PubMed]
73. Budnik, V.; Ruiz-Cañada, C.; Wendler, F. Extracellular vesicles round off communication in the nervous system. *Nat. Rev.* **2016**, *17*, 160–172. [CrossRef] [PubMed]
74. Van Breevoort, D.; Snijders, A.P.; Hellen, N.; Weckhuysen, S.; van Hooren, K.W.; Eikenboom, J.; Valentijn, K.; Fernandez-Borja, M.; Ceulemans, B.; De Jonghe, P.; et al. STXBP1 promotes Weibel-Palade body exocytosis through its interaction with the Rab27A effector Slp4-a. *Blood* **2014**, *123*, 3185–3194. [CrossRef] [PubMed]
75. Yuen, R.K.; Thiruvahindrapuram, B.; Merico, D.; Walker, S.; Tammimies, K.; Hoang, N.; Chrysler, C.; Nalpathamkalam, T.; Pellecchia, G.; Liu, Y.; et al. Whole-genome sequencing of quartet families with autism spectrum disorder. *Nat. Med.* **2015**, *21*, 185–191. [CrossRef] [PubMed]
76. Franceschini, A.; Lin, J.; von Mering, C.; Jensen, L.J. SVD-phy: Improved prediction of protein functional associations through singular value decomposition of phylogenetic profiles. *Bioinformatics* **2016**, *32*, 1085–1087. [CrossRef] [PubMed]

77. Braida, D.; Guerini, F.R.; Ponzoni, L.; Corradini, I.; De Astis, S.; Pattini, L.; Bolognesi, E.; Benfante, R.; Fornasari, D.; Chiappedi, M.; et al. Association between SNAP-25 gene polymorphisms and cognition in autism: Functional consequences and potential therapeutic strategies. *Transl. Psychiatry* **2015**, *5*, e500. [CrossRef] [PubMed]
78. Hong, B.S.; Cho, J.H.; Kim, H.; Choi, E.J.; Rho, S.; Kim, J.; Kim, J.H.; Choi, D.S.; Kim, Y.K.; Hwang, D.; et al. Colorectal cancer cell-derived microvesicles are enriched in cell cycle-related mRNAs that promote proliferation of endothelial cells. *BMC Genom.* **2009**, *10*, 556. [CrossRef] [PubMed]
79. Waites, C.L.; Garner, C.C. Presynaptic function in health and disease. *Trends Neurosci.* **2011**, *34*, 326–337. [CrossRef]
80. Baker, K.; Gordon, S.L.; Grozeva, D.; van Kogelenberg, M.; Roberts, N.Y.; Pike, M.; Blair, E.; Hurles, M.E.; Chong, W.K.; Baldeweg, T.; et al. Identification of a human synaptotagmin-1 mutation that perturbs synaptic vesicle cycling. *J. Clin. Investig.* **2015**, *125*, 1670–1678. [CrossRef] [PubMed]
81. Geppert, M.; Goda, Y.; Hammer, R.E.; Li, C.; Rosahl, T.W.; Stevens, C.F.; Südhof, T.C. Synaptotagmin I: A major Ca2+ sensor for transmitter release at a central synapse. *Cell* **1994**, *79*, 717–727. [CrossRef]
82. Bai, J.; Wang, P.; Chapman, E.R. C2A activates a cryptic Ca (2+)-triggered membrane penetration activity within the C2B domain of synaptotagmin I. *Proc. Natl. Acad. Sci. USA* **2002**, *99*, 1665–1670. [CrossRef]
83. Zoghbi, H.Y.; Bear, M.F. Synaptic dysfunction in neurodevelopmental disorders associated with autism and intellectual disabilities. *Cold Spring Harb. Perspect. Biol.* **2012**, *4*, a009886. [CrossRef]
84. Bacaj, T.; Wu, D.; Yang, X.; Morishita, W.; Zhou, P.; Xu, W.; Malenka, R.C.; Südhof, T.C. Synaptotagmin-1 and synaptotagmin-7 trigger synchronous and asynchronous phases of neurotransmitter release. *Neuron* **2013**, *80*, 947–959. [CrossRef] [PubMed]
85. Pettersen, E.F.; Goddard, T.D.; Huang, C.C.; Couch, G.S.; Greenblatt, D.M.; Meng, E.C.; Ferrin, T.E. UCSF Chimera–a visualization system for exploratory research and analysis. *J. Comput. Chem.* **2004**, *25*, 1605–1612. [CrossRef]
86. Plaisance, V.; Abderrahmani, A.; Perret-Menoud, V.; Jacquemin, P.; Lemaigre, F.; Regazzi, R. MicroRNA-9 controls the expression of Granuphilin/Slp4 and the secretory response of insulin-producing cells. *J. Biol. Chem.* **2006**, *281*, 26932–26942. [CrossRef] [PubMed]
87. Rolland, T.; Taşan, M.; Charloteaux, B.; Pevzner, S.J.; Zhong, Q.; Sahni, N.; Yi, S.; Lemmens, I.; Fontanillo, C.; Mosca, R.; et al. A proteome-scale map of the human interactome network. *Cell* **2014**, *159*, 1212–1226. [CrossRef] [PubMed]
88. Eppig, J.T.; Blake, J.A.; Bult, C.J.; Kadin, J.A.; Richardson, J.E. Mouse Genome Database Group. The mouse genome database (MGD): Facilitating mouse as a model for human biology and disease. *Nucleic Acids Res.* **2015**, *43*, D726–D736. [CrossRef] [PubMed]
89. Feng, R.; Sang, Q.; Zhu, Y.; Fu, W.; Liu, M.; Xu, Y.; Shi, H.; Xu, Y.; Qu, R.; Chai, R.; et al. MiRNA-320 in the human follicular fluid-development in vitro. *Sci. Rep.* **2015**, *5*, 8689. [CrossRef] [PubMed]
90. Fatima, M.; Prajapati, B.; Saleem, K.; Kumari, R.; Mohindar Singh Singal, C.; Seth, P. Novel insights into role of miR-320a-VDAC1 axis in astrocyte-mediated neuronal damage in neuroAIDS. *Glia* **2017**, *65*, 250–263. [CrossRef] [PubMed]
91. Song, H.T.; Sun, X.Y.; Zhang, L.; Zhao, L.; Guo, Z.M.; Fan, H.M.; Zhong, A.F.; Niu, W.; Dai, Y.H.; Zhang, L.Y.; et al. A preliminary analysis of association between the downregulation of microRNA-181b expression and symptomatology improvement in schizophrenia patients before and after antipsychotic treatment. *J. Psychiatr. Res.* **2014**, *54*, 134–140. [CrossRef] [PubMed]
92. Khanzada, N.S.; Butler, M.G.; Manzardo, A.M. GeneAnalytics pathway analysis and genetic overlap among autism spectrum disorder, bipolar disorder and schizophrenia. *Int. J. Mol. Sci.* **2017**, *18*, 527. [CrossRef] [PubMed]
93. Sundararajan, T.; Manzardo, A.M.; Butler, M.G. Functional analysis of schizophrenia genes using GeneAnalytics program and integrated databases. *Gene* **2018**, *641*, 25–34. [CrossRef] [PubMed]
94. Mor, M.; Nardone, S.; Sams, D.S.; Elliott, E. Hypomethylation of miR-142 promoter and upregulation of microRNAs that target the oxytocin receptor gene in the autism prefrontal cortex. *Mol. Autism* **2015**, *6*, 46. [CrossRef] [PubMed]
95. Frattini, S.A.; Zucchi, I.; Patrosso, C.P. Characterization sequence/EST database screening. *Genomics* **1996**, *34*, 323–327.

96. Joyner, A.H.; Cooper Roddey, J.; Bloss, C.S.; Bakken, T.E.; Rimol, L.M.; Melle, I.; Agartz, I.; Djurovic, S.; Topol, E.J.; Schork, N.J.; et al. A common MECP2 haplotype associates with reduced cortical surface area in humans in two independent populations. *Proc. Natl. Acad. Sci. USA* **2009**, *106*, 15483–15488. [CrossRef] [PubMed]
97. Sklar, P.; Smoller, J.W.; Fan, J.; Ferreira, M.A.; Perlis, R.H.; Chambert, K.; Nimgaonkar, V.L.; McQueen, M.B.; Faraone, S.V.; Kirby, A.; et al. Whole-genome association study of bipolar disorder. *Mol. Psychiatry* **2008**, *13*, 558–569. [CrossRef] [PubMed]
98. Erhardt, A.; Akula, N.; Schumacher, J.; Czamara, D.; Karbalai, N.; Müller-Myhsok, B.; Mors, O.; Borglum, A.; Kristensen, A.S.; Woldbye, D.P.; et al. Replication and meta-analysis of TMEM132D gene variants in panic disorder. *Transl. Psychiatry* **2012**, *2*, e156. [CrossRef] [PubMed]
99. Butler, M.G.; Rafi, S.K.; Manzardo, A.M. High-resolution chromosome ideogram representation of currently recognized genes for autism spectrum disorders. *Int. J. Mol. Sci.* **2015**, *16*, 6464–6495. [CrossRef] [PubMed]
100. Roy, A.; Kucukural, A.; Zhang, Y. I-TASSER: A unified platform for automated protein structure and function prediction. *Nat. Protoc.* **2010**, *5*, 725–738. [CrossRef]
101. Yang, J.; Yan, R.; Roy, A.; Xu, D.; Poisson, J.; Zhang, Y. The I-TASSER Suite: Protein structure and function prediction. *Nat. Methods* **2015**, *12*, 7–8. [CrossRef]
102. Wu S, Zhang Y: LOMETS: A local meta-threading-server for protein structure prediction. *Nucleic Acids Res.* **2007**, *35*, 3375–3382. [CrossRef]
103. Rual, J.F.; Venkatesan, K.; Hao, T.; Hirozane-Kishikawa, T.; Dricot, A.; Li, N.; Berriz, G.F.; Gibbons, F.D.; Dreze, M.; Ayivi-Guedehoussou, N.; et al. Towards a proteome-scale map of the human protein-protein interaction network. *Nature* **2005**, *437*, 1173–1178. [CrossRef]
104. Smith, C.M.; Finger, J.H.; Hayamizu, T.F.; McCright, I.J.; Xu, J.; Berghout, J.; Campbell, J.; Corbani, L.E.; Forthofer, K.L.; Frost, P.J. The mouse gene expression database (GXD): 2014 update. *Nucleic Acids Res.* **2014**, *42*, D818–D824. [CrossRef] [PubMed]
105. Gandal, M.J.; Haney, J.R.; Parikshak, N.N.; Leppa, V.; Ramaswami, G.; Hartl, C.; Schork, A.J.; Appadurai, V.; Buil, A.; Werge, T.M.; et al. Shared molecular neuropathology across major psychiatric disorders parallels polygenic overlap. *Science* **2018**, *359*, 693–697. [CrossRef] [PubMed]
106. Schaaf, C.P.; Sabo, A.; Sakai, Y.; Crosby, J.; Muzny, D.; Hawes, A.; Lewis, L.; Akbar, H.; Varghese, R.; Boerwinkle, E.; et al. Oligogenic heterozygosity in individuals with high-functioning autism spectrum disorders. *Hum. Mol. Genet.* **2011**, *20*, 3366–3375. [CrossRef] [PubMed]
107. Guo, H.; Wang, T.; Wu, H.; Long, M.; Coe, B.P.; Li, H.; Xia, K. Inherited and multiple de novo mutations in autism/developmental delay risk genes suggest a multifactorial model. *Mol. Autism* **2018**, *9*, 64. [CrossRef] [PubMed]

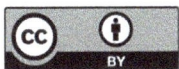

© 2019 by the authors. Licensee MDPI, Basel, Switzerland. This article is an open access article distributed under the terms and conditions of the Creative Commons Attribution (CC BY) license (http://creativecommons.org/licenses/by/4.0/).

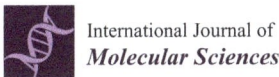

Article

Network-Based Integrative Analysis of Genomics, Epigenomics and Transcriptomics in Autism Spectrum Disorders

Noemi Di Nanni [1,2], Matteo Bersanelli [3,4], Francesca Anna Cupaioli [1], Luciano Milanesi [1], Alessandra Mezzelani [1] and Ettore Mosca [1,*]

1. Institute of Biomedical Technologies, Italian National Research Council, Via Fratelli Cervi 93, 20090 Segrate (MI), Italy
2. Department of Industrial and Information Engineering, University of Pavia, Via Ferrata 5, 27100 Pavia, Italy
3. Department of Physics and Astronomy, University of Bologna, Via B. Pichat 6/2, 40127 Bologna, Italy
4. National Institute of Nuclear Physics (INFN), 40127 Bologna, Italy
* Correspondence: ettore.mosca@itb.cnr.it; Tel.: +39-02-26-42-2614

Received: 14 June 2019; Accepted: 6 July 2019; Published: 9 July 2019

Abstract: Current studies suggest that autism spectrum disorders (ASDs) may be caused by many genetic factors. In fact, collectively considering multiple studies aimed at characterizing the basic pathophysiology of ASDs, a large number of genes has been proposed. Addressing the problem of molecular data interpretation using gene networks helps to explain genetic heterogeneity in terms of shared pathways. Besides, the integrative analysis of multiple omics has emerged as an approach to provide a more comprehensive view of a disease. In this work, we carry out a network-based meta-analysis of the genes reported as associated with ASDs by studies that involved genomics, epigenomics, and transcriptomics. Collectively, our analysis provides a prioritization of the large number of genes proposed to be associated with ASDs, based on genes' relevance within the intracellular circuits, the strength of the supporting evidence of association with ASDs, and the number of different molecular alterations affecting genes. We discuss the presence of the prioritized genes in the SFARI (Simons Foundation Autism Research Initiative) database and in gene networks associated with ASDs by other investigations. Lastly, we provide the full results of our analyses to encourage further studies on common targets amenable to therapy.

Keywords: autism spectrum disorders; biological networks; genomics; multi-omics; network diffusion; data integration

---

1. Introduction

Autism spectrum disorders (ASDs) are among the most common neurodevelopmental disorders. ASDs are characterized by impaired social interactions, repetitive behavior, and restricted interests, and they are often comorbidities with other conditions such as epilepsy, mental retardation, inflammation, and gastrointestinal disorders. Despite the fact that the high heritability of ASDs is well established, the exact underlying causes are unknown in at least 70% of the cases [1]. Large genome-wide association studies (GWAS), Copy Number Variation (CNV) testing and genome sequencing yielded many non-overlapping genes, a fact that underlines the complex genetic heterogeneity of ASDs [1] and reflects the architecture of intracellular networks, in which several possible combinations of genetic variations are likely to lead to a common pathological phenotype [2,3].

The identification of the key molecular pathways that link many ASDs-causing genes is of prominent importance in developing therapeutic interventions [1]. In this context, network-based and pathway-based analyses provide functional explanations to non-overlapping genes and narrow the targets for therapeutic intervention [4]. The rich functional pathway information emerging from such analyses might unearth common targets that are amenable to therapy [1].

One of the challenges that network-based analyses face is the identification of the so-called "disease modules," i.e., gene networks associated with diseases [2]. Under the hypothesis of the "omnigenic model," gene regulatory networks are so interconnected that a large number of genes is liable to affect the function of core genes, i.e., those whose variations are strongly related to disease [3].

The analysis of the human interactome—the complex web of molecular interactions occurring within human cells—is challenging due to its size (e.g., 10^4 genes and 10^5 interactions), and several approaches have been proposed [5]. In the last few decades, the mathematical machinery of network diffusion (ND)—also referred to as network propagation—has been exploited to address several problems in biological data analysis, thanks to its ability to quantify network proximity between query network nodes (e.g., genes) and to simultaneously consider all the possible network paths among them [6]. When applied to studying the large number of genes proposed to be associated with a pathology like ASDs (shortly, disease genes), ND amplifies the relevance of those disease genes that are in close network proximity with other disease genes. In addition, ND predicts the importance of other genes not known a priori but that will probably act as "linkers" (or "silent players"), because they occupy a relevant network position in relation to the network location of disease genes.

In a previous study by our group, the application of ND to genes associated with ASDs from genetic data led to the identification of gene networks and pathways particularly enriched in disease genes [7]. Interestingly, several genes predicted as relevant in such study are now included in the SFARI (Simons Foundation Autism Research Initiative) Gene database [8], which provides curated information on all known human genes associated with ASDs.

In addition to genetics, several reports have suggested a role for epigenetic mechanisms in ASD etiology [9,10]. Recent studies have also demonstrated the utility of integrating gene expression with mutation data for the prioritization of genes disrupted by potentially pathogenic mutations [11,12]. More generally, the integrative analysis of multiple omics has emerged as an approach to provide a more comprehensive view of a disease [13,14].

While the analysis of epigenomics and transcriptomics from brain-derived samples can provide important insights into the potential mechanisms of disease etiology, there are relevant limitations with these types of studies (e.g., the quality of autopsy-derived tissue, sample size, influence of life experience, and cause of death) [10]. These barriers have been overcome by analyzing blood samples, and recent blood-based works have shown the usefulness of this alternative approach to gather insights into ASDs [10,15–17].

In this manuscript, we describe a network-based integrative meta-analysis of the results which have emerged from several studies on ASDs, based on genomics, epigenomics, and transcriptomics. Firstly, following the hypothesis of the omnigenic model [3], we analyzed genetic data to introduce a graduated scale of gene relevance in relation to core genes for ASDs. Subsequently, we identified a gene network significantly enriched in genes supported by one or more of the considered evidence (genomics, epigenomics, and transcriptomics). The gene network involves genes that participate in several pathways relevant to ASDs, which we have distinguished by type (or types) of alteration from which they are affected. Collectively, our network-based meta-analysis provides a prioritization of the large number of genes proposed to be associated with ASDs, based on genes' relevance within the intracellular circuits, the strength of the supporting evidences of association with ASDs, and the number of different molecular alterations affecting genes. We discuss the presence of the prioritized genes in the SFARI database and in gene networks associated with ASDs by other studies [18–22]. Lastly, we provide the full results of our analyses to encourage further studies on common targets amenable to therapy.

2. Results

Firstly, we describe the results obtained regarding the genes associated with ASDs on the basis of genomics. We collected these genes from the SFARI Gene database [8], two recent large studies [23,24], and a series of previous studies summarized by Mosca et al. [7], for a total of 1133 genes (Table 1). Following the criteria adopted by SFARI, we distinguished between the genes with the strongest genomics evidence (334 genes, the "genomics-major" group) from the others (799, the "genomics-minor").

Table 1. Datasets considered in this study. Selected: The number of genes for which at least a high confidence interaction with any other gene is catalogued in the STRING database (see methods). G: Genomics; E: Epigenomics; T: Transcriptomics. ** major evidence; * minor evidence.

Type of Evidence	Description	Subjects	Number of Genes			
			Initial		Selected	
			**	*	**	*
G	SFARI [8].	-	404	1087	334	799
G	Network diffusion-based prioritization of autism risk genes identifies significantly connected gene modules [7].	-				
G	Meta-analysis of GWAS of over 16,000 individuals with autism spectrum disorder [23].	15,954				
G	Synaptic, transcriptional and chromatin genes disrupted in autism [24].	13,808				
E	Case-control meta-analysis of blood DNA methylation and autism spectrum disorder [10].	1654	416	1444	272	955
T	Gene expression profiling differentiates autism case-controls and phenotypic variants of autism spectrum disorders [25].	116	330	3045	256	2131
T	Blood gene expression signatures distinguish autism spectrum disorders from controls [15].	285				
T	Disrupted functional networks in autism underlie early brain mal-development and provide accurate classification. [26].	147				
T	Gene expression in blood of children with autism spectrum disorder [27].	47				

Subsequently, we could describe the multi-omics analysis in which we also considered evidences emerged in studies that focused on epigenomics [10] and transcriptomics [15,25–27]. Additionally in these cases, we distinguished between the genes with the strongest evidences ("epigenomics-major" and "transcriptomics-major") from the others ("epigenomics-minor" and "transcriptomics-minor"), following the indications of the corresponding studies from which we collected the data (Table 1).

2.1. Genomics Analysis

Recently, the "omnigenic model" was proposed to explain the inheritance of complex diseases [3]. In this model, the genes whose genetic damage tend to have the strongest effects on disease risk are considered core genes, while those genes that have a minor impact on disease risk are designated as peripheral. The number of peripheral genes may be large as a consequence of the multiple ways in which these genes may interact with core genes throughout cell regulatory networks. Importantly, such classification may be on a graduated scale rather than simply binary [3].

In this context, ND provides an opportunity to define quantitatively the degree of peripherality of all genes in relation to "seed" genes, exploring all possible network paths among genes in intracellular networks. We applied ND on the human interactome (high confidence functional and biophysical interactions catalogued in STRING), considering as seeds: the core genes for ASDs, among which we included those classified in SFARI as "syndromic," "high confidence," "strong candidate," "suggestive evidence," and "syndromic minimal evidence," for a total of 334 genes; other 799 genes proposed to have a role in ASDs (Supplementary Table S1).

We found several genes with a significant network proximity to core genes (Figure 1A, Supplementary Table S1). From a topological point of view, among these genes, we found both hubs (genes that establish many interactions, such as UBC, ubiquitin C; DYNC1H1, dynein cytoplasmic 1 heavy chain 1; and EP300, E1A binding protein p300) and genes with a lower number of connections (e.g., CHD2, chromodomain helicase DNA binding protein 2; NUDCD2, NudC domain containing 2; and SETD5, SET domain containing 5), which are nevertheless important for the information flow within the network (Figure 1A).

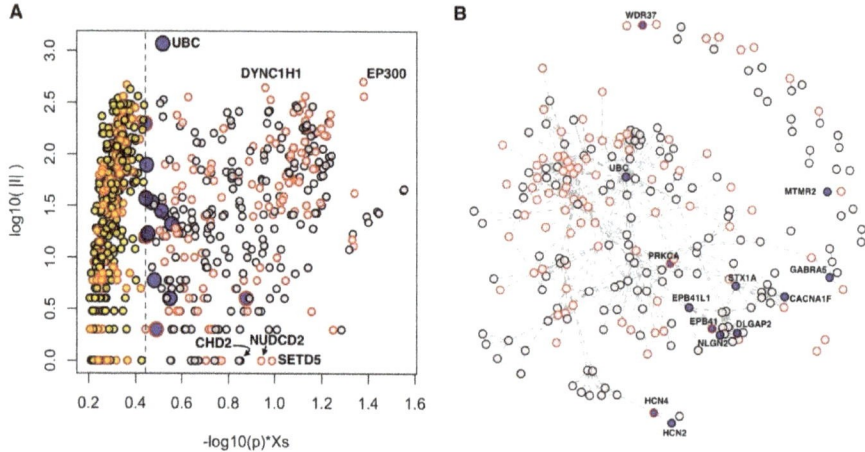

Figure 1. Genes in network proximity to the core genes of autism spectrum disorders (ASDs). (**A**) Diffusion score (Xs) normalized by its empirical p-value (horizontal axis) and number of interactions (|I|, vertical axis); only genes with $p < 0.05$ are shown. (**B**) Connected components of "core+13" network. (**A,B**) Blue points: 13 genes of "core+13"; pink points: core genes; yellow points: Significant genes outside "core+13" genes; red border of points: Genes supported at transcriptomic and/or epigenetic levels.

Interestingly, 13 genes obtained scores comparable to those of core genes (Figure 1). These results indicate that these 13 genes closely interact with the core genes, and, in almost all cases, the number of interactions that these genes establish with the core genes is significant (Table 2, Supplementary Figure S1). From now on, we will call the set of core genes and the 13 genes closely related to the core genes as "core+13." In the core+13 gene network, the 13 genes act as linkers between groups of core genes not directly connected with each other; for instance, *WDR37* (WD repeat domain 37) links *PACS1* (phosphofurin acidic cluster sorting protein 1) and *PACS2* (phosphofurin acidic cluster sorting protein 2). The resulting largest connected component involves 204 genes, while the remaining 143 genes are mostly isolated or form very small modules of two or three genes.

We checked whether any of these 13 genes, currently not included in the highest categories of SFARI, are nevertheless classified in other categories corresponding to a lower degree of evidence or have been reported in other network-based analyses of ASDs data. We found that six genes belong to the categories designated as "minimal evidence" or "hypothesized but untested," and eight genes were proposed as part of gene networks associated with ASDs (Table 2).

Table 2. The 13 genes that closely interact with the core genes of ASDs. |I|: Number of interactors; |Ic|: Number of interactors that are core genes; p: Hypergeometric probability of observing |Ic| in a hypergeometric experiment; G: Genomics; E: Epigenomics; T: Transcriptomics; ** major; * minor; 0: No evidence; SFARI score: "minimal evidence" (4), "hypothesized but untested" (5); other modules: Reference of gene-networks studies of ASDs in which the gene is mentioned. The total number of genes considered is equal to the interactome size: 12,739 genes.

Symbol	Description	|I|	|Ic|	|core|	p	G	E	T	SFARI Score	Other Modules
HCN4	hyperpolarization activated cyclic nucleotide gated potassium channel 4	4	2	334	3.97×10^{-3}	*	*	0	-	-
DLGAP2	DLG associated protein 2	21	8	334	3.10×10^{-8}	*	0	0	4	[18,21,22]
HCN2	hyperpolarization activated cyclic nucleotide gated potassium and sodium channel 2	4	1	334	1.01×10^{-1}	*	0	0	-	-
UBC	ubiquitin C	1168	43	334	1.41×10^{-2}	*	0	0	-	[20]
NLGN2	neuroligin 2	28	8	334	4.04×10^{-7}	*	0	0	4	[18]
WDR37	WD repeat domain 37	2	2	334	6.85×10^{-4}	0	0	*	-	-
MTMR2	myotubularin related protein 2	6	1	334	1.47×10^{-1}	*	0	0	-	-
EPB41L1	erythrocyte membrane protein band 4.1 like 1	34	9	334	1.55×10^{-7}	*	0	0	-	[21]
GABRA5	gamma-aminobutyric acid type A receptor alpha5 subunit	17	4	334	8.43×10^{-4}	*	0	0	5	[21]
STX1A	syntaxin 1A	78	10	334	3.47×10^{-5}	*	0	0	4	[20,21]
EPB41	erythrocyte membrane protein band 4.1	16	5	334	4.14×10^{-5}	*	0	**	-	[20]
CACNA1F	calcium voltage-gated channel subunit alpha1 F	37	6	334	3.63×10^{-4}	*	0	0	4	[21]
PRKCA	protein kinase C alpha	197	11	334	1.48×10^{-2}	*	*	*	4	-

Collectively, we observed that a significant number of "core+13" genes emerged as associated with ASDs at epigenomics level ($p = 2.63 \times 10^{-4}$; hypergeometric test; Table 3) and at transcriptomics level; $p = 1.22 \times 10^{-3}$ hypergeometric test, Table 3).

Table 3. Overlaps among the lists of genes associated with ASDs. G: Genomic; E: Epigenomics; T: Transcriptomics; ** major; * minor; core+13(E) and core+13(T) indicate genes belonging to the core+13 set and which are supported by E and T, respectively.

A	B	|A|	|B|	|U|	|A∩B|	⟨|A∩B|⟩	P(x≥|A∩B|)
core+13	core+13(E)	347	1227	12739	54	3.27	2.63×10^{-4}
core+13	core+13(T)	347	2387	12739	88	6.37	1.22×10^{-3}
G	E	1133	1227	12739	146	109	1.09×10^{-4}
G	T	1133	2387	12739	235	212	3.95×10^{-2}
E	T	1227	2387	12739	243	230	1.66×10^{-1}
G **	E **	334	272	12739	15	7.13	5.47×10^{-3}
G **	T **	334	256	12739	15	6.71	3.12×10^{-3}
E **	T **	272	256	12739	5	5.47	6.42×10^{-1}

The association with ASDs for 12 of the 13 genes is supported at genomic level. In addition, *HCN4* (hyperpolarization activated cyclic nucleotide gated potassium channel 4) was found with epigenetic modifications in a study of Andrews et al. [10], while *PRKCA* (protein kinase C alpha) was found both epigenetically modified [10] and differentially expressed [26]. WDR37 does not have supporting evidences at genomic level, but it was found differentially expressed [25].

2.2. Multi-Omics Analysis

We assessed the significance of the overlaps among the lists of genes associated with ASDs by genomics, epigenomics, and transcriptomics evidences. We observed significant overlaps between the list of genes from genomics and those supported by epigenomics or transcriptomics (Table 3). The intersection among the three gene lists consists of 40 genes, 34 of which are included in the considered interactome (shortly "shared") (Figure 2). Out of the shared genes, 26 do not interact directly with any other shared gene, while eight genes form three connected components composed of: *DYNC1H1*, *TRAPPC6B* (trafficking protein particle complex 6B), *TRAPPC9* (trafficking protein particle complex 9) and *CSNK1D* (casein kinase 1 delta); *GNAS* (GNAS complex locus) and *PRKCA* (protein kinase C alpha); *EP400* and *TRRAP* (transformation/transcription domain associated protein) (Supplementary Figure S2).

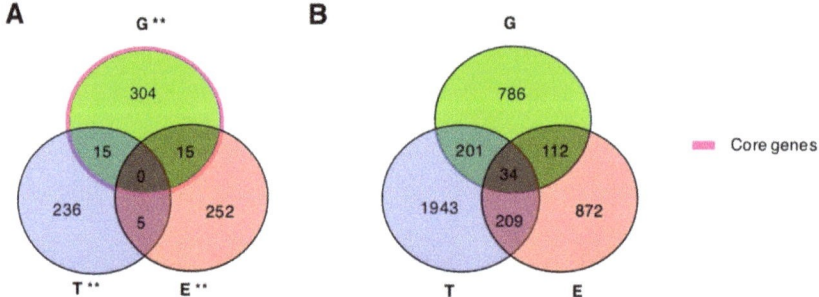

Figure 2. Overlaps among genes associated with ASDs by genomics, epigenomics, and transcriptomics. (**A**,**B**) G: Genomics; E: Epigenomics; T: Transcriptomics. ** major.

In order to find modules of functionally related genes supported by one or more types of evidences ("layers" from now on), we used ND (see methods) and obtained a final diffusion score that summarized the relevance of each gene in relation to its location in the interactome and its network proximity to other genes associated with ASDs in one or more layers (genomics, epigenomics, and transcriptomics). The higher the final diffusion score, the closer the gene to ASDs genes in one or more of the considered layers.

At the top of the resulting genome-wide ranking, we found genes with significant scores (Figure 3, Supplementary Table S2). To assess whether these highly ranked genes formed significantly connected gene modules, we used network resampling [28] and found a multi-omics integrative gene module (INT-MODULE) involving a total of 275 genes (Supplementary Figure S3). The largest connected component (266 genes) of the INT-MODULE connected 22 shared genes which do not establish direct interactions with each other if considered in isolation (Figure 3).

We compared the INT-MODULE with gene networks proposed by other studies on ASDs and found that 157 genes occurred in at least one of such networks (Supplementary Table S3). In addition to the 144 INT-MODULE genes occurring among the highest SFARI categories, we found that 10 genes are classified as "minimal evidence" and "hypothesized but untested" in SFARI (Table 4, Supplementary Figure S4), and seven of these 10 genes were reported by other network-based analyses (Table 4). The INT-MODULE includes also *LRRC46* (leucine rich repeat containing 46), the only gene of the module that does not occur in any of the input gene lists (Figure 3, Supplementary Figure S4).

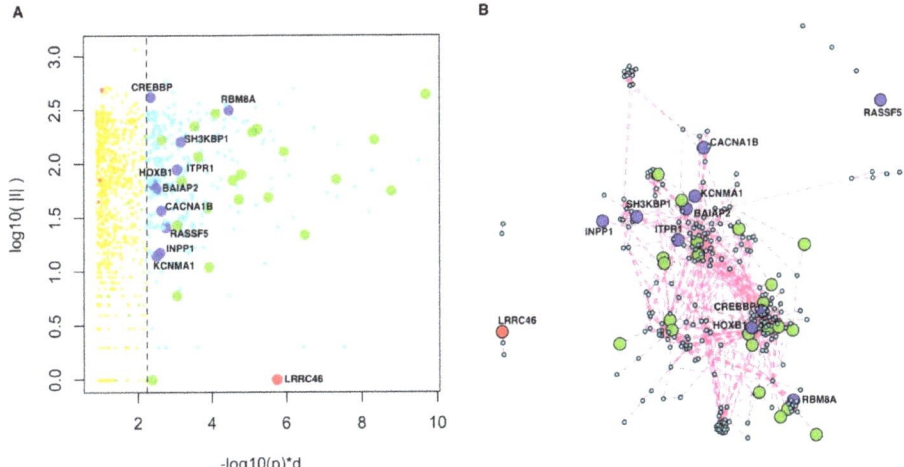

Figure 3. Integrative multi-omics analysis. (**A**) Global network diffusion scores (horizontal axis) and number of interactions (vertical axis) of the top ranking genes; the vertical dashed line separates the top 275 genes belonging to the INT-MODULE (higher scores, on the right) from the other genes (lower scores, on the left). (**B**) Network of the top 275 genes (INT-MODULE). Green circles: shared genes; blue circles: Genes included in SFARI categories 4 and 5; red circle: *LRRC46*.

Table 4. INT-MODULE genes SFARI. G: Genomics; E: Epigenomics; T: Transcriptomics. ** major; * minor. Im: Number of interactors within the INT-MODULE; SFARI score: "minimal evidence" (4), "hypothesized but untested" (5). Other modules: Reference of gene-networks studies that also associated the gene to ASDs.

Symbol	Description	#Im	G	E	T	SFARI Score	Other Modules
BAIAP2	BAI1-associated protein 2	4	*	*	0	5	[19,21]
CACNA1B	calcium voltage-gated channel subunit alpha1 B	7	0	**	0	4	[19,21]
CREBBP	CREB binding protein	43	0	0	**	5	[18,20,21]
HOXB1	homeobox B1	12	0	*	*	5	[18]
INPP1	inositol polyphosphate-1-phosphatase	1	0	**	0	4	[18,21]
ITPR1	inositol 1,4,5-trisphosphate receptor type 1	11	*	*	0	4	[19,21]
KCNMA1	potassium large conductance calcium-activated channel, subfamily M, alpha member 1	1	0	**	0	4	[20]
RASSF5	Ras association domain family member 5	0	0	**	**	4	-
RBM8A	RNA binding motif protein 8A	10	0	**	*	5	-
SH3KBP1	SH3-domain kinase binding protein 1	12	*	0	**	5	-

To functionally characterize the INT-MODULE, we partitioned its largest connected component (266 genes) in topological clusters and assessed both the enrichment of each cluster in terms of molecular pathways and the types of evidences associated with each cluster (Supplementary Tables S2, S4–S6). We explored several community detection strategies and found the highest modularity with a partition of 12 clusters (Figure 4A, Supplementary Figure S5).

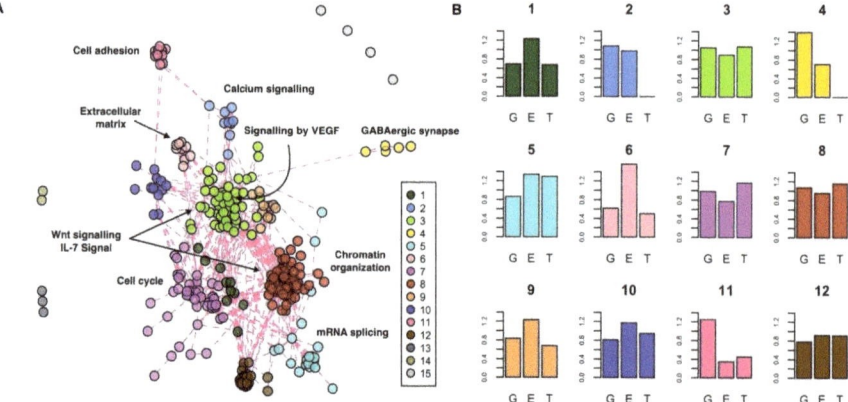

Figure 4. Functional characterization of the INT-MODULE. (**A**) Topological clusters; #1–12: Clusters of the largest connected component; #13,14: Two clusters of three and two genes, respectively; #15: The remaining four genes. (**B**) Enrichment (vertical axis) of each cluster in terms of genes supported by genomics (G), epigenomics (E), and transcriptomics (T): A value of 1 indicates the same proportion within the cluster and in the whole INT-MODULE.

The two largest clusters are composed of 61 (cluster #8) and 53 (cluster #3) genes, and they are characterized by a similar proportion of supporting evidences (Figure 4B). These two central clusters contain genes that are part of the same pathways, such as the Wnt signaling pathway (#8: $q = 1.83 \times 10^{-2}$; #3: $q = 1.79 \times 10^{-5}$) and IL-7 signal transduction (#8: $q = 4.54 \times 10^{-2}$; #3: $q = 6.02 \times 10^{-4}$), but they are also marked by specific pathways. In particular, among the pathways specifically enriched in cluster #8 and #3, we found chromatin organization ($q = 1.27 \times 10^{-27}$) and signaling by VEGF ($q = 5.41 \times 10^{-23}$), respectively. Cluster #7 (41 genes) is the most enriched in differentially expressed genes and significantly associated with pathways involved in cell cycle processes. Cluster #5 is mainly enriched in genes associated with epigenetic and transcriptional changes, and it is marked by mRNA splicing ($q = 1.92 \times 10^{-12}$). Cluster #6 is particularly enriched in genes with epigenetic changes and associated it with extracellular matrix organization ($q = 6.10 \times 10^{-5}$). Cluster #2 (nine genes) is supported at the genomics and epigenomics levels and is enriched in genes of the calcium signaling pathway ($q = 4.88 \times 10^{-12}$). Lastly, clusters #11 and #4 are composed of genes associated with ASDs mainly at the genetic level, which, respectively, control the GABAergic synapse (#4: $q = 3.90 \times 10^{-6}$) and encode for cell adhesion molecules (#11: $q = 1.58 \times 10^{-5}$) active in the neuronal system.

3. Discussion

The integrative analysis of gene related evidence (e.g., DNA polymorphism or mutations, epigenetic changes, transcriptional variations) and gene–gene interaction evidences allows for the extraction of otherwise hidden patterns. In this context, it is worth noting that 68 genes that we proposed as relevant to ASDs in a previous network-based analysis of genetic data are now classified in SFARI (Supplementary Table S7).

In light of the utmost importance of jointly analyzing omics data and intracellular networks, Boyle et al. [3] proposed an explanation for the large number of genes that may be involved in a complex disease as the result of the highly interacting nature of molecular networks. Following the omnigenic model [3], we considered as core genes of ASDs those whose variations are highly scored in SFARI and quantified, by means of network proximity, the degree of peripherality of all other genes in relation to the core genes. This analysis led to the identification of 13 genes significantly connected with the core genes. The strong functional relationship we found between these 13 genes and the core genes suggests that even the former can play an important role in ASDs.

As for the 13 predicted genes (Table 2) that closely interact with the core genes of ASDs, they mainly belong to different neuronal pathways and are especially involved in synaptic function and plasticity that, if impaired, could actively contribute to the pathogenesis of ASDs and/or to their comorbidities. Genes encoding for the ion channel were found among these genes, and the role of various ion channel gene defects (channelopathies) is known in the pathogenesis of ASDs. For instance, *HCN2* and *HCN4* belong to the hyperpolarization-activated cyclic nucleotide-gated (HCN) channels family, encoding for non-selective voltage-gated cation channels, and they are strongly expressed in the brain. These channels establish the slow native pacemaker currents contributing to membrane resting potentials, input resistance, dendritic integration, synaptic transmission, and neuronal excitability. Interestingly, it seems that *SHANK3*, strongly linked to ASDs, works in organization of HCN-channels [29] and that its expression negatively influences those of *HCN2* [30], so variations in the *SHANK3* gene are reflected in pacemaker current abnormalities. In addition, variants in *HCN1*, another member of the HCN family, were detected in patients with epileptic encephalopathy and clinical features of Dravet syndrome, intellectual disability, and autistic features [31].

Some of the predicted genes, such as *EPB41* and *EPB41L1*, take part in cytoskeleton and synaptic structures. *EPB41* is the founding member of the large family of proteins that associate with membrane proteins and cytoskeleton and in neurons is involved in protein–protein interactions at synaptic level. It interacts with NRXN1 and NRXN2, as well as NLGN1, -2, -3, and -4X. These proteins act at the presynaptic and post synaptic level and causative variations in *NRXN1*, -2 [32,33], as well and *NLGN2* (also in core+13 gene set), -3, and -4X [34,35] have already been described in ASDs. Furthermore, EPB41L1 (highly expressed in the brain) and the ionotropic glutamate receptor GRIA1, were listed in the 13 predicted and in core genes, respectively, interact thus contributing to glutamate neurotransmission. An alteration of glutamate neurotransmission was found in ASDs. Interestingly, EPB41L1 is associated with mental retardation, deafness autosomal dominant 11 and autosomal dominant non-syndromic intellectual disability.

Then again, DLGAP2 is a member of the postsynaptic density proteins (as SHANK3), probably involved in molecular organization of synapses and signaling in neuronal cells, with implications in synaptogenesis and plasticity. In particular, DLGAP2 could be an adapter protein linking the ion channel to the sub-synaptic cytoskeleton. Animal models demonstrated that *DLGAP2* has key role in social behaviors and synaptic functions [36]. Case studies also report rare *DLGAP2* duplications in ASDs [37–39]. Then again, the *DLGAP2* gene has an important paralog, *DLGAP1*, already associated with ASDs. DLGAP1 proteins interact with other ASDs-associated proteins such as DLG1, DLG4, SHANK1, SHANK2 and SHANK3 [18]. Moreover, the analysis of rare copy number variants in ASDs found numerous de novo and inherited events in many novel ASDs genes including *DLGAP2* [22].

Among the 13 predicted genes, syntaxin-1A (*STX1A*) is also involved in synaptic signaling. This gene encodes for part of complex of proteins mediating fusion of synaptic vesicles with the presynaptic plasma membrane. A dysregulation of *STX1A* expression [40–42] has been reported in high functioning autism and Asperger syndrome. A significant association between three *STX1A* SNPs (Single Nucleotide Polymorhpisms) and Asperger syndrome was recently described. These SNPs could alter transcription factor binding sites both directly and through other variants in linkage disequilibrium [43].

The list of predicted genes includes *GABRA5*. It transcribes for the subunit 5 of GABA receptor alpha whose reduced expression and reduced protein level have been described in autism [44], and the SNPs of this gene are biomarkers of symptoms and developmental deficit in Han Chinese with autism [45]. The inclusion of this gene in the core list strengthens the evidences of imbalance between excitatory and inhibitory neurotransmission in ASDs and abnormalities in glutamate and GABA signaling as possible causative pathological mechanisms of ASDs.

Few of these predicted genes encode for proteins involved in non-neuronal specific signaling pathways, which are also important for ASDs: *PRKCA*, *WDR37* and *UBC*. PRKCA regulates many signaling pathways such as cell proliferation, apoptosis, differentiation, tumorigenesis, angiogenesis, platelet function, and inflammation. A meta-analysis performed on the de novo mutation data of 10,927 individuals with neurodevelopmental disorders found an excess of missense variants in the *PRKCA* gene [46]. The *WDR37* gene encodes a member of a protein family that is involved in many cellular processes such as cell cycle progression, signal transduction, apoptosis, and gene regulation. WDR37 is a nuclear protein ubiquitous expressed and particularly abundant in the cerebellum and whole brain. There are no direct evidences for ASDs development and WDR37—however, recently, it has been demonstrated that WDR47 shares functional characteristics with PAFAH1B1, which causes lissencephaly. PAFAH1B1 also constitutes a key protein-network interaction node with high-risk ASDs genes expressed in the synapse that can impact synaptogenesis and social behavior [47].

Our analysis confirms the importance of the X-linked gene in the aetiopathogenesis of ASDs. Mutations of *CACNA1F* (located at Xp11.23) mainly cause X-linked eye disorders. Since the role of various ion channel gene defects (channelopathies) in the pathogenesis of ASDs is becoming evident, the deep resequencing of these functional genomic regions has been performed. These studies revealed potentially causative rare variants contributing to ASDs in *CACNA1F*. Then again, *CACNA1D*, an important paralog of *CACNA1F*, displayed de novo missense variants in ASDs probands from the Simons Simplex Collection [48,49]. Moreover, the gene being X-linked could contribute to the sex bias of ASDs.

Out of the 13 genes tightly interconnected with the core, the occurrence in SFARI (six genes in "minimal evidence" or "hypothesized but untested"), the inclusion in networks associated with ASDs by other studies (eight genes) and the presence of epigenetics and/or transcriptional changes modified in ASDs patients vs controls (four genes), constitute further evidences in favor of these genes. A similar reasoning can be extended to peripheral genes, for which we proposed a graduated scale of relevance in relation to the core genes. To this aim, we provided the full results.

Overall, we observed a significant overlap between the lists of genes associated with ASDs by studies of genomics, as well as by studies of epigenomics and transcriptomics from blood samples, with a total of 40 genes supported by all the three types of evidences (of which 34 had high confidence functional interactions). We also observed that a significant number of the core+13 genes has been reported as epigenetically and/or transcriptionally modified in ASDs patients. The observation that different types of alterations refer to the same genes further stresses the role of these genes in ASDs. These results are in line with those of previous studies that suggested the potential role of genetic factors in contributing to DNA methylation differences in ASDs [10]. Moreover, blood-derived epigenetic changes observed in genes whose sequence variations are associated with ASDs are more likely to have a common function across tissues compared to those not related to genetic changes [17].

The existence of molecular relations between altered genes increases the likelihood that such alterations have a role in ASDs, suggesting molecular pathways that encompass such genes and functional relations among different types of alterations. Our analysis highlighted a network of 275 genes, which is strongly supported by genomics, epigenomics, and transcriptomics. Importantly, this network gathers 22 genes not directly linked to each other but supported by all three types of evidences. Interestingly, 157 of the INT-MODULE genes were proposed by other network-based studies on ASDs, different in terms of input data and analysis approach. A total of 144 genes belong to the highest scoring SFARI categories. Ten other genes of the network are currently classified in SFARI as "minimal evidence" and "hypothesized but untested" and are also supported by epigenomics and/or transcriptomics. Therefore, they deserve special attention among the genes of such categories.

The largest connected component of the network (275 genes) can be partitioned in 12 subgroups or topological sub-modules. This analysis suggests a different role of the sub-modules by function and by association with one or more types of alterations. For example, cluster #3, equally supported by all the three types of evidence, includes genes that belong to inflammatory mediator regulation of transient receptor potential (TRP) channels. Inflammation and immune system dysfunctions are in comorbidity with ASDs, and TRP canonical channel 6 (TRPC6) is emerging as a functional element for the control of calcium currents in immune-committed cells and target tissues, influencing leukocytes tasks. Interestingly, TRPC6 is also involved in neuronal development and variants in the *TRPC6* gene (within core gene) were found in patients with ASDs. Moreover, MeCP2, a transcriptional regulator whose mutations cause Rett syndrome, was found abundant in a TRPC6 promoter region resulting a transcriptional regulator of this gene [50] TRPC6, in turn, activates neuronal pathways, including BDNF, CAMKIV, Akt, and CREB signaling pathways, also involved in ASDs [51].

The prioritization of genes in terms of causality is a relevant challenge, especially in a complex and multi-genic disorder like ASDs. Nevertheless, it is possible to distinguish, among the functional themes highlighted by our integrative analysis, possible causative pathways considering their function and/or alteration type. For example, genes of clusters #4 and #11 mainly display genetic alterations and participate, respectively, in neuronal cell adhesion and GABAergic synapses, pathways already associated with brain morpho-functional abnormalities in ASDs.

Our integrative analysis of the large number of genes reported by studies on ASDs that focused on genomics, epigenomics, and transcriptomics prioritized a series of genes interconnected by functional relations and associated with one or more types of molecular alteration. Since this rich information might unearth common targets that are amenable to therapy [1], we have provided the full results of our network-based meta-analyses.

4. Materials and Methods

4.1. Molecular Interactions

Molecular interactions were collected from the STRING database [52] for a total of 12,739 genes and 355,171 links with high confidence (score ≥ 700). Native identifiers were mapped to Entrez Gene [53] identifiers. In case multiple proteins mapped to the same gene identifier, only the pair of gene identifiers with the highest STRING confidence score was considered.

4.2. Genomics

Genes associated with ASDs on the basis of genomics evidences were collected from the SFARI Gene database [8] and previous studies [7,23,24]. The SFARI Gene scoring system classifies genes on the basis of the strength of the supporting evidences as: "Syndromic" (S), "high confidence" (1), "strong candidate" (2), "suggestive evidence" (3), "minimal evidence" (4), "hypothesized but untested" (5), and "Evidence does not support a role" (6). Genes classified as S, 1, 2, 3, 1S, 2S, 3S, and 4S were assigned to the genomics-major evidence group.

Genes belonging to the genomics-minor group were collected from Mosca et al. [7], in which genes associated with SNPs, mutations, and CNV emerging from several large studies were reported, the meta-analysis study of GWAS of over 16,000 individuals with ASDs [23], and the whole-exome sequencing study of rare coding variation in 3871 autism cases and 9937 ancestry-matched or parental controls [24]. Native gene identifiers were converted to Entrez Gene identifiers [53].

4.3. Epigenomics

Genes associated with ASDs at the epigenomics level were collected from a previous study [10] in which the authors performed a case-control meta-analysis of blood DNA methylation among two large case-control studies of autism (796 ASDs cases and 868 controls) using METAL software [54] on the probes that were present in both studies. All genes found by their meta-analysis with $p < 10^{-3}$ were assigned to epigenomics-major group, while the genes with $10^{-3} \leq p < 5 \times 10^{-3}$ were assigned to epigenomics-minor. Native gene identifiers were converted to Entrez Gene [53] identifiers.

4.4. Transcriptomics

Genes associated with ASDs at transcriptomics level were collected from the four studies [15,25–27] reported in [55], in which the original authors generated blood-based gene expression profiles from microarray experiments with sample sizes greater than 40 and provided list of differentially expressed genes. Following the approach by [55], genes reported as differentially expressed in at least two studies were assigned to the transcriptomics-major group, while the other differentially expressed genes were assigned to the transcriptomics-minor group. Native gene identifiers were converted to Entrez Gene [53] identifiers, and only genes occurring in STRING network were considered in network-based analyses.

4.5. Gene Prioritization Based on Network Diffusion

Network diffusion (ND) was performed using an approach previously described [7,28,56,57]. A genes-by-layers input matrix $\mathbf{X}_0 = (\mathbf{x}_1, \mathbf{x}_2, \mathbf{x}_3)$ was defined where each element x_{ij} was set to: 1 if the gene i was member of a "-major" group in layer j; 0.5 if the gene i was member of a "-minor" group in layer j; and 0 if the gene was i was not associated with ASDs in layer j. ND was applied to $\mathbf{X}_0$ using the genome-wide interactome represented by the symmetric normalized adjacency matrix $\mathbf{W}$, according to the following iterative procedure:

$$\mathbf{X}_{t+1} = \alpha \mathbf{W} \mathbf{X}_t + (1-\alpha) \mathbf{X}_0$$

$$\mathbf{X}^{ss} = \lim_{t \to \infty} \mathbf{X}_t$$

where $\alpha \in (0, 1)$ is a scalar that weights the relative importance of the two addends and was set to 0.7, a value that represents a good trade-off between diffusion rate and computational cost and determined consistent results in previous studies [7,28,56–58]. The resulting matrix $\mathbf{X}^{ss}$, containing ND scores, was column-wise normalized by the maximum of each column, obtaining the matrix $\mathbf{X}^*$. Similarly to what was done by Ruffalo et al. [59], a final diffusion score d_i was calculated for each gene i, multiplying the sum of its three scores $(x^*_{i1}, x^*_{i2}, x^*_{i3})$ by the sum of the three averages $(y^*_{i1}, y^*_{i2}, y^*_{i3})$ obtained considering the top 3 direct neighbors of i with the highest diffusion scores in each layer [60]. Statistical significance of gene scores was assessed by empirical p values, calculated using 1000 permutations of the input matrix $\mathbf{X}_0$.

4.6. Functional Characterization of the INT-MODULE

Topological community identification was performed using methods based on different rationales such as modularity/energy function optimization, edge removal, label propagation, leading eigenvector, and random walks. Modularity was quantified using the Newman definition [61]. Community identification and modularity quantification were performed using functions implemented R package igraph [62].

Pathway analysis was carried out using gene-pathway associations from Biosystems [63] and MSigDB Canonical Pathways [64]. Each pathway was assessed for the over-representation of genes from each cluster using the hypergeometric test (R functions "phyper" and "dhyper"). Nominal p values were corrected for multiple testing using the Bonferroni–Hochberg method (R function "p.adjust"), obtaining q values.

The enrichment of each cluster in terms of a type A of evidence (e.g., genomics) was quantified as the ratio between the fraction of genes supported by A in the cluster and the fraction of genes supported by A in the INT-MODULE.

Supplementary Materials: Supplementary materials can be found at http://www.mdpi.com/1422-0067/20/13/3363/s1.

Author Contributions: Conceptualization, N.D.N. and E.M.; data curation, N.D.N. and E.M.; formal analysis, N.D.N., M.B., and E.M.; funding acquisition, L.M., A.M., and E.M.; investigation, N.D.N., M.B., F.A.C., L.M., A.M., and E.M.; methodology, N.D.N., M.B., and E.M.; project administration, E.M.; supervision, L.M., A.M., and E.M.; visualization, N.D.N., M.B., and E.M.; writing—original draft, N.D.N. and E.M.; writing—review and editing, F.A.C., L.M., A.M., and E.M.

Funding: This research was funded by: European Union's Horizon 2020 research and innovation programme, grant GEMMA 825033; Italian Ministry of Education, University and Research, grant INTEROMICS PB05; Fondazione Regionale per la Ricerca Biomedica (Regione Lombardia), grant LYRA 2015-0010.

Conflicts of Interest: The authors declare no conflict of interest.

References

1. Schaaf, C.P.; Zoghbi, H.Y. Solving the autism puzzle a few pieces at a time. *Neuron* **2011**, *70*, 806–808. [CrossRef] [PubMed]
2. Barabási, A.L.; Gulbahce, N.; Loscalzo, J. Network medicine: A network-based approach to human disease. *Nat. Rev. Genet.* **2011**, *12*, 56–68. [CrossRef] [PubMed]
3. Boyle, E.A.; Li, Y.I.; Pritchard, J.K. An Expanded View of Complex Traits: From Polygenic to Omnigenic. *Cell* **2017**, *169*, 1177–1186. [CrossRef] [PubMed]
4. Devlin, B.; Scherer, S.W. Genetic architecture in autism spectrum disorder. *Curr. Opin. Genet. Dev.* **2012**, *22*, 229–237. [CrossRef] [PubMed]
5. Mitra, K.; Carvunis, A.R.; Ramesh, S.K.; Ideker, T. Integrative approaches for finding modular structure in biological networks. *Nat. Rev. Genet.* **2013**, *14*, 719–732. [CrossRef] [PubMed]
6. Cowen, L.; Ideker, T.; Raphael, J.B.; Sharan, R. Network propagation: A universal amplifier of genetic associations. *Nat. Rev.* **2017**, *18*, 551–562. [CrossRef] [PubMed]
7. Mosca, E.; Bersanelli, M.; Gnocchi, M.; Moscatelli, M.; Castellani, G.; Milanesi, L.; Mezzelani, A. Network Diffusion-Based Prioritization of Autism Risk Genes Identifies Significantly Connected Gene Modules. *Front. Genet.* **2017**, *8*, 129. [CrossRef]
8. Abrahams, B.S.; Arking, D.E.; Campbell, D.B.; Mefford, H.C.; Morrow, E.M.; Weiss, L.A.; Menashe, I.; Wadkins, T.; Banerjee-Basu, S.; Packer, A. SFARI Gene 2.0: A community-driven knowledgebase for the autism spectrum disorders (ASDs). *Mol. Autism* **2013**, *4*, 36. [CrossRef]
9. Wiśniowiecka-Kowalnik, B.; Nowakowska, B.A. Genetics and epigenetics of autism spectrum disorder—Current evidence in the field. *J. Appl. Genet.* **2019**, *60*, 37–47. [CrossRef]
10. Andrews, S.V.; Sheppard, B.; Windham, G.C.; Schieve, L.A.; Schendel, D.E.; Croen, L.A.; Chopra, P.; Alisch, R.S.; Newschaffer, C.J.; Warren, S.T.; et al. Case-control meta-analysis of blood DNA methylation and autism spectrum disorder. *Mol. Autism* **2018**, *9*, 40. [CrossRef]
11. Luo, R.; Sanders, S.J.; Tian, Y.; Voineagu, I.; Huang, N.; Chu, S.H.; Klei, L.; Cai, C.; Ou, J.; Lowe, J.K.; et al. Genome-wide transcriptome profiling reveals the functional impact of rare de novo and recurrent CNVs in autism spectrum disorders. *Am. J. Hum. Genet.* **2012**, *91*, 38–55. [CrossRef] [PubMed]
12. Codina-Solà, M.; Rodríguez-Santiago, B.; Homs, A.; Santoyo, J.; Rigau, M.; Aznar-Laín, G.; Campo, M.; Gener, B.; Gabau, E.; Botella, M.P.; et al. Integrated analysis of whole-exome sequencing and transcriptome profiling in males with autism spectrum disorders. *Mol. Autism* **2015**, *6*, 21. [CrossRef] [PubMed]
13. Karczewski, K.J.; Snyder, M.P. Integrative omics for health and disease. *Nat. Rev. Genet.* **2018**, *19*, 299–310. [CrossRef]
14. Higdon, R.; Earl, R.K.; Stanberry, L.; Hudac, C.M.; Montague, E.; Stewart, E.; Janko, I.; Choiniere, J.; Broomall, W.; Kolker, N.; et al. The promise of multi-omics and clinical data integration to identify and target personalized healthcare approaches in autism spectrum disorders. *OMICS* **2015**, *19*, 197–208. [CrossRef] [PubMed]
15. Kong, S.W.; Collins, C.D.; Shimizu-Motohashi, Y.; Holm, I.A.; Campbell, M.G.; Lee, I.H.; Brewster, S.J.; Hanson, E.; Harris, H.K.; Lowe, K.R.; et al. Characteristics and Predictive Value of Blood Transcriptome Signature in Males with Autism Spectrum Disorders. *PLoS ONE* **2012**, *7*, e49475. [CrossRef]
16. Tylee, D.S.; Kawaguchi, D.M.; Glatt, S.J. On the Outside, Looking in: A Review and Evaluation of the Comparability of Blood and Brain "-omes". *Am. J. Med. Genet. Part B* **2013**, *162*, 595–603. [CrossRef]
17. Andrews, S.V.; Ellis, S.E.; Bakulski, K.M.; Sheppard, B.; Croen, L.A.; Hertz-Picciotto, I.; Newschaffer, C.J.; Feinberg, A.P.; Arking, D.E.; Ladd-Acosta, C.; et al. Cross-tissue integration of genetic and epigenetic data offers insight into autism spectrum disorder. *Nat. Commun.* **2017**, *8*, 1011. [CrossRef] [PubMed]
18. Li, J.; Shi, M.; Zhihai Ma, Z.; Zhao, S.; Euskirchen, G.; Ziskin, J.; Urban, A.; Hallmayer, J.; Snyder, M. Integrated systems analysis reveals a molecular network underlying autism spectrum disorders. *Mol. Syst. Biol.* **2014**, *10*, 774. [CrossRef]

19. Gilman, S.R.; Iossifov, I.; Levy, D.; Ronemus, M.; Wigler, M.; Vitkup, D. Rare de novo variants associated with autism implicate a large functional network of genes involved in formation and function of synapses. *Neuron* **2011**, *70*, 898–907. [CrossRef]
20. Hormozdiari, F.; Penn, O.; Borenstein, E.; Eichler, E.E. The discovery of integrated gene networks for autism and related disorders. *Genome Res.* **2015**, *25*, 142–154. [CrossRef]
21. Parikshak, N.N.; Luo, R.; Zhang, A.; Won, H.; Lowe, J.K.; Chandran, V.; Horvath, S.; Geschwind, D.H. Integrative functional genomic analyses implicate specific molecular pathways and circuits in autism. *Cell* **2013**, *155*, 1008–1021. [CrossRef]
22. Pinto, D.; Delaby, E.; Merico, D.; Barbosa, M.; Merikangas, A.; Klei, L.; Thiruvahindrapuram, B.; Xu, X.; Ziman, R.; Wang, Z.; et al. Convergence of genes and cellular pathways dysregulated in autism spectrum disorders. *Am. J. Hum. Genet.* **2014**, *94*, 677–694. [CrossRef] [PubMed]
23. The Autism Spectrum Disorders Working Group of the Psychiatric Genomics Consortium. Meta-analysis of GWAS of over 16,000 individuals with autism spectrum disorder highlights a novel locus at 10q24.32 and a significant overlap with schizophrenia. *Mol. Autism* **2017**, *8*, 21. [CrossRef]
24. De Rubeis, S.; He, X.; Goldberg, A.P.; Poultney, C.S.; Samocha, K.; Cicek, A.E.; Kou, Y.; Liu, L.; Fromer, M.; Walker, S.; et al. Synaptic, transcriptional and chromatin genes disrupted in autism. *Nature* **2014**, *515*, 209–215. [CrossRef]
25. Hu, V.W.; Sarachana, T.; Kim, K.S.; Nguyen, A.; Kulkarni, S.; Steinberg, M.E.; Luu, T.; Lai, Y.; Lee, N.H. Gene Expression Profiling Differentiates Autism Case–Controls and Phenotypic Variants of Autism Spectrum Disorders: Evidence for Circadian Rhythm Dysfunction in Severe Autism. *Autism Res.* **2009**, *2*, 78–97. [CrossRef] [PubMed]
26. Pramparo, T.; Lombardo, M.V.; Campbell, K.; Barnes, C.C.; Marinero, S.; Solso, S.; Young, J.; Mayo, M.; Dale, A.; Ahrens-Barbeau, C.; et al. Cell cycle networks link gene expression dysregulation, mutation, and brain maldevelopment in autistic toddlers. *Mol. Syst. Biol.* **2015**, *11*, 841. [CrossRef] [PubMed]
27. Gregg, J.P.; Lit, L.; Baron, C.A.; Hertz-Picciotto, I.; Walker, W.; Davis, R.A.; Croen, L.A.; Ozonoff, S.; Hansen, R.; Pessah, I.N.; et al. Gene expression changes in children with autism. *Genomics* **2008**, *91*, 22–29. [CrossRef]
28. Bersanelli, M.; Mosca, E.; Remondini, D.; Castellani, G.; Milanesi, L. Network diffusion-based analysis of high-throughput data for the detection of differentially enriched modules. *Sci. Rep.* **2016**, *6*, 34841. [CrossRef]
29. Yi, F.; Danko, T.; Botelho, S.C.; Patzke, C.; Pak, C.; Wernig, M.; Südhof, T.C. Autism-associated SHANK3 haploinsufficiency causes Ih channelopathy in human neurons. *Science* **2016**, *6*, aaf2669. [CrossRef]
30. Zhu, M.; Idikuda, V.K.; Wang, J.; Wei, F.; Kumar, V.; Shah, N.; Waite, C.B.; Liu, Q.; Zhou, L. Shank3-deficient thalamocortical neurons show HCN channelopathy and alterations in intrinsic electrical properties. *J Physiol.* **2018**, *596*, 1259–1276. [CrossRef]
31. Nava, C.; Dalle, C.; Rastetter, A.; Striano, P.; de Kovel, C.G.; Nabbout, R.; Cancès, C.; Ville, D.; Brilstra, E.H.; Gobbi, G.; et al. De novo mutations in HCN1 cause early infantile epileptic encephalopathy. *Nat. Genet.* **2014**, *46*, 640–645. [CrossRef] [PubMed]
32. Feng, J.; Schroer, R.; Yan, J.; Song, W.; Yang, C.; Bockholt, A.; Cook, E.H., Jr.; Skinner, C.; Schwartz, C.E.; Sommer, S.S. High frequency of neurexin 1β signal peptide structural variants in patients with autism. *Neurosci. Lett.* **2006**, *409*, 10–13. [CrossRef] [PubMed]
33. Gauthier, J.; Siddiqui, T.J.; Huashan, P.; Yokomaku, D.; Hamdan, F.F.; Champagne, N.; Lapointe, M.; Spiegelman, D.; Noreau, A.; Lafrenière, R.G.; et al. Truncating mutations in NRXN2 and NRXN1 in autism spectrum disorders and schizophrenia. *Hum. Genet.* **2011**, *130*, 563–573. [CrossRef] [PubMed]
34. Parente, D.J.; Garriga, C.; Baskin, B.; Douglas, G.; Cho, M.T.; Araujo, G.C.; Shinawi, M. Neuroligin 2 nonsense variant associated with anxiety, autism, intellectual disability, hyperphagia, and obesity. *Am. J. Med. Genet. A* **2017**, *173*, 213–216. [CrossRef] [PubMed]
35. Jamain, S.; Quach, H.; Betancur, C.; Råstam, M.; Colineaux, C.; Gillberg, I.C.; Soderstrom, H.; Giros, B.; Leboyer, M.; Gillberg, C.; et al. Paris Autism Research International Sibpair Study. Mutations of the X-linked genes encoding neuroligins NLGN3 and NLGN4 are associated with autism. *Nat. Genet.* **2003**, *34*, 27–29. [CrossRef] [PubMed]
36. Jiang-Xie, L.F.; Liao, H.M.; Chen, C.H.; Chen, Y.T.; Ho, S.Y.; Lu, D.H.; Lee, L.J.; Liou, H.H.; Fu, W.M.; Gau, S.S. Autism-associated gene Dlgap2 mutant mice demonstrate exacerbated aggressive behaviors and orbitofrontal cortex deficits. *Mol. Autism* **2014**, *1*, 32. [CrossRef]

37. Marshall, C.R.; Noor, A.; Vincent, J.B.; Lionel, A.C.; Feuk, L.; Skaug, J.; Shago, M.; Moessner, R.; Pinto, D.; Ren, Y.; et al. Structural variation of chromosomes in autism spectrum disorder. *Am. J. Hum. Genet.* **2008**, *82*, 477–488. [CrossRef]
38. Pinto, D.; Pagnamenta, A.T.; Klei, L.; Anney, R.; Merico, D.; Regan, R.; Conroy, J.; Magalhaes, T.R.; Correia, C.; Abrahams, B.S.; et al. Functional impact of global rare copy number variation in autism spectrum disorders. *Nature* **2010**, *466*, 368–372. [CrossRef]
39. Poquet, H.; Faivre, L.; El Chehadeh, S.; Morton, J.; McMullan, D.; Hamilton, S.; Goel, H.; Isidor, B.; Le Caignec, C.; Andrieux, J.; et al. Further Evidence for Dlgap2 as Strong Autism Spectrum Disorders/Intellectual Disability Candidate Gene. *Autism Open Access* **2017**, *6*, 197. [CrossRef]
40. Nakamura, K.; Anitha, A.; Yamada, K.; Tsujii, M.; Iwayama, Y.; Hattori, E.; Toyota, T.; Suda, S.; Takei, N.; Iwata, Y.; et al. Genetic and expression analyses reveal elevated expression of syntaxin 1A (STX1A) in high functioning autism. *Int. J. Neuropsychopharmacol.* **2008**, *11*, 1073–1084. [CrossRef]
41. Nakamura, K.; Iwata, Y.; Anitha, A.; Miyachi, T.; Toyota, T.; Yamada, S.; Tsujii, M.; Tsuchiya, K.J.; Iwayama, Y.; Yamada, K.; et al. Replication study of Japanese cohorts supports the role of STX1A in autism susceptibility. *Prog. Neuropsychopharmacol. Biol. Psychiatry* **2011**, *35*, 454–458. [CrossRef] [PubMed]
42. Kofuji, T.; Hayashi, Y.; Fujiwara, T.; Sanada, M.; Tamaru, M.; Akagawa, K. A part of patients with autism spectrum disorder has haploidy of HPC-1/syntaxin1A gene that possibly causes behavioral disturbance as in experimentally gene ablated mice. *Neurosci. Lett.* **2017**, *644*, 5–9. [CrossRef] [PubMed]
43. Durdiaková, J.; Warrier, V.; Banerjee-Basu, S.; Baron-Cohen, S.; Chakrabarti, B. STX1A and Asperger syndrome: A replication study. *Mol. Autism.* **2014**, *5*, 14. [CrossRef] [PubMed]
44. Fatemi, S.H.; Reutiman, T.J.; Folsom, T.D.; Rooney, R.J.; Patel, D.H.; Thuras, P.D. mRNA and protein levels for GABAAα4, α5, β1 and GABABR1 receptors are altered in brains from subjects with autism. *J. Autism Dev. Disord.* **2010**, *40*, 743–750. [CrossRef] [PubMed]
45. Yang, S.; Guo, X.; Dong, X.; Han, Y.; Gao, L.; Su, Y.; Dai, W.; Zhang, X. GABA(A) receptor subunit gene polymorphisms predict symptom-based and developmental deficits in Chinese Han children and adolescents with autistic spectrum disorders. *Sci. Rep.* **2017**, *7*, 3290. [CrossRef] [PubMed]
46. Coe, B.P.; Stessman, H.A.F.; Sulovari, A.; Geisheker, M.R.; Bakken, T.E.; Lake, A.M.; Dougherty, J.D.; Lein, E.S.; Hormozdiari, F.; Bernier, R.A.; et al. Neurodevelopmental disease genes implicated by de novo mutation and copy number variation morbidity. *Nat. Genet.* **2019**, *51*, 106–116. [CrossRef] [PubMed]
47. Sudarov, A.; Gooden, F.; Tseng, D.; Gan, W.B.; Ross, M.E. Lis1 controls dynamics of neuronal filopodia and spines to impact synaptogenesis and social behaviour. *EMBO Mol. Med.* **2013**, *5*, 591–607. [CrossRef] [PubMed]
48. O'Roak, B.J.; Vives, L.; Girirajan, S.; Karakoc, E.; Krumm, N.; Coe, B.P.; Levy, R.; Ko, A.; Lee, C.; Smith, J.D.; et al. Sporadic autism exomes reveal a highly interconnected protein network of de novo mutations. *Nature* **2012**, *485*, 246–250. [CrossRef] [PubMed]
49. Iossifov, I.; Ronemus, M.; Levy, D.; Wang, Z.; Hakker, I.; Rosenbaum, J.; Yamrom, B.; Lee, Y.H.; Narzisi, G.; Leotta, A.; et al. De novo gene disruptions in children on the autistic spectrum. *Neuron* **2012**, *2*, 285–299. [CrossRef]
50. Griesi-Oliveira, K.; Acab, A.; Gupta, A.R.; Sunaga, D.Y.; Chailangkarn, T.; Nicol, X.; Nunez, Y.; Walker, M.F.; Murdoch, J.D.; Sanders, S.J.; et al. Modeling non-syndromic autism and the impact of TRPC6 disruption in human neurons. *Mol. Psychiatry* **2015**, *11*, 1350–1365. [CrossRef]
51. Beltrão-Braga, P.C.; Muotri, A.R. Modeling autism spectrum disorders with human neurons. *Brain Res.* **2017**, *1656*, 49–54. [CrossRef] [PubMed]
52. Szklarczyk, D.; Franceschini, A.; Wyder, S.; Forslund, K.; Heller, D.; Huerta-Cepas, J.; Simonovic, M.; Roth, A.; Santos, A.; Tsafou, K.P.; et al. STRING v10: Protein-protein interaction networks, integrated over the tree of life. *Nucleic Acids Res.* **2015**, *43*, D447–D452. [CrossRef] [PubMed]
53. Brown, G.R.; Hem, V.; Katz, K.S.; Ovetsky, M.; Wallin, C.; Ermolaeva, O.; Tolstoy, I.; Tatusova, T.; Pruitt, K.D.; Maglott, D.R.; et al. Gene: A gene-centered information resource at NCBI. *Nucleic Acids Res.* **2015**, *43*, D36–D42. [CrossRef] [PubMed]
54. Willer, C.J.; Li, Y.; Abecasis, G.R. METAL: Fast and efficient meta-analysis of genomewide association scans. *Bioinformatics* **2010**, *26*, 2190–2191. [CrossRef] [PubMed]
55. Saeliw, T.; Tangsuwansri, C.; Thongkorn, S.; Chonchaiya, W.; Suphapeetiporn, K.; Mutirangura, A.; Tencomnao, T.; Hu, V.W.; Sarachana, T. Integrated genome-wide Alu methylation and transcriptome profiling

analyses reveal novel epigenetic regulatory networks associated with autism spectrum disorder. *Mol. Autism* **2018**, *9*, 27. [CrossRef] [PubMed]
56. Vanunu, O.; Magger, O.; Ruppin, E.; Shlomi, T.; Sharan, R. Associating Genes and Protein Complexes with Disease via Network Propagation. *PLoS Comput. Biol.* **2010**, *6*, e1000641. [CrossRef]
57. Mosca, E.; Alfieri, R.; Milanesi, L. Diffusion of Information throughout the Host Interactome Reveals Gene Expression Variations in Network Proximity to Target Proteins of Hepatitis C Virus. *PLoS ONE* **2014**, *9*, e113660. [CrossRef]
58. Hofree, M.; Shen, J.P.; Carter, H.; Gross, A.; Ideker, T. Network-based stratification of tumor mutations. *Nat. Methods* **2013**, *10*, 1108–1115. [CrossRef]
59. Ruffalo, M.; Koyuturk, M.; Sharan, R. Network-Based Integration of Disparate Omic Data to Identify "Silent Players" in Cancer. *PLoS Comput. Biol.* **2015**, *11*, e1004595. [CrossRef]
60. Di Nanni, N.; Gnocchi, M.; Moscatelli, M.; Milanesi, L.; Mosca, E. Gene relevance based on multiple evidences in complex networks. *Bioinformatics*. under review.
61. Newman, M.E.J. Modularity and community structure in networks. *Proc. Natl. Acad. Sci. USA* **2006**, *103*, 8577–8582. [CrossRef] [PubMed]
62. Csardi, G.; Nepusz, T. The igraph software package for complex network research. *InterJ. Complex Syst.* **2006**, *1695*, 1–9.
63. Geer, L.Y.; Marchler-Bauer, A.; Geer, R.C.; Han, L.; He, J.; He, S.; Liu, C.; Shi, W.; Stephen, H.; Bryant, S.H. The NCBI BioSystems database. *Nucleic Acids Res.* **2010**, *38*, D492–D496. [CrossRef] [PubMed]
64. Liberzon, A.; Subramanian, A.; Pinchback, R.; Thorvaldsdóttir, H.; Tamayo, P.; Mesirov, J.P. Molecular signatures database (MSigDB) 3.0. *Bioinformatics* **2011**, *27*, 1739–1740. [CrossRef] [PubMed]

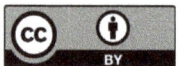

© 2019 by the authors. Licensee MDPI, Basel, Switzerland. This article is an open access article distributed under the terms and conditions of the Creative Commons Attribution (CC BY) license (http://creativecommons.org/licenses/by/4.0/).

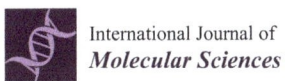

Review

Risk Factors for Unhealthy Weight Gain and Obesity among Children with Autism Spectrum Disorder

Khushmol K. Dhaliwal [1], Camila E. Orsso [2], Caroline Richard [2], Andrea M. Haqq [1,2,*,†] and Lonnie Zwaigenbaum [1,*,†]

1. Department of Pediatrics, Faculty of Medicine and Dentistry, University of Alberta, 11405 87 Avenue, Edmonton, AB T6G 1C9, Canada
2. Department of Agricultural, Food and Nutritional Science, Faculty of Agricultural, Life & Environmental Sciences, University of Alberta, 2-06 Agriculture Forestry Centre, Edmonton, AB T6G 2P5, Canada
* Correspondence: haqq@ualberta.ca (A.M.H.); lonniez@ualberta.ca (L.Z.); Tel.: +1-780-492-0015 (A.M.H.); +1-780-735-8280 (L.Z.)
† Co-senior authors.

Received: 7 June 2019; Accepted: 3 July 2019; Published: 4 July 2019

Abstract: Autism Spectrum Disorder (ASD) is a developmental disorder characterized by social and communication deficits and repetitive behaviors. Children with ASD are also at a higher risk for developing overweight or obesity than children with typical development (TD). Childhood obesity has been associated with adverse health outcomes, including insulin resistance, diabetes, heart disease, and certain cancers. Importantly some key factors that play a mediating role in these higher rates of obesity include lifestyle factors and biological influences, as well as secondary comorbidities and medications. This review summarizes current knowledge about behavioral and lifestyle factors that could contribute to unhealthy weight gain in children with ASD, as well as the current state of knowledge of emerging risk factors such as the possible influence of sleep problems, the gut microbiome, endocrine influences and maternal metabolic disorders. We also discuss some of the clinical implications of these risk factors and areas for future research.

Keywords: Autism spectrum disorder; ASD; Obesity; Overweight; Body mass index; BMI

1. Introduction

Autism Spectrum Disorder (ASD) is a developmental disorder characterized by social and communication impairments and repetitive behaviors [1,2]; the global prevalence is estimated at 1 in 160 children [3], although current North American estimates are around 1 in 60 children [4,5]. Children with ASD are also often at an increased risk for becoming obese (i.e., body mass index [BMI]-for-age ≥95th percentile) or overweight (i.e., BMI-for-age ≥85th percentile) than children with typical development (TD) [6–8]. These BMI levels are associated with adverse health outcomes, including insulin resistance, diabetes, heart disease, and certain cancers [9,10]. Obesity in childhood can also adversely affect physical, emotional, and social functioning, as well as academic performance [11], which might compound disability and reduced quality of life associated with ASD.

Some known key factors that may play a mediating role in the higher rates of obesity observed in children with ASD include eating behaviors [12], lifestyle [13], secondary comorbidities [14], and medications usage [15]. There is also evidence showing that reduced gut microbiota diversity [16,17], hormonal imbalances [18–20], and maternal metabolic disorders [21,22] may influence the development of either ASD or childhood obesity alone. However, it is yet not clear whether and to what extent these emerging factors are contributors for unhealthy weight gain and obesity among children with ASD. We define emerging risk factors as factors independently associated with increased risk for both obesity and ASD that have not yet been studied as risk factors for unhealthy weight gain and obesity among children with ASD.

Preventing unhealthy weight gain and obesity among children with ASD is crucial, as obesity affects overall children's health and well-being and often persists into adulthood [23]. To develop appropriate strategies with increased efficacy, a comprehensive understanding of the risk factors for obesity development in ASD is required. Therefore, the purpose of this narrative review is to critically summarize current knowledge of behavioral, lifestyle, and biological factors potentially contributing to unhealthy weight gain in children with ASD. We also discuss the current state of knowledge of novel emerging risk factors for pediatric obesity in ASD.

Briefly, studies discussed in this manuscript were obtained after conducting a literature search in the main databases MEDLINE, CINAHL, and Google Scholar from inception to May 2019. We searched for multiple variations of the disorder (e.g., autism, autism spectrum disorder, Asperger syndrome) and keywords related to each section of this manuscript (e.g., obesity, overweight, weight gain, oral sensitivities, food selectivity, physical activity, recreational activities). Search was limited to articles in English and reference lists of selected articles, systematic reviews, and meta-analyses were manually reviewed to identify additional relevant articles. A critical synthesis of the literature is presented throughout the main text, describing the limitations of included articles.

2. Feeding Behavior

Reported rates of atypical behavior related to sensory experiences are high among children with ASD [24]. Compared to sex- and age-matched controls, individuals with autism aged 3 to 56 years old exhibited an abnormal oral sensory processing, characterized by either greater oral seeking (e.g., child putting everything into their mouth) or oral defensiveness (e.g., avoidance of certain textures and tastes and/or only eating a limited variety of foods) [25,26]. Interestingly, age-group analyses revealed reductions in the differences of sensory processing difficulties between ASD and TD children over time, suggesting that children are the most affected ones [25]. These sensory difficulties can lead to atypical eating behaviors and feeding practices in ASD, as children may avoid certain foods due to texture and/or taste and only eat a limited variety of foods (i.e., food selectivity). In fact, a recent meta-analysis identified that children with ASD experienced about five times more feeding problems and exhibited lower intake of calcium than TD children [27]. Thus, children with ASD may be at risk for inadequate micronutrient intake [28].

Although several studies characterizing feeding behaviors in children with ASD have evaluated the prevalence of overweight and obesity, few have attempted to investigate whether differences in feeding behavior are related to body weight categories. To our knowledge, only one study found that male children with ASD, who were overweight or obese, had more problematic mealtime and feeding behaviors than overweight or obese TD children, as indicated by the higher scores on a Behavior Pediatrics Feeding Assessment Scale (BPFA) in the ASD group [29]. There were no differences in BPFA scores between children with ASD and TD children, of either thin or adequate weight status [29]. However, another study of younger male and female children described no differences in feeding behaviors (assessed by questionnaire depicting oral function, eating problems, and others) across weight categories [30]. It is important to note that the sample populations in these two studies differed by age, sex, and cultural origins (Brazilian vs. Chinese), limiting comparison. Moreover, the second study found that children with ASD actually had lower mean BMI z-scores than TD children. Another approach to assessing whether feeding behaviors play a role in obesity is to examine within sample correlations. For example, one study found no significant association between dietary patterns and BMI z-score in children with ASD aged 3 to 11 years [31]. Therefore, it is not clear from the current literature whether feeding behavior is, and to what degree, a contributor to excess weight gain in children and adolescents with ASD. We speculate that abnormal feeding behaviors and/or dietary intake could influence weight status. For example, a study found children with ASD tended to consume more sweetened beverages and snacks foods (chips, candy, etc.) [31]. Thus, although children may be eating a limited variety of foods, these may be unhealthier overall (driving weight gain). However, picky eating could also result in weight loss [32].

Overall total energy intake and macronutrient distribution could also contribute to weight gain among children with ASD. With regard to total energy intake, two recent meta-analyses included three-day food record and food frequency questionnaires (FFQs) data from six prospective studies [27] and 14 observational studies [27,33]. No significant overall differences in total energy intake were detected between children with ASD and TD children [33]. It is also important to consider macronutrient distribution, which can lead to variations in body weight and cardiometabolic risk profiles [34,35]. However, the optimal macronutrient distribution for improving the weight status of children and adolescents is not yet understood [36]. Data from the same two meta-analyses that examined energy intake also assessed macronutrient intake, finding no significant difference in the intake of carbohydrates and fats between children with ASD and TD children [27,33]. Intake also tended to be within the acceptable macronutrient distribution range (AMDR) [8,33]. Children with ASD consumed less protein than TD children [27,33], but both groups were consuming more protein than currently recommended for a healthy diet [33].

Micronutrients are also integral to maintaining healthy body weight and have important functions in various metabolic pathways [37]. Children with ASD are often placed on restrictive diets, such as the gluten-free, casein-free (GFCF) diet [38], which may reduce intake of certain micronutrients. GFCF diets have been considered as a possible therapeutic intervention for some of the behavioral symptoms of ASD; however, evidence is lacking [39]. A recent systematic review identified three studies showing that nutrient inadequacies tended to remain among children with ASD even after controlling for common elimination diets, such as GFCF regimens [27,40–42]. Evidence suggests that deficiencies of vitamin A, vitamin D, B-complex vitamins, calcium, and zinc may be associated with increased fat deposition [43]. Findings from a meta-analysis confirm intake deficiencies in calcium and vitamin D in children with ASD relative to TD children and dietary intake recommendations [33]. However, the causality in the relationship between micronutrient intake and fat deposition remains unestablished [43]. Future studies should also take into account the use of dietary supplements, which are commonly offered to children with ASD [39].

In addition to these feeding behaviors and patterns, anecdotal reports indicate that children with ASD may limit their intake of fruits and vegetables due to factors such as taste and texture [42]. The consumption of fruits and vegetables has shown to be inversely associated with weight change and body adiposity [44,45]. However, studies based on prospective three-day food records generally demonstrate no difference in the intake of vegetables or fruits between children with ASD and TD children [40,46], with both groups consuming below the recommendations for vegetable intake [46]. In contrast, a systematic review of studies using FFQs (which assess subjective, longer-term eating patterns) indicated that children with ASD consume fewer daily servings of fruits and vegetables [31]. Likewise, Bandini et al. found that FFQ data revealed children with ASD refuse more vegetables than TD children [42]. In agreement with this, a study found that food refusal in children with ASD may in some cases be due to a bitter taste sensitivity associated with the TAS2R38 genotype [47]. Although little research has investigated the implications of polymorphisms in taste receptors and feeding behaviors in ASD, previous research has demonstrated that TD children exhibit two sensitive alleles for bitter taste had a lower threshold concentration to detected sucrose and a greater sugar consumption compared to children with less sensitive alleles [48]. Thus, future research into the prevalence of genetic variants of taste receptors in ASD may help to provide further insight into particular eating behavior differences, such as vegetable intake, among groups [49].

Overall, much of the recent literature seems to suggest that among those with ASD, overall intake of energy and macronutrients is fairly comparable to the TD population. These findings, however, must be interpreted with caution, because methods for collecting dietary information are often limited by variances in day-to-day food intake [50], under-reporting of energy intake [51], and behavioral reactions to measurement (e.g., changes in food intake, especially in individuals with obesity) [52].

Furthermore, although FFQs are designed to capture long-term eating habits, they include a limited number of foods and both FFQs and three-day food recalls are prone to recall bias [53]. Thus, the relationship between dietary intake and obesity rates may be clouded by limitations in these commonly used measures. In addition, parents of children with ASD may be more attuned to their children's food selectivity behaviors, than parents of TD children, influencing diet data collection. Future studies using direct methods, such as doubly labeled water, to measure energy expenditure and energy intake, may be more informative [52,54]. Additionally, researchers should further elucidate differences in dietary intake within the ASD group based on oral sensitivities, dietary restrictions, and secondary comorbidities (e.g., GI disorders), and take into account age- and possibly sex-related differences. Eating disorders, such as anorexia nervosa, can also impact feeding behaviors and studies have found comorbidities between eating disorders and ASD, specifically among females [55,56]. Studies suggest that specific behavioral phenotypes, such as rigid and repetitive behaviors and social anhedonia, overlap among both conditions [56,57]. This further highlights the importance of stratifying feeding behaviors based on sex differences.

3. Physical Activity and Sedentary Behavior

School-based or extracurricular programs provide opportunities for children to be physically active and engage with peers. Physical activity (PA) is considered a protective factor in maintaining a healthy body weight and preventing obesity [58]. However, opportunities for PA may be limited in children with ASD due to social and behavioral challenges [59,60], as well as motor deficits [61–63].

For optimal health benefits [64], the U.S. Department of Health and Human Services Office of Disease Prevention and Health Promotion suggests that children between the ages of 6 and 17 years should engage in moderate- to vigorous-intensity physical activity (MVPA) for at least 60 min, 3 days per week [65]. Studies that have assessed intensity and frequency of PA in children and adolescents with ASD are summarized in Table 1. Studies comparing the daily time spent in MVPA, as measured by accelerometers, between children with and without ASD have yielded mixed findings. For example, while Bandini et al. reported similar daily MVPA in children with ASD and TD children [66], Stanish et al. found that children with ASD who are younger than 16 years old spent less time engaged in MVPA; but for those adolescents over 16 years, the difference in MVPA was not significant [67]. In contrast, a systematic review found a consistently negative association between PA and age [68]. The discrepancies in these findings suggest that longitudinal studies would enhance the understanding on whether age influences PA patterns. Notably, both children with ASD [67] and TD children [69] were unlikely to meet the recommendations for MVPA.

Table 1. Physical activity.

Study	Design	Study Group	Control Group	Measure	Result	BMI
Bandini et al. [66]	Cross-sectional	53 male and female children with ASD (age: 3–11 years)	58 male and female TD children (age: 3–11 years)	Accelerometer data Questionnaire (parent report on type and frequency)	Similar daily MVPA for both groups (ASD: 50.0 min/day; TD: 57.1 min/day). Children with ASD participate in significantly fewer types of physical activities (6.9 vs. 9.6, $p < 0.0001$) and spend less time annually participating in these activities than TD children (158 vs. 225 h per year, $p < 0.0001$).	No significant difference between the two groups BMI-z score not significantly associated with percent time spent in MVPA
Stanish et al. [67]	Cross-sectional	35 male and female children with ASD (age: 13–21 years)	60 male and female TD children (age: 13–18 years)	Accelerometer data (total average daily PA) Questionnaire (type and frequency of PA)	Children with ASD who are younger than 16 spend less time in MVPA (ASD: 26 min/day vs. 51 min/day) and participate in fewer activities. No significant difference in MVPA among individuals older than 16 years.	N/A
Must et al. [70]	Cross-sectional	53 children with ASD (age: 3–11 years)	58 TD children (age: 3–11 years)	Parent report questionnaire (type and frequency)	An inverse correlation between the total number of barriers reported and the number of PA hours per year (ASD: 119 h; TD 169 h; $p < 0.05$).	No significant difference in BMI percentiles
McCoy et al. [71]	Cross-sectional	915 male and female children with ASD (age: 10–17 years)	41,879 male and female TD children from the 2011–2012 National Survey of Children's Health (age: 10–17 years)	Parent report questionnaire (type and frequency)	Adolescents with ASD are less likely to engage in PA ($p < 0.05$) Higher autism severity is associated with increased odds of being obese (OR: 2.8; 95% CI: 1.39, 3.74), and decreased odds of PA (OR: 0.30; 95% CI: 0.20, 0.46).	Adolescents with ASD are more likely to be overweight and obese (ASD: 22%; TD 14.1%; $p < 0.05$).
Healy et al. [72]	Cross-sectional	67 male and female children with ASD (age: 13 years)	74 randomly selected male and female TD children (age: 13 years)	Parent report questionnaire (type and frequency)	Significantly lower participation in MVPA ($p < 0.001$) and sports reported for children with ASD ($p < 0.001$).	No statistically significant difference between the two groups in mean BMI and overweight/obese status.

Abbreviations: ASD, Autism Spectrum Disorder; TD, Typically Developing; MVPA, Medium–Vigorous Physical Activity; BMI, Body Mass Index.

Studies utilizing parent report questionnaires generally show that children with ASD spend less time engaged in PA than TD children [70–72]. Although questionnaires are more feasible than objective measures given the associated time demands and costs, parent-reports often underestimate PA [73]. In the Bandini et al. study, parents reported that their children with ASD spent significantly less time in PA annually (158 vs. 225 h per year) and participated in fewer types of PA, but no differences in PA between children with ASD and TD children were observed based on accelerometry data [66]. Parents of children with ASD also report more barriers to PA (e.g., increased needs for supervision), which could influence their estimates of overall PA [70]. Moreover, a weak to moderate correlation has been found between parent reports of children's PA and accelerometer-measured activity, depending on type of activity and age group [73]. It is possible that children react to being monitored by increasing their PA [74]; on the other hand, social desirability bias could cause parents to under- or over-report their children's PA based on weight status [75].

Another important variable to consider is sedentary behavior (SB), which is defined as resting behavior with very little expenditure of energy [76]. Factors contributing to prolonged SB in children may include increased access to television, computers, and phones [77,78]. Prolonged SB has long-term health consequences, such as increased body weight, cardiovascular diseases, and type 2 diabetes [79,80]. In a recent systematic review, only two of six studies comparing the prevalence rates of SB reported greater participation in SB by children with ASD than TD children [68]. However, children with ASD (aged 8–18 years old) spent 62% more time on screen activities compared to their TD siblings, as reported by parents [81]. Furthermore, children with ASD spent more hours per day playing video games (both boys and girls), but spent less time using social media or playing interactive video games [81,82].

Overall, the relationships between time spent in MVPA or SB and the propensity for children with ASD to be overweight or obese were not directly investigated in the reviewed studies. It is important to note that ASD severity may influence these relationships by affecting behavior as well as social and motor functioning [83]. Indeed, McCoy et al. found an association between higher parent-reported levels of autism severity, increased odds of being obese, and decreased odds of PA [71]. In the future, research based on objective measures of MVPA and SB (e.g., accelerometer data) could yield insights into differences in these variables between children with ASD and TD children. Further sample stratification based on ASD severity could further clarify how symptoms moderate the relationship between PA and SB among children with ASD.

4. Genetics

Genetic vulnerabilities and syndromic causes of ASD and obesity have been explored extensively, albeit independently. Both conditions are heritable; thus, understanding possible shared genetic links may yield insights into their interplay. Specifically, sibling and twin studies have shown that ASD tends to run in families [84,85]. Likewise, genetics also play a role in childhood obesity [86]. When compared to adopted siblings, the risk of being obese is higher among individuals with affected siblings and parents who are already obese [87]. Because both ASD and obesity have heritable components, investigation of any genetic overlap in their pathways may help explain the higher rates of obesity among individuals with ASD.

Sharma et al. hypothesized that a common molecular pathway may contribute to the pathogenesis of ASD and obesity, as a pathway-based analysis revealed 36 common genes between these two conditions [88]. Specifically, one study has shown that ASD, Attention Deficit Hyperactivity Disorder (ADHD), developmental delays and obesity are highly associated with a microdeletion involving 11p14.1 [89]. Furthermore, deletions in 16p11.2 were associated with genetic vulnerabilities related to both obesity and ASD [90,91]. More recently, in a genetic analysis of very obese children with ASD, Cortes and Wevrick focused on de novo mutations and found that very obese ASD probands had loss of function mutations in DNMT3A and POGZ [92].

In addition, Prader-Willi Syndrome (PWS) is a genetic disorder caused by paternal 15q11–13 deletions [93]. PWS is characterized by hyperphagia, elevated ghrelin concentrations, and increased risk for obesity [93,94]. PWS is also associated with higher rates of social-communication impairments and repetitive behaviors [95], although the degree to which symptoms meet diagnostic criteria for ASD varies across studies, emphasizing that ASD symptom measures require careful consideration of developmental profile and overall clinical context [95,96]. That said, genetic mechanisms underlying the association between Prader Willi and ASD may underlie obesity risk related to hyperphagia in a subset of individuals with ASD [97].

In summary, although evidence indicates that certain genetic vulnerabilities are associated with both ASD and obesity, there is a need to further investigation, such as pathway-based analyses to reveal how genetics influence the complex etiologies of both conditions. In addition, it is not currently clear what proportion of children with ASD and obesity would be accounted for by these rare genetic variants; future efforts to parse the relative contribution of genetic versus non-genetic associations would provide important insights into this topic. Genetic testing, in the form of clinical microarrays, are increasingly becoming standard of practice for ASD diagnosis [98] and determining whether there are deletions in areas such as 16p11.2 may allow for early interventions and targeted molecular therapy, with potential to prevent obesity in children with ASD.

5. Medications

Comorbid conditions, such as ADHD and depression, often manifest in ASD [99]. To manage these and other behavioral symptoms, psychotropics including stimulants, selective serotonin reuptake inhibitors (SSRIs), and antipsychotics are often prescribed [100]. The prescription rate of these drugs in children with ASD has been reported at 27–64% (median 41.9%) [101–104].

A 2016 meta-analysis by Park found that 1 in 6 children with ASD were prescribed anti-psychotic medication [105]. Second-generation anti-psychotics (SGA) such as risperidone and aripiprazole, are often prescribed to alleviate behavioral symptoms comorbid with ASD such as hyperactivity, irritability and aggression [106,107], but are associated with substantial weight gain [15,106]. A systematic review of seven randomized controlled trials (RCTs) of risperidone use among children and adolescents with ASD, revealed weight gain as an adverse event [15]. Furthermore, dose-related increases in blood glucose, insulin, and leptin have been reported [108] and metabolic changes (e.g., leptin) track closely with changes in fat mass [109]. Furthermore, a systematic review looking at two RCTs of apriprazole use in children with ASD reported a mean difference of 1.13 kg of weight gain in children using apriprazole compared to a placebo after 8 weeks of treatment [110]. Other commonly prescribed antipsychotics in ASD are olanzapine and clozapine [111,112]. A 2014 meta-analysis found that olanzapine and clozapine were also both associated with severe weight gain [113]. The mechanism of action behind weight gain associated with atypical antipsychotics relates in part to serotonin receptor blockade and reduction in dopamine (D2) receptor-mediated neurotransmission [114], implicated in weight regulation [115]. Thus, monitoring adverse effects of antipsychotics are important to alleviate behavioral symptoms without detrimental effects on metabolic health [116].

Selective serotonin reuptake inhibitors (SSRIs) are another class of medications commonly prescribed to children with ASD for comorbid anxiety, depression and obsessive-compulsive behaviors [117,118]. Previous research on the efficacy of citalopram [119] and fluoxetine [120] in children with ASD have not examined changes in weight gain. However, other research has suggested SSRIs such as citalopram may cause weight gain [121]. The degree and persistence of weight gain with these medications, particularly from long term use, are not known in children with ASD, and thus would benefit from further study.

6. Emerging Factors

6.1. Breastfeeding

Breast milk provides energy, nutrients and antibodies, and reduces risks for various infections during infancy [122]. Researchers have also studied how breastfeeding affects children's cognitive development. The rate and duration of exclusive breastfeeding also appears to be a potential risk factor for ASD [123]. For example, Boucher et al. found associations between longer durations of breastfeeding and better cognitive development and fewer autistic traits in children, after controlling for relevant demographic and social confounding variables [124]. Tseng et al. also reported that children with ASD were significantly less likely to have been breastfed than children without ASD [123]. Tseng et al. highlighted some proposed explanations for the role of breastfeeding in ASD pathophysiology, such as the nutrition theory [125], oxytocin stimulation [126], and the secretion of neurotrophic factors [123,127].

Researchers have also found that breastfeeding may lower the risk of childhood obesity [128,129]. In their meta-analysis, Yan et al. showed a dose-response effect between breastfeeding duration and reduced risk of childhood obesity [130]. These studies highlight that reduced breastfeeding may be a contributing factor to obesity, although they did not specifically examine these relationships in ASD. Thus, future studies could examine how breastfeeding affects the growth patterns and long-term weight status of children with ASD.

6.2. Sleep

Evidence suggests that sleep duration and quality of sleep are risk factors for becoming overweight or obese [131]. Numerous studies have confirmed an inverse correlation between sleep quantity, BMI, and the risk for overweight and obesity [132,133]. A 2016 meta-analysis found an association between poor sleep quality (independent of sleep duration) and overweight and obesity in children [134]. Decreased quality of sleep can lead to endocrine changes affecting appetite regulation and glucose metabolism, with implications on body weight gain [135]. As such, an inverse relationship between total sleep and ghrelin levels has been reported, as well as a positive relationship between total sleep and leptin levels [136]. Ghrelin and leptin are appetite regulating hormones that influence food intake. Childhood obesity can present with sleeping problems such as obstructive sleep apnea (OSA) [137]. OSA is associated with inadequate duration and poorer quality of sleep and may be associated with specific metabolic markers such as insulin resistance and hypertension [137].

Studies have found that children with ASD have higher rates of sleep problems when compared to TD controls [138]. One study found associations between poor sleep quality and weight status among children with ASD, with 86% of the obese group presenting with clinically significant sleep problems compared to 76% of those with healthy weight [139]. Children with ASD are more likely to be diagnosed with insomnia, circadian rhythm disorder, or sleep-disordered breathing such as OSA [140]. Metabolic risk factors, as well as day-time sleepiness, may reduce daytime activity levels, contributing to unhealthy weight gain [139]. Although many findings suggest that children with ASD are at greater risk for sleep problems, associations with BMI remain underexplored within this population. However, sleep duration and quality are important factors to consider, because increased findings of sleep problems may be compounding the risk for unhealthy weight gain in children with ASD.

6.3. Microbiota

Gastrointestinal (GI) disorders, such as diarrhea, chronic constipation [141], and abdominal pain are common in ASD [142]. In a study including 163 preschoolers with ASD, 25.8% of the participants reported having at least one severe GI symptom [143]. Studies have also shown that children with ASD and GI problems have higher levels of affective problems, including anxiety, than children with ASD who have normal GI functioning [14,143,144]. This link between GI and behavior disorders suggests that gut microbiota may influence developmental course in ASD [145].

Data from several pediatric studies reveals a unique gut microbiota profile in children with ASD compared to those with TD, but inconsistent findings on the characterization of the bacterial communities [146]. While one study reported decreased bacteria of the genera *Prevotella*, *Coprococcus* and *Veillonellaceae*, other studies found increased *Lactobacillus*, *Clostridium*, *Candida* spp., and the Firmicutes/Bacteroidetes ratio [16,146–148]. Similar to what has been seen in ASD, studies exploring the gut microbiome in obesity have reported an increased Firmicutes/Bacteroidetes ratio, and this ratio could be positively associated with BMI in children and adults with obesity [149–151]. To further understand the implications of obesity on gut composition, animal studies comparing lean, wild-type, and obese mice (leptin-deficient) have demonstrated an increase in the Firmicutes/Bacteroidetes ratio in obese mice, independent of diet [152]. Indeed, a high-fat diet was shown to promote more profound increases in Firmicutes [153]. Certain features of the gut microbiota, such as individual variability, may explain the lack of a consistent microbiota signature in ASD and obesity. As the gut microbiota is assembled mainly during infancy, before the age of 2 years, diverse factors including birth mode, antibiotics, feeding practices, and environmental exposure to bacteria shape the gut community and contribute to this individual variability [154]. Thus, characterizing the microbiome from an ecological perspective (bacterial diversity, abundance, community interactions, metabolic profiles), may be more informative in understanding the interplay between gut microbiota, ASD prognosis, and weight gain.

Growing evidence suggests that decreased gut microbiota diversity in ASD [16,155] may be associated with behavioral and GI symptoms. Sharon et al. took this hypothesis a step forward, reporting that offspring of germ-free mice receiving gut microbiota from individuals with ASD indeed exhibited behaviors related to those observed in ASD [156]. This finding, however, must be interpreted with caution given the small sample size used in the experiments and relevance to behavioral expression in the human condition.

Gut microbiome dysbiosis, which refers to changes in the composition and function of gut microbiome especially early in life, are associated with increased production of pro-inflammatory cytokines and alterations in the dynamics of the communication between the gut and brain, known as the gut-brain axis [157–159]. These cytokines affect the inflammation pathways, which have been implicated in ASD development [158–160]. Inflammatory cytokines and an increased gut permeability also promote metabolic endotoxemia [161], which plays a role in the development of obesity and metabolic diseases [162]. Indeed, gut microbiome dysbiosis has also been reported in obesity [163].

A much-debated topic is whether gut permeability contributes to ASD development [159], with evidence remaining limited and controversial. To our knowledge, only three studies have investigated gut permeability in children with ASD using varied biomarkers [164–166]. Specifically, children with ASD exhibited greater gut permeability than TD children, as assessed by zonulin concentrations [164] or sugar probes (lactulose and mannitol) [165]. In contrast, no difference in gut permeability using the lactulose and rhamnose probe was observed in children with ASD compared to TD children [166]. There were marked differences in the design of these studies; in particular, with respect to the selection of comparison groups. One study included children with and without GI complaints in both study (i.e., children with ASD) and control (i.e., children with TD) groups; another study excluded children with GI symptoms from the control group only; and in the third study, all children (study and control groups) had mild GI disorders. Thus, it is not clear whether gut permeability is increased due to the presence of ASD or GI-associated disorders per se. Furthermore, studies have shown significantly lower short-chain fatty acids (SCFAs) in ASD [167]. As SCFAs are produced by gut microbiota (from dietary fiber fermentation), and their production promotes gut barrier and mucosal integrity [168], it could be speculated that individuals with ASD may have decreased ability to repair the intestinal barrier.

Dietary intake has a direct impact not only on obesity development, but also on the microbiome composition [169]; the role of diets in ASD could thereby be explored as a possible way to alleviate both irritable bowel syndrome symptoms and some ASD problem behaviors. An interesting avenue to explore would be fiber interventions in ASD, especially in those children with concomitant obesity. Many studies have found that fiber intake in children with ASD, as well as TD, does not meet recommended levels [8,42]. Fiber-rich foods can alleviate GI symptoms, such as chronic constipation and increase feelings of fullness, as these foods take longer to digest [170]. Fiber intake could also promote a healthier metabolic profile by mediating the gut microbiota [171,172]. Our bodies produce SCFAs by degrading fiber in the gut, which results in the release of anorexigenic gut hormones [173], improvements of the gut barrier [174], and triggering of anti-inflammatory cytokines [175,176]. More specifically, the SCFA propionate was shown to promote increases in peptide YY (PYY) and glucagon like peptide-1 (GLP-1) levels in an in vitro study using human colonic cells [177]. Subsequent in vivo studies were conducted in human adults; while acute intake of inulin-propionate ester reduced energy intake by ≈14% with increases in plasma PYY and GLP-1, supplementation over 24 weeks reduced rate of weight gain and intra-abdominal adiposity [177]. In addition to alleviating GI symptoms associated with ASD, SCFAs thus also prevented obesity and its comorbidities [178]. However, sensory aversions (e.g., to food texture) associated with ASD may create challenges with increasing intake of fiber rich foods.

Further delineating the microbial signature of individuals with comorbid ASD and obesity may provide further insight into the complex etiologies of both conditions. Although more studies are needed, there is emerging evidence of a dysbiotic gut microbiome influencing children with ASD. If supported by more definitive studies (e.g., metagenomics), evaluation of novel therapeutic strategies would be warranted, such as dietary interventions and fecal transplantations. Some challenges in this area include the need for approaches to directly sample the gut mucosa in order to reliably characterize the microbiome in various group and regions [179]. Furthermore, animal studies remain difficult to translate because of the precise control over genetics, the environment, and diet; which is not possible in human studies, making the human microbiome a lot more heterogeneous [179].

6.4. Endocrine Influences

Researchers have also begun to explore the role of endocrine factors in the pathogenesis of ASD. It has been hypothesized that specific chemical messengers, such as endocrine hormones, and neuropeptides work together with neurotransmitters (e.g., dopamine and serotonin) to influence the developing fetal brain [20]. Thus, imbalances in the chemical transmissions could lead to defective encoding, which could in turn lead to some of the social behaviors exhibited by those with ASD [20]. Research in this area has been focused on understanding how hormonal imbalances and differences may contribute to the pathogenesis of ASD. In this section, we review evidence related to specific appetite hormones, leptin, adiponectin and ghrelin.

6.5. Leptin

Leptin is an anorexigenic (satiety) hormone that regulates how much one consumes and inhibits appetite [180]. Produced by adipose tissue in amounts proportionate to fat mass [181], leptin is an important hormone involved in energy homeostasis and growth [182]. Evidence suggests that obese individuals exhibit leptin resistance, whereby the brain no longer responds to leptin by inhibiting energy intake and increasing energy expenditure [183,184].

Several studies have reported higher circulating concentrations of leptin in individuals with ASD compared to control groups [18,19,185–188], summarized in Table 2. Ashwood et al. found higher concentrations of peripheral blood leptin in individuals with ASD compared to age-matched controls, despite no group differences in BMI [18]. Leptin plays an important role in growth [182] and rapid growth has also been independently implicated as a risk factor for ASD [189]. One study found that children born small-for-gestational age (SGA) had lower leptin cord levels; among those born SGA, children with the most rapid weight gain had the highest childhood leptin levels and were more likely to be diagnosed with ASD [187], suggesting differences in early weight trajectories between children with ASD and TD children [7]. Hasan et al. measured fasting serum concentrations for 20 children with ASD and 20 TD children; the BMI of the group with ASD was significantly lower compared to the control group; however, no children in either group were found to be of obese status [188]. The study found that the children with ASD had higher leptin concentrations and lower BMI [188], suggesting that leptin concentrations could be higher among individuals with ASD, regardless of weight status. The studies summarized in Table 2 have consistently found higher concentrations of leptin in children with ASD when compared to TD children. In the future, leptin concentrations could be analyzed based on BMI percentile stratifications to explore relationship to obesity among children with ASD.

Table 2. Leptin in ASD.

Study	Design	Study Group	Control Group	Measure	Result	BMI
Ashwood et al. [18]	Case control	70 male and female children with ASD (age: 2–15 years)	50 age matched TD children	Peripheral plasma concentrations of leptin	Leptin levels were higher in children with autism compared with typically developing non-ASD controls ($p < 0.006$)	No statistical differences in BMI or z-scores between ASD or controls
Blardi et al. [19]	Case control	35 male and female children with ASD (mean age 14.1 years)	35 TD sex and age matched children	Baseline: 6 mL blood sample after an overnight fast 1 year after: 6 mL blood sample after an overnight fast	Leptin concentrations of children with ASD were significantly higher than TD children at baseline ($p < 0.001$) and after a year ($p < 0.001$)	No significant difference between children with ASD and TD children on weight or height at baseline or after 1 year BMI z-score not provided
Al-Zaid et al. [185]	Case control	31 male children with ASD (age: 3–8 years)	28 age- and sex-matched TD children (age: 3–8 years)	7 mL of venous blood samples were collected after an overnight fast	Leptin concentrations were higher in the group with ASD when compared to the TD group ($p \leq 0.01$)	Weight was higher in the children with ASD (19.3 kg in TD children and to 22.7 kg in children with ASD) ($p = 0.05$) No significant difference in BMI between groups ($p = 0.28$)
Rodrigues et al. [186]	Case control	30 male and female children with ASD (ages not provided)	19 TD children matched for age, gender, maternal age at child birth	10 mL plasma blood samples	Plasma levels of leptin were higher ($p < 0.01$) in children with ASD, compared to TD children	Article suggests differences in BMI (unclear of significance and values)
Raghavan et al. [187]	Prospective cohort	39 male and female children with ASD	616 male and female TD children	Plasma umbilical cord blood sample and non-fasting childhood (median age= 18.4 months) venous blood sample	Mean cord leptin was lower in children later diagnosed with ASD ($p = 0.05$) Children with the highest leptin levels had an increased ASD risk (OR: 5.41; 95% CI: 1.53, 19.05)	Birthweight was greater in TD children and compared to children with ASD ($p = 0.03$) Extremely rapid weight gain was associated with greater ASD risk
Hasan et al. [188]	Case control	20 children with ASD (16 males and 4 females) (mean age: 5.9 years)	20 age matched TD children (13 males and 7 females) (mean age: 6.0 years)	5 mL blood samples from participants (serum)	Serum levels of leptin were higher in children with ASD compared to TD children ($p = 0.038$)	TD children had greater mean weight ($p < 0.001$), height ($p < 0.001$), and BMI ($p < 0.05$), compared to children with ASD

Abbreviations: ASD, Autism Spectrum Disorder; TD, Typically Developing; BMI, Body Mass Index

6.6. Adiponectin

Adiponectin is a protein hormone secreted by the adipocytes [190]. Plasma adiponectin levels and BMI are strongly negatively correlated in both men and women [191]. Adiponectin is an anti-inflammatory protein [192]; decreased levels may lead to increased expression of adhesion molecules and inflammatory molecules, resulting in higher risk for cardiovascular diseases associated with obesity [193]. Therefore, adiponectin and its receptors may be therapeutic targets for individuals who are obese or overweight [193,194].

Disturbances in immunoinflammatory factors and adipocytokines have been reported among individuals with ASD relative to age- and weight-matched TD controls [195]. Table 3 summarizes published data on adiponectin concentrations in children with ASD compared to controls [19,186,196,197]. One study reported lower serum adiponectin levels among individuals with ASD relative to age- and sex-matched healthy controls [196], but two other studies showed no significant differences [19,186]. Differences in findings among the three studies may be explained by differences in exclusion and inclusion criteria and sample composition, particularly by sex and age. For example, Rodrigues et al. and Blardi et al. included both males and females, whereas Fujita-Shimizu et al. only included males [19,186,196]. Past studies have found sex differences in adiponectin levels and body composition [198,199], whereby adiponectin concentrations decrease into late puberty and become significantly lower in males by adulthood [199]. Furthermore, recent findings also suggest a link between a high leptin/adiponectin ratio (i.e., higher concentrations of leptin and lower concentrations of adiponectin) and abdominal obesity [200]. Although higher concentrations of leptin among individuals with ASD is a relatively consistent finding, the role of adiponectin is less clear. Exploring the relationship between these two hormones and its potential role in the propensity for individuals with ASD to become overweight or obese warrants further examination.

6.7. Ghrelin

Ghrelin is an appetite-stimulating hormone [201], but its exact role in obesity is poorly understood, as, counterintuitively, ghrelin is often suppressed in obese individuals, and concentrations increase with weight loss [202]. Evidence about the role of this hunger hormone in children with ASD is also unclear. Researchers have explored serum ghrelin concentrations in two case control studies of children with ASD (see Table 4). One study found that male children with ASD had significantly lower concentrations of acylated, des-acylated, and total ghrelin [185]. However, findings from a more recent study, that included both boys and girls, showed a trend towards lower concentrations of ghrelin, although not significant, in children with ASD when compared to age-matched TD children [188]. Previous studies have found that ghrelin levels can be modified by an increase in sex hormone [203], whereby testosterone can lead to marked decreases in ghrelin [203], which may contribute to differences in findings between these two studies. Future studies should examine ghrelin levels relative to weight status as well as ASD diagnosis and consider sex differences.

Table 3. Adiponectin in ASD.

Study	Design	Study Group	Control Group	Measure	Result	BMI
Blardi et al. [19]	Case control	35 male and female children with ASD (mean age 14.1 years)	35 TD sex and age matched children	Baseline: 6 mL blood sample after an overnight fast 1 year after: 6 mL blood sample after an overnight	Adiponectin levels in autistic patients were not significantly different from those found in controls at each time.	No significant difference between children with ASD and TD children on weight or height at baseline or after 1 year BMI z-score not provided
Fujita-Shimizu et al. [196]	Case-control	31 male children with ASD (age: 6–19 years)	31 age-matched male TD children (age: 6–19 years)	Fasting blood samples	Serum levels of adiponectin in the group with ASD were significantly lower ($p = 0.005$) than the TD group	No significant difference in weight, height, waist circumference, and BMI between the two groups BMI z-score or BMI weight categories not provided
Rodrigues et al. [186]	Case control	30 male and female children with ASD (ages not provided)	19 TD children matched for age, gender, maternal age at child birth	10 mL of blood (plasma)	No difference in the plasma concentration of adiponectin in children with ASD compared to TD children	Articles suggests differences in BMI (unclear of significance) BMI z-score or BMI weight categories not provided
Raghavan et al. [197]	Prospective cohort	55 male and female children with ASD	792 male and female TD children	Plasma umbilical cord blood sample and non-fasting childhood (median age = 19.03 months) venous blood sample	Mean cord blood adiponectin was higher in TD children compared to the group with ASD ($p = 0.01$) No significant difference in early childhood adiponectin	Birthweight was greater in TD children and compared to children with ASD ($p = 0.03$) Extremely rapid weight gain was associated with greater ASD risk

Abbreviations: ASD, Autism Spectrum Disorder; TD, Typically Developing; BMI, Body Mass Index.

Table 4. Ghrelin in ASD.

Study	Design	Study Group	Control Group	Measure	Result	BMI
Al-Zaid et al. [185]	Case control	31 male children with ASD (age: 3–8 years)	28 age- and sex-matched TD children (age: 3–8 years)	7 mL of venous blood samples were collected after an overnight fast	Acylated ghrelin concentrations were lower in the group with ASD than TD children ($p \leq 0.001$) Deacylated ghrelin concentrations were lower in group with ASD compared to TD children ($p \leq 0.005$)	Weight was higher in the children with ASD (19.3 kg in TD children and to 22.7 kg in children with ASD) ($p = 0.05$) No significant difference in BMI or height BMI z-score or BMI weight categories not provided
Hasan et al. [188]	Case control	20 male and female children with ASD (16 males and 4 females) (mean age: 5.9 years)	20 age-matched healthy control children (13 males and 7 females) (mean age: 6.0 years)	5 mL blood samples from participants (serum)	Serum levels of ghrelin were lower in children with ASD compared to TD children, but not statistically significant ($p = 0.32$)	TD children had a greater mean weight (31.17 kg), height (1.32 m^2), and BMI (17.6 kg/m^2) compared to children with ASD with a mean weight of 21.26 kg, height of 1.17 m^2, and BMI of 15.5 kg/m^2 BMI z-score or BMI weight categories not provided

Abbreviations: ASD, Autism Spectrum Disorder; TD, Typically Developing; BMI, Body Mass Index.

Although researchers have begun to explore the role of hormones in contributing to higher rates of obesity among children with ASD, they have focused primarily on hormonal differences in relation to ASD pathogenesis. Furthermore, some of the studies discussed above did not report a difference in BMI or weight status among children with ASD, when compared to TD children. However, the relatively smaller sample sizes, compared to larger scale studies (which have reported greater rates of obesity in children with ASD), may have contributed to these differences in findings [6,7]. Future studies, which stratify study groups based on weight status (overweight, obese, etc.), sex, and age would help to understand whether there are potential biological differences associated with specific weight status. Therefore, further research into possible differences in these hormones' concentrations, in children with ASD, may yield insights into hormonal impacts on unhealthy weight gain and obesity.

6.8. Maternal Metabolic Disorders

Although maternal metabolic disorders such as diabetes, hypertension and obesity could place children with ASD at higher risk for becoming overweight or obese, this hypothesis has not been explored directly. Instead, researchers have focused on examining maternal metabolic disorders as potential risk factors for ASD in children; separately, others have studied how maternal metabolic disorders may increase risk of obesity in children.

Maternal obesity prior to pregnancy is a risk factor for ASD [21,204,205]. Evidence has also shown significant associations between maternal diabetes and hypertension and ASD risk [206–208]. Several mechanisms may contribute to these in-utero effects. In a systematic review, Xu et al. suggested several potential pathways through which maternal diabetes may increase the risk for ASD in offspring: (a) maternal hyperglycemia can result in hypoxia and impair neural development in the fetus [209–211] (b) maternal hyperglycemia can cause oxidative stress associated with ASD risk [212,213], and (c) increased maternal adiposity can cause chronic inflammation that can affect neuronal development [206,214].

Concurrently, there has been considerable research on how maternal metabolic disorders may increase children's obesity risk. In their systematic review, Wang et al. found a strong positive association between parental and child obesity and overweight status across various countries, indicating a genetic predisposition toward obesity, with other factors playing a mediating role, such as obesogenic lifestyles and behaviors [22]. In another recent systematic review and meta-analysis, Kawasaki et al. reported an association between gestational diabetes mellitus and higher BMI z-scores among offspring [215]. Deierlein et al. found an association between fetal exposure to maternal glucose concentration in the high–normal range and children being overweight or obese at 3 years of age, independent of maternal pre-pregnancy BMI [216]. Furthermore, Lawlor et al. conducted a sibling analysis to control for shared genetics and environment and reported that children exposed to diabetes in utero had higher BMI than their unexposed siblings [217].

These findings may help explain how certain maternal metabolic disorders increase risk for obesity. Factors such as lifestyle behaviors and genetic predisposition may have compounded effects on weight gain for children with ASD. Additional research on in-utero effects of maternal metabolic disorders may help explain why many children with ASD tend to become overweight or obese. Longitudinal studies to assess parental weight status and track neurodevelopmental outcomes and weight in offspring would provide important insights into the extent to which parental obesity status influences the development of obesity in children with ASD. A better conceptualization of the role of maternal metabolic disorders and any shared pathophysiology between ASD and obesity would help mothers understand how to best reduce their children's risk for both health conditions.

7. Future Directions and Perspectives

The current treatments for childhood obesity generally involve a combination of (1) non-pharmacological interventions (e.g., behavioral treatments, weight-reducing diets), (2) pharmacological interventions, (3) and surgical treatments [23]. Typically, behavioral treatments and weight-reducing diets, such as family-based interventions, are the first therapeutic steps [218].

However, these may be problematic for children with ASD, who struggle with social and behavioral communication, changes in routine, and sensory processing difficulties [24,68]. Furthermore, challenges with self-management and, in many cases, impairments in decision-making skills play an important role in the challenges associated with this first line of treatment in children with ASD [219]. The second line of intervention is through common pharmacological treatments for childhood obesity, such as orlistat, sibutramine, and metformin. These, however, may cause abdominal pain, fecal incontinence, nausea, and vomiting [220,221]. Administering medications that can cause GI problems to children with ASD, who typically already have co-morbid GI disorders, may cause additional difficulties [222]. Moreover, because many children already take medication to manage symptoms of ASD and other comorbid medical conditions, additional medications may increase the risk of side effects, as well as pharmacological interactions and medication burden [223,224]. Finally, severe and morbid forms of pediatric obesity may warrant surgical interventions such as bariatric surgery [225]. Although the prevalence of severe morbid obesity (that would warrant consideration of bariatric surgery) among children with ASD is unclear, a study reported that children with the de novo 16p11.2 deletion, which is associated with autism, were also severely obese (BMI ≥ 120% of 95th percentile) [226]. Bariatric surgery, however, also comes with its risks and complications associated with Roux-en-Y gastric bypass, such as pulmonary embolism, shock, intestinal obstruction, postoperative bleeding, staple line leaks and severe malnutrition [23]. Furthermore, adolescents are more likely to have remission of type 2 diabetes and hypertension after bariatric surgery, when compared to adults [227], emphasizing that optimal timing for surgery in order to reverse metabolic complications of obesity is still unclear. Furthermore, little research has been done in this area to address treatment needs that may be specific to this population [219]. A systematic review looking more broadly at children with intellectual disabilities suggested the need for further research into how obesity treatment can be more specifically tailored for children with intellectual disabilities [219]. Finding more intensive treatments and combination of techniques are warranted for children with intellectual disabilities, such as more training for parents to support children with defiant behaviors [219,228].

Furthermore, although much is known about behavioral and lifestyle factors, little is known about possible biological drivers of obesity among children with ASD. There is also a need to identify whether specific biological drivers can be monitored and assessed at an earlier age, such as at the time of ASD diagnosis. Research in this area is particularly important, because evidence suggests that weight trajectories, at an earlier age, may be different among children with ASD. Therefore, clinical health surveillance of these weight trajectories in ASD and monitoring of growth patterns may serve as a useful method in preventing unhealthy weight gain and obesity. Based on this review, biological factors (gut microbiota, endocrine hormones, maternal metabolic disorders) may be driving increased propensity to become overweight, but further research is needed. Finally, given some of the unique challenges faced by children with ASD, results from pediatric obesity trials in the general population may not generalize to patients with ASD. Thus, as a field, we may require more targeted treatment options and ASD-specific randomized, controlled trials. In an era of precision medicine, there is a need to take into account the interplay between behavioral and biological characteristics influencing unhealthy weight gain in ASD.

8. Conclusion and Recommendations

Body weight is determined by energy balance, which is influenced by environmental (e.g., nutrition), behavioral (e.g., food selectivity, PA, SB), and biological (e.g., genetics, metabolic dysfunction) factors. Because the etiologies of ASD and obesity are so complex, risk factors specifically associated with one condition or the other are difficult to disentangle. Nevertheless, it is important to understand that many risk factors for becoming obese or overweight are heightened in individuals with ASD, as suggested by growing evidence. Figure 1 summarizes the risk factors discussed within this review. A limitation of this narrative review is that we compared various risk factors for unhealthy weight gain and obesity in children with ASD to TD children. Although similarities were found with regard to specific risk factors between children with ASD and TD children (i.e., physical activity, etc.), this does not necessarily mean these are not clinically relevant to children with ASD and should still be taken into account in future studies, including clinical trials.

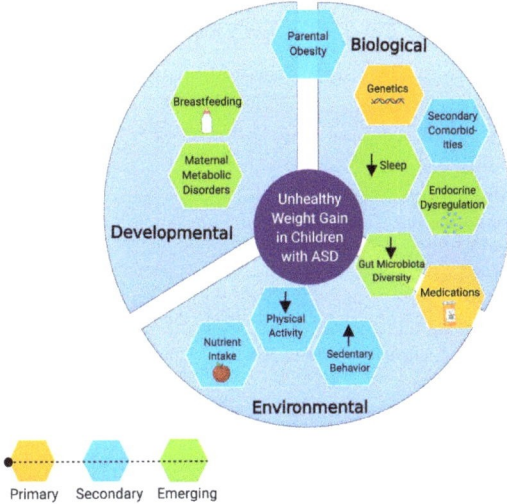

Figure 1. Risk factors for becoming obese or overweight among individuals with ASD. Primary factors include risk factors which have been directly implicated in obesity and/or unhealthy weight gain, in children with ASD. Secondary factors are those which are not specific to children with ASD but could result in unhealthy weight gain. Emerging factors are those on which we have postulated hypotheses based on indirect evidence. *Created with BioRender.

Overall, evidence suggests that oral sensitivities may mediate food selectivity and food and nutrient intake and other factor such as PA, SB, sleep, genetics, and medication usage may all contribute to some degree, and ultimately have a compounded effect on weight gain in ASD. Additionally, researchers have begun to investigate the roles of sleep problems, the gut microbiome, the endocrine system, and developmental risk factors. Going forward, studies of obesity in ASD should incorporate assessment of both biological and lifestyle-related factors, as well as test for mediating and moderating relationships such as ASD severity, oral sensitivities, and sex and age differences. It is important to consider these multiple factors in conjunction with individual factors to clarify whether unhealthy weight gain affects children across the entire ASD spectrum, or whether certain children are more vulnerable than others. Understanding each of these individual risk factors and components is important to effectively prevent and treat unhealthy weight gain among children with ASD and to facilitate the development of potential early intervention strategies. An understanding of individual risk factors would enable the development of personalized approaches to help children with ASD manage their weight, including dietary recommendations, medical therapies, and nutrition and exercise regimens. Overall in conjunction with the clinical guidelines for pediatric obesity [229] and ASD care [98], clinicians should consider more tailored medical surveillance in children with ASD that considers the above factors in a care and management plan.

Author Contributions: K.K.D., A.M.H., and L.Z. devised the main conceptual ideas and outline of the review. K.K.D. wrote the review and conducted the literature search. C.E.O. contributed additional support in writing to specific subsections. C.E.O., A.M.H., and L.Z. provided their expertise and contributed to revising the article critically for important intellectual content and editing. C.R. provided her expertise in nutrition and contributions to revisions. All authors read and approved the final manuscript.

Acknowledgments: The authors express sincerely thanks to Autism Edmonton and the Autism Research Centre (at the Glenrose Rehabilitation Hospital in Edmonton, AB). This work was supported by the Autism Edmonton and Autism Research Centre Graduate Student Pilot Grant, the Glenrose Rehabilitation Hospital Foundation Clinical Research Grant, the Stollery Children's Hospital Foundation Chair in Autism, and the Alberta Diabetes Institute. C.E.O is a recipient of the 2018 Alberta SPOR Graduate Studentship in Patient-Oriented Research, which is jointly funded by Alberta Innovates and the Canadian Institutes of Health Research. L.Z is supported by the Stollery Children's Hospital Foundation in Autism and the Stollery Science Lab.

Conflicts of Interest: The authors declare no conflicts of interest.

Abbreviations

ADHD	Attention Deficit Hyperactivity Disorder
AMDR	Acceptable Macronutrient Distribution Range
ASD	Autism Spectrum Disorder
BMI	Body Mass Index
BPFA	Behavior Pediatrics Feeding Assessment Scale
FFQ	Food Frequency Questionnaire
GFCF	Gluten-Free Casein-Free
GI	Gastrointestinal
GLP-1	Glucagon-Like Peptide-1
MVPA	Moderate- to Vigorous-intensity Physical Activity
OSA	Obstructive Sleep Apnea
PA	Physical Activity
PYY	Peptide YY
PWS	Prader-Willi Syndrome
RCT	Randomized Controlled Trial
SB	Sedentary Behavior
SCFA	Short-Chain Fatty Acid
SGA	Second Generation Antipsychotic
SSRI	Selective Serotonin Reuptake Inhibitors
TD	Typically Developing

References

1. Lai, M.-C.; Lombardo, M.V.; Baron-Cohen, S. Autism. *Lancet* **2014**, *383*, 896–910. [CrossRef]
2. American Psychiatric Association. *Diagnostic and Statistical Manual of Mental Disorders (DSM-5)*, 5th ed.; American Psychiatric Association: Arlington, VA, USA, 2013.
3. World Health Organization. Autism spectrum disorders. Available online: https://www.who.int/news-room/fact-sheets/detail/autism-spectrum-disorders (accessed on 26 May 2019).
4. Baio, J.; Wiggins, L.; Christensen, D.L.; Maenner, M.J.; Daniels, J.; Warren, Z.; Kurzius-Spencer, M. Prevalence of Autism Spectrum Disorder Among Children Aged 8 Years—Autism and Developmental Disabilities Monitoring Network, 11 Sites, United States, 2014. *MMWR Surveill. Summ.* **2018**, *67*, 1–23. [CrossRef] [PubMed]
5. Ofner, M.; Coles, A.; Decou, M.L.; Do, M.T.; Bienek, A.; Snider, J.; Ugnat, A.-M. Autism spectrum disorder among children and youth in Canada 2018: A report of the National Autism Spectrum Disorder Surveillance System. Available online: https://www.canada.ca/en/public-health/services/publications/diseases-conditions/autism-spectrum-disorder-children-youth-canada-2018.html (accessed on 5 May 2019).
6. Zheng, Z.; Zhang, L.; Li, S.; Zhao, F.; Wang, Y.; Huang, L.; Huang, J.; Zou, R.; Qu, Y.; Mu, D. Association among obesity, overweight and autism spectrum disorder: A systematic review and meta-analysis. *Sci. Rep.* **2017**, *7*, 11697. [CrossRef] [PubMed]
7. Hill, A.P.; Zuckerman, K.E.; Fombonne, E. Obesity and Autism. *Pediatrics* **2015**, *136*, 1051–1061. [CrossRef]
8. Hyman, S.L.; Stewart, P.A.; Schmidt, B.; Cain, U.; Lemcke, N.; Foley, J.T.; Peck, R.; Clemons, T.; Reynolds, A.; Johnson, C.; et al. Nutrient intake from food in children with autism. *Pediatrics* **2012**, *130*, S145–S153. [CrossRef] [PubMed]
9. Steinberger, J.; Daniels, S.R. Obesity, insulin resistance, diabetes, and cardiovascular risk in children. *Circulation* **2003**, *107*, 1448–1453. [CrossRef] [PubMed]

10. Weihrauch-Blüher, S.; Schwarz, P.; Klusmann, J.-H. Childhood obesity: Increased risk for cardiometabolic disease and cancer in adulthood. *Metab. Clin. Exp.* **2019**, *92*, 147–152. [CrossRef]
11. Khodaverdi, F.; Alhani, F.; Kazemnejad, A.; Khodaverdi, Z. The Relationship between Obesity and Quality of Life in School Children. *Iran. J. Public Health* **2011**, *40*, 96–101.
12. Bandini, L.; Curtin, C.; Phillips, S.; Anderson, S.E.; Maslin, M.; Must, A. Changes in food selectivity in children with autism spectrum disorder. *J. Autism Dev. Disord.* **2017**, *47*, 439–446. [CrossRef]
13. Askari, S.; Anaby, D.; Bergthorson, M.; Majnemer, A.; Elsabbagh, M.; Zwaigenbaum, L. Participation of Children and Youth with Autism Spectrum Disorder: A Scoping Review. *Rev. J. Autism Dev. Disord.* **2015**, *2*, 103–114. [CrossRef]
14. Ferguson, B.J.; Marler, S.; Altstein, L.L.; Lee, E.B.; Akers, J.; Sohl, K.; McLaughlin, A.; Hartnett, K.; Kille, B.; Mazurek, M.; et al. Psychophysiological Associations with Gastrointestinal Symptomatology in Autism Spectrum Disorder. *Autism Res.* **2017**, *10*, 276–288. [CrossRef] [PubMed]
15. Maneeton, N.; Maneeton, B.; Puthisri, S.; Woottiluk, P.; Narkpongphun, A.; Srisurapanont, M. Risperidone for children and adolescents with autism spectrum disorder: A systematic review. Available online: https://www.dovepress.com/risperidone-for-children-and-adolescents-with-autism-spectrum-disorder-peer-reviewed-fulltext-article-NDT (accessed on 20 May 2019).
16. Kang, D.-W.; Park, J.G.; Ilhan, Z.E.; Wallstrom, G.; Labaer, J.; Adams, J.B.; Krajmalnik-Brown, R. Reduced incidence of Prevotella and other fermenters in intestinal microflora of autistic children. *PLoS ONE* **2013**, *8*, e68322. [CrossRef] [PubMed]
17. Castaner, O.; Goday, A.; Park, Y.-M.; Lee, S.-H.; Magkos, F.; Shiow, S.-A.T.E.; Schröder, H. The Gut Microbiome Profile in Obesity: A Systematic Review. *Int. J. Endocrinol.* **2018**, 1–9. [CrossRef] [PubMed]
18. Ashwood, P.; Kwong, C.; Hansen, R.; Hertz-Picciotto, I.; Croen, L.; Krakowiak, P.; Walker, W.; Pessah, I.N.; Van de Water, J. Brief report: Plasma leptin levels are elevated in autism: Association with early onset phenotype? *J. Autism Dev. Disord.* **2008**, *38*, 169–175. [CrossRef] [PubMed]
19. Blardi, P.; de Lalla, A.; Ceccatelli, L.; Vanessa, G.; Auteri, A.; Hayek, J. Variations of plasma leptin and adiponectin levels in autistic patients. *Neurosci. Lett.* **2010**, *479*, 54–57. [CrossRef] [PubMed]
20. Tareen, R.S.; Kamboj, M.K. Role of endocrine factors in autistic spectrum disorders. *Pediatr. Clin. N. Am.* **2012**, *59*, 75–88. [CrossRef] [PubMed]
21. Reynolds, L.C.; Inder, T.E.; Neil, J.J.; Pineda, R.G.; Rogers, C.E. Maternal obesity and increased risk for autism and developmental delay among very preterm infants. *J. Perinatol.* **2014**, *34*, 688–692. [CrossRef]
22. Wang, Y.; Min, J.; Khuri, J.; Li, M. A Systematic Examination of the Association between Parental and Child Obesity across Countries123. *Adv. Nutr.* **2017**, *8*, 436–448. [CrossRef]
23. Han, J.C.; Lawlor, D.A.; Kimm, S.Y.S. Childhood Obesity—2010: Progress and Challenges. *Lancet* **2010**, *375*, 1737–1748. [CrossRef]
24. Leekam, S.R.; Nieto, C.; Libby, S.J.; Wing, L.; Gould, J. Describing the Sensory Abnormalities of Children and Adults with Autism. *J. Autism Dev. Disord.* **2007**, *37*, 894–910. [CrossRef]
25. Kern, J.K.; Trivedi, M.H.; Garver, C.R.; Grannemann, B.D.; Andrews, A.A.; Savla, J.S.; Johnson, D.G.; Mehta, J.A.; Schroeder, J.L. The pattern of sensory processing abnormalities in autism. *Autism* **2006**, *10*, 480–494. [CrossRef] [PubMed]
26. Cermak, S.A.; Curtin, C.; Bandini, L.G. Food selectivity and sensory sensitivity in children with autism spectrum disorders. *J. Am. Diet. Assoc.* **2010**, *110*, 238–246. [CrossRef] [PubMed]
27. Sharp, W.G.; Berry, R.C.; McCracken, C.; Nuhu, N.N.; Marvel, E.; Saulnier, C.A.; Klin, A.; Jones, W.; Jaquess, D.L. Feeding Problems and Nutrient Intake in Children with Autism Spectrum Disorders: A Meta-analysis and Comprehensive Review of the Literature. *J. Autism Dev. Disord.* **2013**, *43*, 2159–2173. [CrossRef] [PubMed]
28. Shmaya, Y.; Eilat-Adar, S.; Leitner, Y.; Reif, S.; Gabis, L. Nutritional deficiencies and overweight prevalence among children with autism spectrum disorder. *Res. Dev. Disabil.* **2015**, *38*, 1–6. [CrossRef] [PubMed]
29. Castro, K.; Faccioli, L.S.; Baronio, D.; Gottfried, C.; Perry, I.S.; Riesgo, R. Feeding behavior and dietary intake of male children and adolescents with autism spectrum disorder: A case-control study. *Int. J. Dev. Neurosci.* **2016**, *53*, 68–74. [CrossRef] [PubMed]
30. Liu, X.; Liu, J.; Xiong, X.; Yang, T.; Hou, N.; Liang, X.; Chen, J.; Cheng, Q.; Li, T. Correlation between Nutrition and Symptoms: Nutritional Survey of Children with Autism Spectrum Disorder in Chongqing, China. *Nutrients* **2016**, *8*, 294. [CrossRef] [PubMed]

31. Evans, E.W.; Must, A.; Anderson, S.E.; Curtin, C.; Scampini, R.; Maslin, M.; Bandini, L. Dietary Patterns and Body Mass Index in Children with Autism and Typically Developing Children. *Res. Autism Spectr. Disord.* **2012**, *6*, 399–405. [CrossRef]
32. Chao, H.-C. Association of Picky Eating with Growth, Nutritional Status, Development, Physical Activity, and Health in Preschool Children. *Front. Pediatr.* **2018**, *6*, 22. [CrossRef]
33. Esteban-Figuerola, P.; Canals, J.; Fernández-Cao, J.C.; Arija Val, V. Differences in food consumption and nutritional intake between children with autism spectrum disorders and typically developing children: A meta-analysis. *Autism* **2018**, *23*, 1079–1095. [CrossRef]
34. Wan, Y.; Wang, F.; Yuan, J.; Li, J.; Jiang, D.; Zhang, J.; Huang, T.; Zheng, J.; Mann, J.; Li, D. Effects of Macronutrient Distribution on Weight and Related Cardiometabolic Profile in Healthy Non-Obese Chinese: A 6-month, Randomized Controlled-Feeding Trial. *EBioMedicine* **2017**, *22*, 200–207. [CrossRef]
35. Hjorth, M.F.; Ritz, C.; Blaak, E.E.; Saris, W.H.; Langin, D.; Poulsen, S.K.; Larsen, T.M.; Sørensen, T.I.; Zohar, Y.; Astrup, A. Pretreatment fasting plasma glucose and insulin modify dietary weight loss success: Results from 3 randomized clinical trials. *Am. J. Clin. Nutr.* **2017**, *106*, 499–505. [CrossRef] [PubMed]
36. Gow, M.L.; Ho, M.; Burrows, T.L.; Baur, L.A.; Stewart, L.; Hutchesson, M.J.; Cowell, C.T.; Collins, C.E.; Garnett, S.P. Impact of dietary macronutrient distribution on BMI and cardiometabolic outcomes in overweight and obese children and adolescents: A systematic review. *Nutr. Rev.* **2014**, *72*, 453–470. [CrossRef] [PubMed]
37. Via, M. The Malnutrition of Obesity: Micronutrient Deficiencies That Promote Diabetes. *ISRN Endocrinol.* **2012**, *2012*, 103472. [CrossRef] [PubMed]
38. Hyman, S.L.; Stewart, P.A.; Foley, J.; Cain, U.; Peck, R.; Morris, D.D.; Wang, H.; Smith, T. The gluten-free/casein-free diet: A double-blind challenge trial in children with autism. *J. Autism Dev. Disord.* **2016**, *46*, 205–220. [CrossRef] [PubMed]
39. Sathe, N.; Andrews, J.C.; McPheeters, M.L.; Warren, Z.E. Nutritional and dietary interventions for autism spectrum disorder: A systematic review. *Pediatrics* **2017**, *139*, e20170346. [CrossRef] [PubMed]
40. Herndon, A.C.; DiGuiseppi, C.; Johnson, S.L.; Leiferman, J.; Reynolds, A. Does nutritional intake differ between children with autism spectrum disorders and children with typical development? *J. Autism Dev. Disord.* **2009**, *39*, 212–222. [CrossRef]
41. Zimmer, M.H.; Hart, L.C.; Manning-Courtney, P.; Murray, D.S.; Bing, N.M.; Summer, S. Food variety as a predictor of nutritional status among children with autism. *J. Autism Dev. Disord.* **2012**, *42*, 549–556. [CrossRef] [PubMed]
42. Bandini, L.G.; Anderson, S.E.; Curtin, C.; Cermak, S.; Evans, E.W.; Scampini, R.; Maslin, M.; Must, A. Food selectivity in children with autism spectrum disorders and typically developing children. *J. Pediatr.* **2010**, *157*, 259–264. [CrossRef]
43. García, O.P.; Long, K.Z.; Rosado, J.L. Impact of micronutrient deficiencies on obesity. *Nutr. Rev.* **2009**, *67*, 559–572. [CrossRef]
44. Yu, Z.M.; DeClercq, V.; Cui, Y.; Forbes, C.; Grandy, S.; Keats, M.; Parker, L.; Sweeney, E.; Dummer, T.J.B. Fruit and vegetable intake and body adiposity among populations in Eastern Canada: The Atlantic Partnership for Tomorrow's Health study. *BMJ Open* **2018**, *8*, e018060. [CrossRef]
45. Bertoia, M.L.; Mukamal, K.J.; Cahill, L.E.; Hou, T.; Ludwig, D.S.; Mozaffarian, D.; Willett, W.C.; Hu, F.B.; Rimm, E.B. Changes in intake of fruits and vegetables and weight change in united states men and women followed for up to 24 years: Analysis from three prospective cohort studies. *PLoS Med.* **2015**, *12*, e1001878. [CrossRef] [PubMed]
46. Graf-Myles, J.; Farmer, C.; Thurm, A.; Royster, C.; Kahn, P.; Soskey, L.; Rothschild, L.; Swedo, S. Dietary adequacy of children with autism compared to controls and the impact of restricted diet. *J. Dev. Behav. Pediatr.* **2013**, *34*, 449–459. [CrossRef] [PubMed]
47. Riccio, M.P.; Franco, C.; Negri, R.; Ferrentino, R.I.; Maresca, R.; D'alterio, E.; Greco, L.; Bravaccio, C. Is food refusal in autistic children related to TAS2R38 genotype? *Autism Res.* **2018**, *11*, 531–538. [CrossRef] [PubMed]
48. Joseph, P.V.; Reed, D.R.; Mennella, J.A. Individual Differences Among Children in Sucrose Detection Thresholds: Relationship with Age, Gender, and Bitter Taste Genotype. *Nurs. Res.* **2016**, *65*, 3–12. [CrossRef] [PubMed]
49. Mennella, J.A.; Bobowski, N.K. The sweetness and bitterness of childhood: Insights from basic research on taste preferences. *Physiol. Behav.* **2015**, *152*, 502–507. [CrossRef] [PubMed]

50. Yang, Y.J.; Kim, M.K.; Hwang, S.H.; Ahn, Y.; Shim, J.E.; Kim, D.H. Relative validities of 3-day food records and the food frequency questionnaire. *Nutr. Res. Pract.* **2010**, *4*, 142–148. [CrossRef]
51. Macdiarmid, J.; Blundell, J. Assessing dietary intake: Who, what and why of under-reporting. *Nutr. Res. Rev.* **1998**, *11*, 231–253. [CrossRef]
52. Subar, A.F.; Freedman, L.S.; Tooze, J.A.; Kirkpatrick, S.I.; Boushey, C.; Neuhouser, M.L.; Thompson, F.E.; Potischman, N.; Guenther, P.M.; Tarasuk, V.; et al. Addressing current criticism regarding the value of self-report dietary data. *J. Nutr.* **2015**, *145*, 2639–2645. [CrossRef]
53. Naska, A.; Lagiou, A.; Lagiou, P. Dietary assessment methods in epidemiological research: Current state of the art and future prospects. *F1000 Res.* **2017**, *6*, 926. [CrossRef]
54. Westerterp, K.R. Doubly labelled water assessment of energy expenditure: Principle, practice, and promise. *Eur. J. Appl. Physiol.* **2017**, *117*, 1277–1285. [CrossRef]
55. Dudova, I.; Kocourkova, J.; Koutek, J. Early-onset anorexia nervosa in girls with Asperger syndrome. *Neuropsychiatr. Dis. Treat.* **2015**, *11*, 1639–1643. [CrossRef] [PubMed]
56. Baron-Cohen, S.; Jaffa, T.; Davies, S.; Auyeung, B.; Allison, C.; Wheelwright, S. Do girls with anorexia nervosa have elevated autistic traits? *Mol. Autism* **2013**, *4*, 24. [CrossRef] [PubMed]
57. Kirkovski, M.; Enticott, P.G.; Fitzgerald, P.B. A Review of the Role of Female Gender in Autism Spectrum Disorders. *J. Autism Dev. Disord.* **2013**, *43*, 2584–2603. [CrossRef] [PubMed]
58. Goran, M.I.; Reynolds, K.D.; Lindquist, C.H. Role of physical activity in the prevention of obesity in children. *Int. J. Obes.* **1999**, *23*, S18–S33. [CrossRef]
59. Andari, E.; Duhamel, J.-R.; Zalla, T.; Herbrecht, E.; Leboyer, M.; Sirigu, A. Promoting social behavior with oxytocin in high-functioning autism spectrum disorders. *Proc. Natl. Acad. Sci. USA* **2010**, *107*, 4389–4394. [CrossRef] [PubMed]
60. Bishop, S.L.; Havdahl, K.A.; Huerta, M.; Lord, C. Sub-dimensions of social-communication impairment in autism spectrum disorder. *J. Child Psychol. Psychiatry* **2016**, *57*, 909–916. [CrossRef] [PubMed]
61. National Institute of Mental Health. Autism Spectrum Disorder. Available online: https://www.nimh.nih.gov/health/topics/autism-spectrum-disorders-asd/index.shtml (accessed on 6 May 2019).
62. McPhillips, M.; Finlay, J.; Bejerot, S.; Hanley, M. Motor deficits in children with autism spectrum disorder: A cross-syndrome study. *Autism Res.* **2014**, *7*, 664–676. [CrossRef]
63. Serdarevic, F.; Ghassabian, A.; van Batenburg-Eddes, T.; White, T.; Blanken, L.M.E.; Jaddoe, V.W.V.; Verhulst, F.C.; Tiemeier, H. Infant muscle tone and childhood autistic traits: A longitudinal study in the general population. *Autism Res.* **2017**, *10*, 757–768. [CrossRef]
64. World Health Organization. Physical Activity and Young People. Available online: https://www.who.int/dietphysicalactivity/factsheet_young_people/en/ (accessed on 2 May 2019).
65. U.S. Department of Health and Human Services. Current Guidelines. Available online: https://health.gov/paguidelines/second-edition/ (accessed on 28 May 2019).
66. Bandini, L.G.; Gleason, J.; Curtin, C.; Lividini, K.; Anderson, S.E.; Cermak, S.A.; Maslin, M.; Must, A. Comparison of physical activity between children with autism spectrum disorders and typically developing children. *Autism* **2013**, *17*, 44–54. [CrossRef]
67. Stanish, H.I.; Curtin, C.; Must, A.; Phillips, S.; Maslin, M.; Bandini, L.G. Physical activity levels, frequency, and type among adolescents with and without autism spectrum disorder. *J. Autism Dev. Disord.* **2017**, *47*, 785–794. [CrossRef]
68. Jones, R.A.; Downing, K.; Rinehart, N.J.; Barnett, L.M.; May, T.; McGillivray, J.A.; Papadopoulos, N.V.; Skouteris, H.; Timperio, A.; Hinkley, T. Physical activity, sedentary behavior and their correlates in children with Autism Spectrum Disorder: A systematic review. *PLoS ONE* **2017**, *12*, e0172482. [CrossRef]
69. Griffiths, L.J.; Cortina-Borja, M.; Sera, F.; Pouliou, T.; Geraci, M.; Rich, C.; Cole, T.J.; Law, C.; Joshi, H.; Ness, A.R.; et al. How active are our children? Findings from the Millennium Cohort Study. *BMJ Open* **2013**, *3*, e002893. [CrossRef] [PubMed]
70. Must, A.; Phillips, S.; Curtin, C.; Bandini, L.G. Barriers to physical activity in children with autism spectrum disorders: Relationship to physical activity and screen time. *J. Phys. Act. Health* **2015**, *12*, 529–534. [CrossRef] [PubMed]
71. McCoy, S.M.; Jakicic, J.M.; Gibbs, B.B. Comparison of obesity, physical activity, and sedentary behaviors between adolescents with autism spectrum disorders and without. *J. Autism Dev. Disord.* **2016**, *46*, 2317–2326. [CrossRef]

72. Healy, S.; Haegele, J.A.; Grenier, M.A.; Garcia, J.M. Physical activity, screen-time behavior, and obesity among 13-year-olds in Ireland with and without autism spectrum disorder. *J. Autism Dev. Disord.* **2017**, *47*, 49–57. [CrossRef] [PubMed]
73. Sarker, H.; Anderson, L.N.; Borkhoff, C.M.; Abreo, K.; Tremblay, M.S.; Lebovic, G.; Maguire, J.L.; Parkin, P.C.; Birken, C.S. Validation of parent-reported physical activity and sedentary time by accelerometry in young children. *BMC Res. Notes* **2015**, *8*, 1–8. [CrossRef]
74. Dössegger, A.; Ruch, N.; Jimmy, G.; Braun-Fahrländer, C.; Mäder, U.; Hänggi, J.; Hofmann, H.; Puder, J.J.; Kriemler, S.; Bringolf-Isler, B. Reactivity to accelerometer measurement of children and adolescents. *Med. Sci. Sports Exerc.* **2014**, *46*, 1140–1146. [CrossRef]
75. Koning, M.; de Jong, A.; de Jong, E.; Visscher, T.L.S.; Seidell, J.C.; Renders, C.M. Agreement between parent and child report of physical activity, sedentary and dietary behaviours in 9–12-year-old children and associations with children's weight status. *BMC Psychol.* **2018**, *6*, 14. [CrossRef] [PubMed]
76. Owen, N.; Sparling, P.B.; Healy, G.N.; Dunstan, D.W.; Matthews, C.E. Sedentary behavior: Emerging evidence for a new health risk. *Mayo Clin. Proc.* **2010**, *85*, 1138–1141. [CrossRef]
77. Matthews, C.E.; Chen, K.Y.; Freedson, P.S.; Buchowski, M.S.; Beech, B.M.; Pate, R.R.; Troiano, R.P. Amount of time spent in sedentary behaviors in the United States, 2003–2004. *Am. J. Epidemiol.* **2008**, *167*, 875–881. [CrossRef]
78. Dunton, G.F.; Liao, Y.; Intille, S.S.; Spruijt-Metz, D.; Pentz, M. Investigating children's physical activity and sedentary behavior using ecological momentary assessment with mobile phones. *Obesity* **2011**, *19*, 1205–1212. [CrossRef] [PubMed]
79. Biswas, A.; Oh, P.I.; Faulkner, G.E.; Bajaj, R.R.; Silver, M.A.; Mitchell, M.S.; Alter, D.A. Sedentary time and its association with risk for disease incidence, mortality, and hospitalization in adults: A systematic review and meta-analysis. *Ann. Intern. Med.* **2015**, *162*, 123. [CrossRef] [PubMed]
80. Ekelund, U.; Brage, S.; Besson, H.; Sharp, S.; Wareham, N.J. Time spent being sedentary and weight gain in healthy adults: Reverse or bidirectional causality? *Am. J. Clin. Nutr.* **2008**, *88*, 612–617. [CrossRef] [PubMed]
81. Mazurek, M.O.; Wenstrup, C. Television, video game and social media use among children with ASD and typically developing siblings. *J. Autism Dev. Disord.* **2013**, *43*, 1258–1271. [CrossRef] [PubMed]
82. Mazurek, M.O.; Shattuck, P.T.; Wagner, M.; Cooper, B.P. Prevalence and correlates of screen-based media use among youths with autism spectrum disorders. *J. Autism Dev. Disord.* **2012**, *42*, 1757–1767. [CrossRef] [PubMed]
83. MacDonald, M.; Lord, C.; Ulrich, D.A. Motor skills and calibrated autism severity in young children with autism spectrum disorder. *Adapt. Phys. Activ. Q* **2014**, *31*, 95–105. [CrossRef] [PubMed]
84. Constantino, J.N.; Zhang, Y.; Frazier, T.; Abbacchi, A.M.; Law, P. Sibling recurrence and the genetic epidemiology of autism. *Am. J. Psychiatry* **2010**, *167*, 1349–1356. [CrossRef]
85. Sandin, S.; Lichtenstein, P.; Kuja-Halkola, R.; Hultman, C.; Larsson, H.; Reichenberg, A. The heritability of autism spectrum disorder. *JAMA* **2017**, *318*, 1182–1184. [CrossRef]
86. Chesi, A.; Grant, S.F.A. The genetics of pediatric obesity. *Trends Endocrinol. Metab.* **2015**, *26*, 711–721. [CrossRef]
87. Sørensen, T.I.; Stunkard, A.J. Does obesity run in families because of genes? An adoption study using silhouettes as a measure of obesity. *Acta Psychiatr. Scand. Suppl.* **1993**, *370*, 67–72. [CrossRef]
88. Sharma, J.R.; Arieff, Z.; Sagar, S.; Kaur, M. Autism and obesity: Prevalence, molecular basis and potential therapies. *Autism Insights* **2012**, *4*, 1–13.
89. Shinawi, M.; Sahoo, T.; Maranda, B.; Skinner, S.A.; Skinner, C.; Chinault, C.; Zascavage, R.; Peters, S.U.; Patel, A.; Stevenson, R.E.; et al. 11p14.1 microdeletions associated with ADHD, autism, developmental delay, and obesity. *Am. J. Med. Genet. A* **2011**, *155A*, 1272–1280. [CrossRef] [PubMed]
90. Walters, R.G.; Jacquemont, S.; Valsesia, A.; de Smith, A.J.; Martinet, D.; Andersson, J.; Falchi, M.; Chen, F.; Andrieux, J.; Lobbens, S.; et al. A new highly penetrant form of obesity due to deletions on chromosome 16p11.2. *Nature* **2010**, *463*, 671–675. [CrossRef] [PubMed]
91. Bachmann-Gagescu, R.; Mefford, H.C.; Cowan, C.; Glew, G.M.; Hing, A.V.; Wallace, S.; Bader, P.I.; Hamati, A.; Reitnauer, P.J.; Smith, R.; et al. Recurrent 200-kb deletions of 16p11.2 that include the SH2B1 gene are associated with developmental delay and obesity. *Genet. Med.* **2010**, *12*, 641–647. [CrossRef] [PubMed]
92. Cortes, H.D.; Wevrick, R. Genetic analysis of very obese children with autism spectrum disorder. *Mol. Genet. Genom.* **2018**, *293*, 725–736. [CrossRef] [PubMed]

93. Dykens, E.M.; Lee, E.; Roof, E. Prader–Willi syndrome and autism spectrum disorders: An evolving story. *J. Neurodev. Disord.* **2011**, *3*, 225–237. [CrossRef] [PubMed]
94. Haqq, A.M.; Grambow, S.C.; Muehlbauer, M.; Newgard, C.B.; Svetkey, L.P.; Carrel, A.L.; Yanovski, J.A.; Purnell, J.Q.; Freemark, M. Ghrelin concentrations in Prader-Willi syndrome (PWS) infants and children. *Clin. Endocrinol. (Oxf.)* **2008**, *69*, 911–920. [CrossRef] [PubMed]
95. Bennett, J.A.; Hodgetts, S.; Mackenzie, M.L.; Haqq, A.M.; Zwaigenbaum, L. Investigating Autism-Related Symptoms in Children with Prader-Willi Syndrome: A Case Study. *Int. J. Mol. Sci.* **2017**, *18*, 517. [CrossRef] [PubMed]
96. Dykens, E.M.; Roof, E.; Hunt-Hawkins, H.; Dankner, N.; Lee, E.B.; Shivers, C.M.; Daniell, C.; Kim, S.-J. Diagnoses and characteristics of autism spectrum disorders in children with Prader-Willi syndrome. *J. Neurodev. Disord.* **2017**, *9*, 18. [CrossRef]
97. Ramos-Molina, B.; Molina-Vega, M.; Fernández-García, J.C.; Creemers, J.W. Hyperphagia and Obesity in Prader–Willi Syndrome: PCSK1 Deficiency and Beyond? *Genes (Basel)* **2018**, *9*, 288. [CrossRef]
98. Anagnostou, E.; Zwaigenbaum, L.; Szatmari, P.; Fombonne, E.; Fernandez, B.A.; Woodbury-Smith, M.; Brian, J.; Bryson, S.; Smith, I.M.; Drmic, I.; et al. Autism spectrum disorder: advances in evidence-based practice. *CMAJ* **2014**, *186*, 509–519. [CrossRef] [PubMed]
99. Linke, A.C.; Olson, L.; Gao, Y.; Fishman, I.; Müller, R.-A. Psychotropic medication use in autism spectrum disorders may affect functional brain connectivity. *Biol. Psychiatry Cogn. Neurosci. Neuroimaging* **2017**, *2*, 518–527. [CrossRef] [PubMed]
100. Nihalani, N.; Schwartz, T.L.; Siddiqui, U.A.; Megna, J.L. Weight gain, obesity, and psychotropic prescribing. *J. Obes.* **2011**, *2011*, 893629. [CrossRef] [PubMed]
101. Coury, D.L.; Anagnostou, E.; Manning-Courtney, P.; Reynolds, A.; Cole, L.; McCoy, R.; Whitaker, A.; Perrin, J.M. Use of psychotropic medication in children and adolescents with autism spectrum disorders. *Pediatrics* **2012**, *130*, S69–S76. [CrossRef] [PubMed]
102. Frazier, T.W.; Shattuck, P.T.; Narendorf, S.C.; Cooper, B.P.; Wagner, M.; Spitznagel, E.L. Prevalence and correlates of psychotropic medication use in adolescents with an autism spectrum disorder with and without caregiver-reported attention-deficit/hyperactivity disorder. *J. Child. Adolesc. Psychopharmacol.* **2011**, *21*, 571–579. [CrossRef] [PubMed]
103. Spencer, D.; Marshall, J.; Post, B.; Kulakodlu, M.; Newschaffer, C.; Dennen, T.; Azocar, F.; Jain, A. Psychotropic medication use and polypharmacy in children with autism spectrum disorders. *Pediatrics* **2013**, *132*, 833–840. [CrossRef]
104. Jobski, K.; Höfer, J.; Hoffmann, F.; Bachmann, C. Use of psychotropic drugs in patients with autism spectrum disorders: A systematic review. *Acta Psychiatr. Scand.* **2017**, *135*, 8–28. [CrossRef]
105. Park, S.Y.; Cervesi, C.; Galling, B.; Molteni, S.; Walyzada, F.; Ameis, S.H.; Gerhard, T.; Olfson, M.; Correll, C.U. Antipsychotic use trends in youth with autism spectrum disorder and/or intellectual disability: A meta-analysis. *J. Am. Acad. Child. Adolesc. Psychiatry* **2016**, *55*, 456–468.e4. [CrossRef]
106. Fallah, M.S.; Shaikh, M.R.; Neupane, B.; Rusiecki, D.; Bennett, T.A.; Beyene, J. Atypical antipsychotics for irritability in pediatric autism: A systematic review and network meta-analysis. *J. Child. Adolesc. Psychopharmacol.* **2019**, *29*, 168–180. [CrossRef]
107. Fung, L.K.; Mahajan, R.; Nozzolillo, A.; Bernal, P.; Krasner, A.; Jo, B.; Coury, D.; Whitaker, A.; Veenstra-Vanderweele, J.; Hardan, A.Y. Pharmacologic Treatment of Severe Irritability and Problem Behaviors in Autism: A Systematic Review and Meta-analysis. *Pediatrics* **2016**, *137*, S124–135. [CrossRef]
108. Srisawasdi, P.; Vanwong, N.; Hongkaew, Y.; Puangpetch, A.; Vanavanan, S.; Intachak, B.; Ngamsamut, N.; Limsila, P.; Sukasem, C.; Kroll, M.H. Impact of risperidone on leptin and insulin in children and adolescents with autistic spectrum disorders. *Clin. Biochem.* **2017**, *50*, 678–685. [CrossRef] [PubMed]
109. Shimizu, H.; Shimomura, Y.; Hayashi, R.; Ohtani, K.; Sato, N.; Futawatari, T.; Mori, M. Serum leptin concentration is associated with total body fat mass, but not abdominal fat distribution. *Int. J. Obes. Relat. Metab. Disord.* **1997**, *21*, 536–541. [CrossRef] [PubMed]
110. Hirsch, L.E.; Pringsheim, T. Aripiprazole for autism spectrum disorders (ASD). *Cochrane Database Syst. Rev.* **2016**, *6*. [CrossRef] [PubMed]
111. Hsia, Y.; Wong, A.Y.S.; Murphy, D.G.M.; Simonoff, E.; Buitelaar, J.K.; Wong, I.C.K. Psychopharmacological prescriptions for people with autism spectrum disorder (ASD): A multinational study. *Psychopharmacology* **2014**, *231*, 999–1009. [CrossRef] [PubMed]

112. Murray, M.L.; Hsia, Y.; Glaser, K.; Simonoff, E.; Murphy, D.G.M.; Asherson, P.J.; Eklund, H.; Wong, I.C.K. Pharmacological treatments prescribed to people with autism spectrum disorder (ASD) in primary health care. *Psychopharmacology* **2014**, *231*, 1011–1021. [CrossRef] [PubMed]
113. Bak, M.; Fransen, A.; Janssen, J.; van Os, J.; Drukker, M. Almost all antipsychotics result in weight gain: A meta-analysis. *PLoS ONE* **2014**, *9*, e94112. [CrossRef]
114. Meltzer, H.Y.; Massey, B.W. The role of serotonin receptors in the action of atypical antipsychotic drugs. *Curr. Opin. Pharm.* **2011**, *11*, 59–67. [CrossRef] [PubMed]
115. Roerig, J.L.; Steffen, K.J.; Mitchell, J.E. Atypical antipsychotic-induced weight gain: Insights into mechanisms of action. *CNS Drugs* **2011**, *25*, 1035–1059. [CrossRef]
116. Pringsheim, T.; Panagiotopoulos, C.; Davidson, J.; Ho, J. Evidence-based recommendations for monitoring safety of second-generation antipsychotics in children and youth. *Paediatr. Child. Health* **2011**, *16*, 581–589. [CrossRef]
117. Williams, K.; Brignell, A.; Randall, M.; Silove, N.; Hazell, P. Selective serotonin reuptake inhibitors (SSRIs) for autism spectrum disorders (ASD). *Cochrane Database Syst. Rev.* **2013**, *8*, CD004677. [CrossRef]
118. Reekie, J.; Hosking, S.P.M.; Prakash, C.; Kao, K.-T.; Juonala, M.; Sabin, M.A. The effect of antidepressants and antipsychotics on weight gain in children and adolescents: Antidepressants/psychotics and weight in youth. *Obes. Rev.* **2015**, *16*, 566–580. [CrossRef] [PubMed]
119. King, B.H.; Hollander, E.; Sikich, L.; McCracken, J.T.; Scahill, L.; Bregman, J.D.; Donnelly, C.L.; Anagnostou, E.; Dukes, K.; Sullivan, L.; et al. Lack of Efficacy of Citalopram in Children with Autism Spectrum Disorders and High Levels of Repetitive Behavior: Citalopram Ineffective in Children with Autism. *Arch. Gen. Psychiatry* **2009**, *66*, 583–590. [CrossRef] [PubMed]
120. Hollander, E.; Soorya, L.; Chaplin, W.; Anagnostou, E.; Taylor, B.P.; Ferretti, C.J.; Wasserman, S.; Swanson, E.; Settipani, C. A Double-Blind Placebo-Controlled Trial of Fluoxetine for Repetitive Behaviors and Global Severity in Adult Autism Spectrum Disorders. *AJP* **2012**, *169*, 292–299. [CrossRef] [PubMed]
121. Blumenthal, S.R.; Castro, V.M.; Clements, C.C.; Rosenfield, H.R.; Murphy, S.N.; Fava, M.; Weilburg, J.B.; Erb, J.L.; Churchill, S.E.; Kohane, I.S.; et al. An Electronic Health Records Study of Long-Term Weight Gain Following Antidepressant Use. *JAMA Psychiatry* **2014**, *71*, 889–896. [CrossRef] [PubMed]
122. Stolzer, J.M. Breastfeeding and obesity: A meta-analysis. *Open J. Prev. Med.* **2011**, *1*, 88–93. [CrossRef]
123. Tseng, P.-T.; Chen, Y.-W.; Stubbs, B.; Carvalho, A.F.; Whiteley, P.; Tang, C.-H.; Yang, W.-C.; Chen, T.-Y.; Li, D.-J.; Chu, C.-S.; et al. Maternal breastfeeding and autism spectrum disorder in children: A systematic review and meta-analysis. *Nutr. Neurosci.* **2019**, *22*, 354–362. [CrossRef]
124. Boucher, O.; Julvez, J.; Guxens, M.; Arranz, E.; Ibarluzea, J.; Sánchez de Miguel, M.; Fernández-Somoano, A.; Tardon, A.; Rebagliato, M.; Garcia-Esteban, R.; et al. Association between breastfeeding duration and cognitive development, autistic traits and ADHD symptoms: A multicenter study in Spain. *Pediatr. Res.* **2017**, *81*, 434–442. [CrossRef]
125. Al-Farsi, Y.M.; Al-Sharbati, M.M.; Waly, M.I.; Al-Farsi, O.A.; Al-Shafaee, M.A.; Al-Khaduri, M.M.; Trivedi, M.S.; Deth, R.C. Effect of suboptimal breast-feeding on occurrence of autism: A case-control study. *Nutrition* **2012**, *28*, e27–32. [CrossRef]
126. Shafai, T.; Mustafa, M.; Hild, T.; Mulari, J.; Curtis, A. The association of early weaning and formula feeding with autism spectrum disorders. *Breastfeed. Med.* **2014**, *9*, 275–276. [CrossRef]
127. Steinman, G. Can the chance of having twins be modified by diet? *Lancet* **2006**, *367*, 1461–1462. [CrossRef]
128. Umer, A.; Hamilton, C.; Britton, C.M.; Mullett, M.D.; John, C.; Neal, W.; Lilly, C.L. Association between breastfeeding and childhood obesity: Analysis of a linked longitudinal study of rural Appalachian fifth-grade children. *Child. Obes.* **2015**, *11*, 449–455. [CrossRef] [PubMed]
129. Ortega-García, J.A.; Kloosterman, N.; Alvarez, L.; Tobarra-Sánchez, E.; Cárceles-Álvarez, A.; Pastor-Valero, R.; López-Hernández, F.A.; Sánchez-Solis, M.; Claudio, L. Full breastfeeding and obesity in children: A prospective study from birth to 6 years. *Child. Obes.* **2018**, *14*, 327–337. [CrossRef] [PubMed]
130. Yan, J.; Liu, L.; Zhu, Y.; Huang, G.; Wang, P.P. The association between breastfeeding and childhood obesity: A meta-analysis. *BMC Public Health* **2014**, *14*, 1267. [CrossRef] [PubMed]
131. Beccuti, G.; Pannain, S. Sleep and obesity. *Curr. Opin. Clin. Nutr. Metab. Care* **2011**, *14*, 402–412. [CrossRef] [PubMed]
132. Patel, S.R.; Hu, F.B. Short sleep duration and weight gain: A systematic review. *Obesity (Silver Spring)* **2008**, *16*, 643–653. [CrossRef] [PubMed]

133. Chen, X.; Beydoun, M.A.; Wang, Y. Is Sleep Duration Associated with Childhood Obesity? A Systematic Review and Meta-analysis. *Obesity* **2008**, *16*, 265–274. [CrossRef]
134. Fatima, Y.; Doi, S.A.; Mamun, A.A. Sleep quality and obesity in young subjects: A meta-analysis. *Obes. Rev.* **2016**, *17*, 1154–1166. [CrossRef]
135. Knutson, K.L. Does inadequate sleep play a role in vulnerability to obesity? *Am. J. Hum. Biol.* **2012**, *24*, 361–371. [CrossRef]
136. Chaput, J.-P.; Lambert, M.; Gray-Donald, K.; McGrath, J.J.; Tremblay, M.S.; O'Loughlin, J.; Tremblay, A. Short Sleep Duration Is Independently Associated with Overweight and Obesity in Quebec Children. *Can. J. Public Health* **2011**, *102*, 369–374.
137. Narang, I.; Mathew, J.L. Childhood obesity and obstructive sleep apnea. *J. Nutr. Metab.* **2012**, *2012*, 134202. [CrossRef]
138. Maxwell-Horn, A.; Malow, B.A. Sleep in Autism. *Semin. Neurol.* **2017**, *37*, 413–418. [PubMed]
139. Zuckerman, K.E.; Hill, A.P.; Guion, K.; Voltolina, L.; Fombonne, E. Overweight and Obesity: Prevalence and Correlates in a Large Clinical Sample of Children with Autism Spectrum Disorder. *J. Autism Dev. Disord.* **2014**, *44*, 1708–1719. [CrossRef] [PubMed]
140. Elrod, M.G.; Nylund, C.M.; Susi, A.L.; Gorman, G.H.; Hisle-Gorman, E.; Rogers, D.J.; Erdie-Lalena, C. Prevalence of Diagnosed Sleep Disorders and Related Diagnostic and Surgical Procedures in Children with Autism Spectrum Disorders. *J. Dev. Behav. Pediatr.* **2016**, *37*, 377–384. [CrossRef] [PubMed]
141. Bresnahan, M.; Hornig, M.; Schultz, A.F.; Gunnes, N.; Hirtz, D.; Lie, K.K.; Magnus, P.; Reichborn-Kjennerud, T.; Roth, C.; Schjølberg, S.; et al. Association of maternal report of infant and toddler gastrointestinal symptoms with autism: Evidence from a prospective birth cohort. *JAMA Psychiatry* **2015**, *72*, 466–474. [CrossRef] [PubMed]
142. McElhanon, B.O.; McCracken, C.; Karpen, S.; Sharp, W.G. Gastrointestinal Symptoms in Autism Spectrum Disorder: A Meta-analysis. *Pediatrics* **2014**, *133*, 872–883. [CrossRef] [PubMed]
143. Prosperi, M.; Santocchi, E.; Balboni, G.; Narzisi, A.; Bozza, M.; Fulceri, F.; Apicella, F.; Igliozzi, R.; Cosenza, A.; Tancredi, R.; et al. Behavioral phenotype of ASD preschoolers with gastrointestinal symptoms or food selectivity. *J. Autism Dev. Disord.* **2017**, *47*, 3574–3588. [CrossRef]
144. Mazefsky, C.A.; Borue, X.; Day, T.N.; Minshew, N.J. Emotion Regulation Patterns in Adolescents with High-Functioning Autism Spectrum Disorder: Comparison to Typically Developing Adolescents and Association With Psychiatric Symptoms. *Autism Res.* **2014**, *7*, 344–354. [CrossRef] [PubMed]
145. Mayer, E.A.; Padua, D.; Tillisch, K. Altered brain-gut axis in autism: Comorbidity or causative mechanisms? *Bioessays* **2014**, *36*, 933–939. [CrossRef]
146. Strati, F.; Cavalieri, D.; Albanese, D.; De Felice, C.; Donati, C.; Hayek, J.; Jousson, O.; Leoncini, S.; Renzi, D.; Calabrò, A.; et al. New evidences on the altered gut microbiota in autism spectrum disorders. *Microbiome* **2017**, *5*, 24. [CrossRef]
147. Williams, B.L.; Hornig, M.; Buie, T.; Bauman, M.L.; Paik, M.C.; Wick, I.; Bennett, A.; Jabado, O.; Hirschberg, D.L.; Lipkin, W.I. Impaired carbohydrate digestion and transport and mucosal dysbiosis in the intestines of children with autism and gastrointestinal disturbances. *PLoS ONE* **2011**, *6*, e24585. [CrossRef]
148. Zhang, M.; Ma, W.; Zhang, J.; He, Y.; Wang, J. Analysis of gut microbiota profiles and microbe-disease associations in children with autism spectrum disorders in China. *Sci. Rep.* **2018**, *8*, 13981. [CrossRef] [PubMed]
149. Chakraborti, C.K. New-found link between microbiota and obesity. *World J. Gastrointest. Pathophysiol.* **2015**, *6*, 110–119. [CrossRef] [PubMed]
150. Koliada, A.; Syzenko, G.; Moseiko, V.; Budovska, L.; Puchkov, K.; Perederiy, V.; Gavalko, Y.; Dorofeyev, A.; Romanenko, M.; Tkach, S.; et al. Association between body mass index and firmicutes/bacteroidetes ratio in an adult Ukrainian population. *BMC Microbiol.* **2017**, *17*, 120. [CrossRef] [PubMed]
151. Indiani, C.M.D.S.P.; Rizzardi, K.F.; Castelo, P.M.; Ferraz, L.F.C.; Darrieux, M.; Parisotto, T.M. Childhood obesity and firmicutes/bacteroidetes ratio in the gut microbiota: A systematic review. *Child. Obes.* **2018**, *14*, 501–509. [CrossRef] [PubMed]
152. Ley, R.E.; Bäckhed, F.; Turnbaugh, P.; Lozupone, C.A.; Knight, R.D.; Gordon, J.I. Obesity alters gut microbial ecology. *Proc. Natl. Acad. Sci. USA* **2005**, *102*, 11070–11075. [CrossRef] [PubMed]

153. Murphy, E.F.; Cotter, P.D.; Healy, S.; Marques, T.M.; O'Sullivan, O.; Fouhy, F.; Clarke, S.F.; O'Toole, P.W.; Quigley, E.M.; Stanton, C.; et al. Composition and energy harvesting capacity of the gut microbiota: Relationship to diet, obesity and time in mouse models. *Gut* **2010**, *59*, 1635–1642. [CrossRef]
154. Bäckhed, F.; Roswall, J.; Peng, Y.; Feng, Q.; Jia, H.; Kovatcheva-Datchary, P.; Li, Y.; Xia, Y.; Xie, H.; Zhong, H.; et al. Dynamics and stabilization of the human gut microbiome during the first year of life. *Cell Host Microbe* **2015**, *17*, 690–703. [CrossRef]
155. Liu, F.; Li, J.; Wu, F.; Zheng, H.; Peng, Q.; Zhou, H. Altered composition and function of intestinal microbiota in autism spectrum disorders: A systematic review. *Transl. Psychiatry* **2019**, *9*, 43. [CrossRef]
156. Sharon, G.; Cruz, N.J.; Kang, D.-W.; Gandal, M.J.; Wang, B.; Kim, Y.-M.; Zink, E.M.; Casey, C.P.; Taylor, B.C.; Lane, C.J.; et al. Human Gut Microbiota from Autism Spectrum Disorder Promote Behavioral Symptoms in Mice. *Cell* **2019**, *177*, 1600–1618. [CrossRef]
157. Jazani, N.H.; Savoj, J.; Lustgarten, M.; Lau, W.L.; Vaziri, N.D. Impact of gut dysbiosis on neurohormonal pathways in chronic kidney disease. *Diseases* **2019**, *7*, 21. [CrossRef]
158. Siniscalco, D.; Brigida, A.L.; Antonucci, N. Autism and neuro-immune-gut link. *Molecular* **2018**, *5*, 166–172. [CrossRef]
159. Siniscalco, D.; Schultz, S.; Brigida, A.L.; Antonucci, N. Inflammation and Neuro-Immune Dysregulations in Autism Spectrum Disorders. *Pharmaceuticals* **2018**, *11*, 56. [CrossRef] [PubMed]
160. Fiorentino, M.; Sapone, A.; Senger, S.; Camhi, S.S.; Kadzielski, S.M.; Buie, T.M.; Kelly, D.L.; Cascella, N.; Fasano, A. Blood-brain barrier and intestinal epithelial barrier alterations in autism spectrum disorders. *Mol. Autism* **2016**, *7*, 49. [CrossRef] [PubMed]
161. Cani, P.D.; Amar, J.; Iglesias, M.A.; Poggi, M.; Knauf, C.; Bastelica, D.; Neyrinck, A.M.; Fava, F.; Tuohy, K.M.; Chabo, C.; et al. Metabolic endotoxemia initiates obesity and insulin resistance. *Diabetes* **2007**, *56*, 1761–1772. [CrossRef]
162. Boulangé, C.L.; Neves, A.L.; Chilloux, J.; Nicholson, J.K.; Dumas, M.-E. Impact of the gut microbiota on inflammation, obesity, and metabolic disease. *Genome Med.* **2016**, *8*, 42. [CrossRef]
163. Kang, Y.; Cai, Y. Gut microbiota and obesity: Implications for fecal microbiota transplantation therapy. *Hormones (Athens)* **2017**, *16*, 223–234. [CrossRef]
164. Esnafoglu, E.; Cırrık, S.; Ayyıldız, S.N.; Erdil, A.; Ertürk, E.Y.; Dağlı, A.; Noyan, T. Increased Serum Zonulin Levels as an Intestinal Permeability Marker in Autistic Subjects. *J. Pediatr.* **2017**, *188*, 240–244. [CrossRef]
165. De Magistris, L.; Familiari, V.; Pascotto, A.; Sapone, A.; Frolli, A.; Iardino, P.; Carteni, M.; De Rosa, M.; Francavilla, R.; Riegler, G.; et al. Alterations of the intestinal barrier in patients with autism spectrum disorders and in their first-degree relatives. *J. Pediatr. Gastroenterol. Nutr.* **2010**, *51*, 418–424. [CrossRef]
166. Kushak, R.I.; Buie, T.M.; Murray, K.F.; Newburg, D.S.; Chen, C.; Nestoridi, E.; Winter, H.S. Evaluation of Intestinal Function in Children with Autism and Gastrointestinal Symptoms. *J. Pediatr. Gastroenterol. Nutr.* **2016**, *62*, 687–691. [CrossRef]
167. Adams, J.B.; Johansen, L.J.; Powell, L.D.; Quig, D.; Rubin, R.A. Gastrointestinal flora and gastrointestinal status in children with autism—comparisons to typical children and correlation with autism severity. *BMC Gastroenterol.* **2011**, *11*, 22. [CrossRef]
168. Morrison, D.J.; Preston, T. Formation of short chain fatty acids by the gut microbiota and their impact on human metabolism. *Gut Microbes* **2016**, *7*, 189–200. [CrossRef] [PubMed]
169. Valdes, A.M.; Walter, J.; Segal, E.; Spector, T.D. Role of the gut microbiota in nutrition and health. *BMJ* **2018**, *361*, k2179. [CrossRef] [PubMed]
170. Yang, J.; Wang, H.-P.; Zhou, L.; Xu, C.-F. Effect of dietary fiber on constipation: A meta analysis. *World J. Gastroenterol.* **2012**, *18*, 7378–7383. [CrossRef] [PubMed]
171. Zou, J.; Chassaing, B.; Singh, V.; Pellizzon, M.; Ricci, M.; Fythe, M.D.; Kumar, M.V.; Gewirtz, A.T. Fiber-Mediated Nourishment of Gut Microbiota Protects against Diet-Induced Obesity by Restoring IL-22-Mediated Colonic Health. *Cell Host Microbe* **2018**, *23*, 41–53. [CrossRef] [PubMed]
172. Deehan, E.C.; Walter, J. The Fiber Gap and the Disappearing Gut Microbiome: Implications for Human Nutrition. *Trends Endocrinol. Metab.* **2016**, *27*, 239–242. [CrossRef] [PubMed]
173. Larraufie, P.; Martin-Gallausiaux, C.; Lapaque, N.; Dore, J.; Gribble, F.M.; Reimann, F.; Blottiere, H.M. SCFAs strongly stimulate PYY production in human enteroendocrine cells. *Sci. Rep.* **2018**, *8*, 74. [CrossRef] [PubMed]

174. Willemsen, L.E.M.; Koetsier, M.A.; van Deventer, S.J.H.; van Tol, E.A. Short chain fatty acids stimulate epithelial mucin 2 expression through differential effects on prostaglandin E(1) and E(2) production by intestinal myofibroblasts. *Gut* **2003**, *52*, 1442–1447. [CrossRef]
175. Macia, L.; Tan, J.; Vieira, A.T.; Leach, K.; Stanley, D.; Luong, S.; Maruya, M.; Ian McKenzie, C.; Hijikata, A.; Wong, C.; et al. Metabolite-sensing receptors GPR43 and GPR109A facilitate dietary fibre-induced gut homeostasis through regulation of the inflammasome. *Nat. Commun.* **2015**, *6*, 6734. [CrossRef]
176. Mirmonsef, P.; Zariffard, M.R.; Gilbert, D.; Makinde, H.; Landay, A.L.; Spear, G.T. Short Chain Fatty Acids Induce Pro-Inflammatory Cytokine Production Alone and in Combination with Toll-like Receptor Ligands. *Am. J. Reprod. Immunol.* **2012**, *67*, 391–400. [CrossRef]
177. Chambers, E.S.; Viardot, A.; Psichas, A.; Morrison, D.J.; Murphy, K.G.; Zac-Varghese, S.E.K.; MacDougall, K.; Preston, T.; Tedford, C.; Finlayson, G.S.; et al. Effects of targeted delivery of propionate to the human colon on appetite regulation, body weight maintenance and adiposity in overweight adults. *Gut* **2015**, *64*, 1744–1754. [CrossRef]
178. De Vadder, F.; Kovatcheva-Datchary, P.; Goncalves, D.; Vinera, J.; Zitoun, C.; Duchampt, A.; Bäckhed, F.; Mithieux, G. Microbiota-generated metabolites promote metabolic benefits via gut-brain neural circuits. *Cell* **2014**, *156*, 84–96. [CrossRef] [PubMed]
179. Zmora, N.; Soffer, E.; Elinav, E. Transforming medicine with the microbiome. *Sci. Transl. Med.* **2019**, *11*, eaaw1815. [CrossRef] [PubMed]
180. Ahima, R.S. Revisiting leptin's role in obesity and weight loss. *J. Clin. Invest.* **2008**, *118*, 2380–2383. [CrossRef] [PubMed]
181. Klein, S.; Coppack, S.W.; Mohamed-Ali, V.; Landt, M. Adipose tissue leptin production and plasma leptin kinetics in humans. *Diabetes* **1996**, *45*, 984–987. [CrossRef] [PubMed]
182. Park, H.-K.; Ahima, R.S. Physiology of leptin: Energy homeostasis, neuroendocrine function and metabolism. *Metabolism* **2015**, *64*, 24–34. [CrossRef] [PubMed]
183. Mazor, R.; Friedmann-Morvinski, D.; Alsaigh, T.; Kleifeld, O.; Kistler, E.B.; Rousso-Noori, L.; Huang, C.; Li, J.B.; Verma, I.M.; Schmid-Schönbein, G.W. Cleavage of the leptin receptor by matrix metalloproteinase-2 promotes leptin resistance and obesity in mice. *Sci. Transl. Med.* **2018**, *10*, eaah6324. [CrossRef] [PubMed]
184. Myers, M.G.; Leibel, R.L.; Seeley, R.J.; Schwartz, M.W. Obesity and leptin resistance: Distinguishing cause from effect. *Trends Endocrinol. Metab.* **2010**, *21*, 643–651. [CrossRef] [PubMed]
185. Al-Zaid, F.S.; Alhader, A.A.; Al-Ayadhi, L.Y. Altered ghrelin levels in boys with autism: A novel finding associated with hormonal dysregulation. *Sci. Rep.* **2014**, *4*, 6478. [CrossRef]
186. Rodrigues, D.H.; Rocha, N.P.; Sousa, L.F.; Barbosa, I.G.; Kummer, A.; Teixeira, A.L. Changes in adipokine levels in autism spectrum disorders. *Neuropsychobiology* **2014**, *69*, 6–10. [CrossRef]
187. Raghavan, R.; Zuckerman, B.; Hong, X.; Wang, G.; Yuelong, J.; Paige, D.; DiBari, J.; Zhang, C.; Fallin, M.D.; Wang, X. Fetal and infancy growth pattern, cord and early childhood plasma leptin, and development of autism spectrum disorder in the Boston birth cohort. *Autism Res.* **2018**, *11*, 1416–1431. [CrossRef]
188. Hasan, Z.A.; Al-Kafaji, G.; Al-Sherawi, M.I.; Razzak, R.A.; Eltayeb, D.; Skrypnk, C.; Bakhiet, M. Investigation of serum levels of leptin, ghrelin and growth hormone in Bahraini children with autism. *Int. Arch. Transl. Med.* **2019**, *5*, 7. [CrossRef]
189. Chawarska, K.; Campbell, D.; Chen, L.; Shic, F.; Klin, A.; Chang, J. Early Generalized Overgrowth in Boys with Autism. *Arch. Gen. Psychiatry* **2011**, *68*, 1021–1031. [CrossRef] [PubMed]
190. Lihn, A.S.; Pedersen, S.B.; Richelsen, B. Adiponectin: Action, regulation and association to insulin sensitivity. *Obes. Rev.* **2005**, *6*, 13–21. [CrossRef] [PubMed]
191. Arita, Y.; Kihara, S.; Ouchi, N.; Takahashi, M.; Maeda, K.; Miyagawa, J.; Hotta, K.; Shimomura, I.; Nakamura, T.; Miyaoka, K.; et al. Paradoxical decrease of an adipose-specific protein, adiponectin, in obesity. *Biochem. Biophys. Res. Commun.* **1999**, *257*, 79–83. [CrossRef] [PubMed]
192. Ouchi, N.; Walsh, K. Adiponectin as an anti-inflammatory factor. *Clin. Chim. Acta* **2007**, *380*, 24–30. [CrossRef] [PubMed]
193. Kawano, J.; Arora, R. The role of adiponectin in obesity, diabetes, and cardiovascular disease. *J. Cardiometab. Syndr.* **2009**, *4*, 44–49. [CrossRef]
194. Achari, A.E.; Jain, S.K. Adiponectin, a Therapeutic Target for Obesity, Diabetes, and Endothelial Dysfunction. *Int. J. Mol. Sci.* **2017**, *18*, 1321. [CrossRef]

195. Ghaffari, M.A.; Mousavinejad, E.; Riahi, F.; Mousavinejad, M.; Afsharmanesh, M.R. Increased Serum Levels of Tumor Necrosis Factor-Alpha, Resistin, and Visfatin in the Children with Autism Spectrum Disorders: A Case-Control Study. *Neurol. Res. Int.* **2016**, *2016*, 7. [CrossRef]
196. Fujita-Shimizu, A.; Suzuki, K.; Nakamura, K.; Miyachi, T.; Matsuzaki, H.; Kajizuka, M.; Shinmura, C.; Iwata, Y.; Suda, S.; Tsuchiya, K.J.; et al. Decreased serum levels of adiponectin in subjects with autism. *Prog. Neuropsychopharmacol. Biol. Psychiatry* **2010**, *34*, 455–458. [CrossRef]
197. Raghavan, R.; Fallin, M.D.; Hong, X.; Wang, G.; Ji, Y.; Stuart, E.A.; Paige, D.; Wang, X. Cord and Early Childhood Plasma Adiponectin Levels and Autism Risk: A Prospective Birth Cohort Study. *J. Autism Dev. Disord.* **2019**, *49*, 173–184. [CrossRef]
198. Song, H.J.; Oh, S.; Quan, S.; Ryu, O.-H.; Jeong, J.-Y.; Hong, K.-S.; Kim, D.-H. Gender differences in adiponectin levels and body composition in older adults: Hallym aging study. *BMC Geriatr.* **2014**, *14*, 8. [CrossRef] [PubMed]
199. Ohman-Hanson, R.A.; Cree-Green, M.; Kelsey, M.M.; Bessesen, D.H.; Sharp, T.A.; Pyle, L.; Pereira, R.I.; Nadeau, K.J. Ethnic and Sex Differences in Adiponectin: From Childhood to Adulthood. *J. Clin. Endocrinol. Metab.* **2016**, *101*, 4808–4815. [CrossRef] [PubMed]
200. Rueda-Clausen, C.F.; Lahera, V.; Calderón, J.; Bolivar, I.C.; Castillo, V.R.; Gutiérrez, M.; Carreño, M.; Oubiña, M.d.P.; Cachofeiro, V.; López-Jaramillo, P. The presence of abdominal obesity is associated with changes in vascular function independently of other cardiovascular risk factors. *Int. J. Cardiol.* **2010**, *139*, 32–41. [CrossRef] [PubMed]
201. Cummings, D.E.; Shannon, M.H. Roles for Ghrelin in the Regulation of Appetite and Body Weight. *Arch. Surg.* **2003**, *138*, 389–396. [CrossRef] [PubMed]
202. Makris, C.M.; Alexandrou, A.; Papatsoutsos, G.E.; Malietzis, G.; Tsilimigras, I.D.; Guerron, D.A.; Moris, D. Ghrelin and obesity: Identifying gaps and dispelling myths a reappraisal. *Vivo* **2017**, *31*, 1047–1050.
203. Lebenthal, Y.; Gat-Yablonski, G.; Shtaif, B.; Padoa, A.; Phillip, M.; Lazar, L. Effect of sex hormone administration on circulating ghrelin levels in peripubertal children. *J. Clin. Endocrinol. Metab.* **2006**, *91*, 328–331. [CrossRef] [PubMed]
204. Sanchez, C.E.; Barry, C.; Sabhlok, A.; Russell, K.; Majors, A.; Kollins, S.H.; Fuemmeler, B.F. Maternal pre-pregnancy obesity and child neurodevelopmental outcomes: A meta-analysis. *Obes. Rev.* **2018**, *19*, 464–484. [CrossRef]
205. Li, Y.-M.; Ou, J.-J.; Liu, L.; Zhang, D.; Zhao, J.-P.; Tang, S.-Y. Association Between Maternal Obesity and Autism Spectrum Disorder in Offspring: A Meta-analysis. *J. Autism Dev. Disord.* **2016**, *46*, 95–102. [CrossRef]
206. Xu, G.; Jing, J.; Bowers, K.; Liu, B.; Bao, W. Maternal Diabetes and the Risk of Autism Spectrum Disorders in the Offspring: A Systematic Review and Meta-Analysis. *J. Autism Dev. Disord.* **2014**, *44*, 766–775. [CrossRef]
207. Wan, H.; Zhang, C.; Li, H.; Luan, S.; Liu, C. Association of maternal diabetes with autism spectrum disorders in offspring. *Medicine (Baltimore)* **2018**, *97*, e9438. [CrossRef]
208. Krakowiak, P.; Walker, C.K.; Bremer, A.A.; Baker, A.S.; Ozonoff, S.; Hansen, R.L.; Hertz-Picciotto, I. Maternal metabolic conditions and risk for autism and other neurodevelopmental disorders. *Pediatrics* **2012**, *129*, e1121–e1128. [CrossRef] [PubMed]
209. Eidelman, A.I.; Samueloff, A. The pathophysiology of the fetus of the diabetic mother. *Semin. Perinatol.* **2002**, *26*, 232–236. [CrossRef] [PubMed]
210. Burstyn, I.; Wang, X.; Yasui, Y.; Sithole, F.; Zwaigenbaum, L. Autism spectrum disorders and fetal hypoxia in a population-based cohort: Accounting for missing exposures via Estimation-Maximization algorithm. *BMC Med. Res. Methodol.* **2011**, *11*, 2. [CrossRef] [PubMed]
211. Kolevzon, A.; Gross, R.; Reichenberg, A. Prenatal and Perinatal Risk Factors for Autism: A Review and Integration of Findings. *Arch. Pediatr. Adolesc. Med.* **2007**, *161*, 326–333. [CrossRef] [PubMed]
212. Ming, X.; Stein, T.P.; Brimacombe, M.; Johnson, W.G.; Lambert, G.H.; Wagner, G.C. Increased excretion of a lipid peroxidation biomarker in autism. *Prostaglandins Leukot. Essent. Fat. Acids* **2005**, *73*, 379–384. [CrossRef] [PubMed]
213. Chen, X.; Scholl, T.O. Oxidative stress: Changes in pregnancy and with gestational diabetes mellitus. *Curr. Diab. Rep.* **2005**, *5*, 282–288. [CrossRef]
214. Onore, C.; Careaga, M.; Ashwood, P. The role of immune dysfunction in the pathophysiology of autism. *Brain Behav. Immun.* **2012**, *26*, 383–392. [CrossRef]

215. Kawasaki, M.; Arata, N.; Miyazaki, C.; Mori, R.; Kikuchi, T.; Ogawa, Y.; Ota, E. Obesity and abnormal glucose tolerance in offspring of diabetic mothers: A systematic review and meta-analysis. *PLoS ONE* **2018**, *13*, e0190676. [CrossRef]
216. Deierlein, A.L.; Siega-Riz, A.M.; Chantala, K.; Herring, A.H. The Association Between Maternal Glucose Concentration and Child BMI at Age 3 Years. *Diabetes Care* **2011**, *34*, 480–484. [CrossRef]
217. Lawlor, D.A.; Lichtenstein, P.; Långström, N. Association of maternal diabetes mellitus in pregnancy with offspring adiposity into early adulthood: Sibling study in a prospective cohort of 280,866 men from 248,293 families. *Circulation* **2011**, *123*, 258–265. [CrossRef]
218. Ash, T.; Agaronov, A.; Young, T.; Aftosmes-Tobio, A.; Davison, K.K. Family-based childhood obesity prevention interventions: A systematic review and quantitative content analysis. *Int. J. Behav. Nutr. Phys. Act.* **2017**, *14*, 113. [CrossRef] [PubMed]
219. Bennett, E.A.; Kolko, R.; Chia, L.; Elliott, J.P.; Kalarchian, M.A. Treatment of Obesity among Youth with Intellectual and Developmental Disabilities: An Emerging Role for Telenursing. *West. J. Nurs. Res.* **2017**, *39*, 1008–1027. [CrossRef] [PubMed]
220. Freemark, M. Pharmacotherapy of Childhood Obesity: An evidence-based, conceptual approach. *Diabetes Care* **2007**, *30*, 395–402. [CrossRef] [PubMed]
221. Heck, A.M.; Yanovski, J.A.; Calis, K.A. Orlistat, a new lipase inhibitor for the management of obesity. *Pharmacotherapy* **2000**, *20*, 270–279. [CrossRef] [PubMed]
222. Wang, L.W.; Tancredi, D.J.; Thomas, D.W. The prevalence of gastrointestinal problems in children across the United States with autism spectrum disorders from families with multiple affected members. *J. Dev. Behav. Pediatr.* **2011**, *32*, 351–360. [CrossRef] [PubMed]
223. Mohammed, M.A.; Moles, R.J.; Chen, T.F. Medication-related burden and patients' lived experience with medicine: A systematic review and metasynthesis of qualitative studies. *BMJ Open* **2016**, *6*, e010035. [CrossRef]
224. Taylor, V.H. Implementing antiobesity treatment in a patient with a mood disorder. *J. Psychiatry Neurosci.* **2008**, *33*, E1–E2. [PubMed]
225. Canoy, D.; Yang, T.O. Obesity in children: Bariatric surgery. *BMJ Clin. Evid.* **2015**, *2015*, 325.
226. Bochukova, E.G.; Huang, N.; Keogh, J.; Henning, E.; Purmann, C.; Blaszczyk, K.; Saeed, S.; Hamilton-Shield, J.; Clayton-Smith, J.; O'Rahilly, S.; et al. Large, rare chromosomal deletions associated with severe early-onset obesity. *Nature* **2010**, *463*, 666–670. [CrossRef]
227. Inge, T.H.; Courcoulas, A.P.; Jenkins, T.M.; Michalsky, M.P.; Brandt, M.L.; Xanthakos, S.A.; Dixon, J.B.; Harmon, C.M.; Chen, M.K.; Xie, C.; et al. Five-Year Outcomes of Gastric Bypass in Adolescents as Compared with Adults. *N. Engl. J. Med.* **2019**, *380*, 2136–2145. [CrossRef]
228. Maiano, M.C.; Normand, C.L.; Aime, A.; Begarie, J. Lifestyle interventions targeting changes in body weight and composition among youth with an intellectual disability: A systematic review. *Res. Dev. Disabil.* **2014**, *35*, 1914–1926. [CrossRef] [PubMed]
229. Styne, D.M.; Arslanian, S.A.; Connor, E.L.; Farooqi, I.S.; Murad, M.H.; Silverstein, J.H.; Yanovski, J.A. Pediatric obesity—Assessment, treatment, and prevention: An endocrine society clinical practice guideline. *J. Clin. Endocrinol. Metab.* **2017**, *102*, 709–757. [CrossRef] [PubMed]

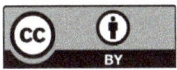 © 2019 by the authors. Licensee MDPI, Basel, Switzerland. This article is an open access article distributed under the terms and conditions of the Creative Commons Attribution (CC BY) license (http://creativecommons.org/licenses/by/4.0/).

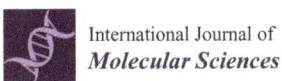

Article

ASD Phenotype—Genotype Associations in Concordant and Discordant Monozygotic and Dizygotic Twins Stratified by Severity of Autistic Traits

Valerie W. Hu *, Christine A. Devlin † and Jessica J. Debski ‡

Department of Biochemistry and Molecular Medicine, School of Medicine and Health Sciences, The George Washington University, Washington, DC 20037, USA
* Correspondence: valhu@gwu.edu; Tel.: +1-202-994-8431
† Current address: Department of Biochemistry, University of Illinois at Urbana-Champaign, Urbana, IL 61801, USA.
‡ Current address: Rowan University School of Osteopathic Medicine, 1 Medical Center Dr., Stratford, NJ 08084, USA.

Received: 13 July 2019; Accepted: 31 July 2019; Published: 3 August 2019

Abstract: Autism spectrum disorder (ASD) is a highly heterogeneous neurodevelopmental disorder characterized by impaired social communication coupled with stereotyped behaviors and restricted interests. Despite the high concordance rate for diagnosis, there is little information on the magnitude of genetic contributions to specific ASD behaviors. Using behavioral/trait severity scores from the Autism Diagnostic Interview-Revised (ADI-R) diagnostic instrument, we compared the phenotypic profiles of mono- and dizygotic twins where both co-twins were diagnosed with ASD or only one twin had a diagnosis. The trait distribution profiles across the respective twin populations were first used for quantitative trait association analyses using publicly available genome-wide genotyping data. Trait-associated single nucleotide polymorphisms (SNPs) were then used for case-control association analyses, in which cases were defined as individuals in the lowest (Q1) and highest (Q4) quartiles of the severity distribution curves for each trait. While all of the ASD-diagnosed twins exhibited similar trait severity profiles, the non-autistic dizygotic twins exhibited significantly lower ADI-R item scores than the non-autistic monozygotic twins. Case-control association analyses of twins stratified by trait severity revealed statistically significant SNPs with odds ratios that clearly distinguished individuals in Q4 from those in Q1. While the level of shared genomic variation is a strong determinant of the severity of autistic traits in the discordant non-autistic twins, the similarity of trait profiles in the concordantly autistic dizygotic twins also suggests a role for environmental influences. Stratification of cases by trait severity resulted in the identification of statistically significant SNPs located near genes over-represented within autism gene datasets.

Keywords: autism; genetics; quantitative traits; stratification by trait severity; heterogeneity reduction; case-control association analysis

---

1. Introduction

Autism spectrum disorder (ASD) is a highly heritable and heterogeneous neurodevelopmental disorder which is characterized by deficits in social communication and reciprocal interactions as well as by stereotyped behavior and restricted interests, often accompanied by language difficulties, especially in the area of pragmatics [1]. ASD is often comorbid with disorders such as anxiety, attention-deficit/hyperactivity disorder, and intellectual disability, and some affected individuals also suffer from gastrointestinal, immune system, and sleep disorders, suggestive of systemic dysregulation.

Severity levels of autism vary broadly with some cases having only mild deficits in social interactions, while other cases exhibit severe deficits in social behaviors and manifest noticeably aberrant stereotypic behaviors, including self-injury. Boys are four times more likely than girls to have an ASD diagnosis and treatment options are limited in part due to the heterogeneity of the disorder as well as a lack of knowledge of the underlying biology [2].

Ever since the twin study of Bailey et al. [3] reported a concordance rate for autism of 60% for genetically identical monozygotic (MZ) twins and 0% for dizygotic (DZ) twins, autism has been perceived as a strongly genetic disorder. However, a review of twin studies conducted between 1977 and 2011 suggests that concordance rates for autism are quite variable ranging from 36% to 96% for MZ twins, depending in part on sex as well as whether or not the diagnosis was narrowly defined (i.e., strict autism) or more broadly defined as autism spectrum disorder (ASD) [4]. The differences in concordance rates and the incomplete penetrance have been attributed to undefined environmental factors. To tease out the contributions of genetics and environment, there have been increased efforts to assemble large twin cohorts not only for genetic analyses but also for studies on the associated phenotypes of autism, including neurodevelopmental differences [5–8]. In fact, heritability rates of ASD vary greatly in different studies conducted since 2011, with Hallmayer et al. reporting a moderate genetic effect of 38% [9], Gaugler et al. reporting a narrow-sense (strictly defined) autism heritability of 52% [10], and Tick et al. estimating heritability at 64–91% in a meta-analysis of twin studies [11], with each study acknowledging the effects of shared environment to explain the non-genetic component of ASD. Heritability studies that included subclinical (i.e., broad autism phenotype) diagnoses also indicate that heritability is determined by both genetics and non-shared environment, but that concordance rates are somewhat dependent on diagnostic method [12]. Using three different diagnostic methods, Colvert et al. showed that concordance rates among monozygotic twins ranged from 62% to 75%, while the rate varied from 5% to 40% among dizygotic twins. More recently, several studies using monozygotic and dizygotic twins have investigated the association between autistic traits and specific phenotypes, such as atypical sensory reactivity [13], face identify recognition [14], and social cognition [15], with all of these studies reinforcing genetic links to these phenotypes. However, few studies have used a broad range of specific phenotypic differences among clinically discordant non-autistic twins to determine how zygosity influences the severity of autistic traits.

While twin studies make it apparent that genetics plays a significant role in ASD and associated phenotypes, no one genetic profile emerges due to the heterogeneity of ASD. In order to overcome this issue, some groups have attempted to reduce the heterogeneity by clustering individuals according to clinical, behavioral, or molecular subphenotypes. Previously, we used cluster analyses of severity scores on a broad spectrum of traits and behaviors probed by the Autism Diagnostic Interview-Revised (ADI-R) instrument [16] to identify four phenotypic subgroups of individuals which were qualitatively described as severely language-impaired, intermediate, mild, and savant [17]. In addition, transcriptomic analyses of lymphoblastoid cell lines derived from individuals in three of the four subgroups showed that the ASD subgroups could be distinguished from a group of non-autistic controls as well as from each other, suggesting the contribution of different biological processes to specific subphenotypes of ASD [18]. Furthermore, case-control association analyses based upon the four ASD phenotypic subgroups using SNPs derived from quantitative trait association analyses which were based on ADI-R scores for multiple traits identified novel and statistically significant SNPs that were subtype-dependent [19]. Similarly, a linkage analysis based on these subphenotypes revealed novel genetic loci with highly significant LOD scores that were not detected in the absence of subtyping in addition to intra-family phenotypic and genetic heterogeneity [20]. Another study used a cohort of ASD individuals with extreme sleep onset delay as a means to decrease heterogeneity of cases to tease out significant variants in genes for melatonin pathway enzymes [21]. Recently, subgrouping of females with autism using X chromosome inactivation status as an epigenetic marker revealed a novel alternatively-spliced isoform of an X-linked chromatin gene, KDM5C, which contained the 3′UTR from a retrotransposed gene and was differentially expressed in this subgroup of autistic females relative to controls [22]. Collectively, these studies based on reducing heterogeneity among cases suggest the potential for relating genotype as well as gene structure with specific subphenotypes of ASD. However, there is little information on the relationship between genotype and the specific traits or subphenotypes observed in ASD.

The goals of this study were to: (1) investigate how genetics influences specific autism-associated behaviors and traits among monozygotic versus dizygotic twins, either concordant or discordant for autism diagnosis; (2) utilize ASD trait distribution profiles based on individual ADI-R scores in quantitative trait association analyses to identify single nucleotide polymorphisms (SNPs or quantitative trait nucleotides [QTNs]) that associate with specific traits; (3) determine whether the QTNs can differentiate cases from controls using individuals with ASD at the extremes of each trait distribution profile to reduce the phenotypic heterogeneity of cases for case-control association analyses; and (4) identify genes, pathways, and biological functions associated with specific traits. The results of these deep phenotyping analyses suggest that while shared genotype is a strong determinant of the severity of autistic traits in discordant monozygotic twins, the similarity of trait profiles of genetically distinct dizygotic twins concordant for diagnosis of ASD also suggests a role for shared environment. Moreover, genetic analyses which utilize both quantitative trait and case-control association analyses in which clinical or phenotypic heterogeneity is reduced by limiting the cases to those at the extremes of trait severities reveal highly significant SNPs associated with genes enriched in autism datasets and over-represented in neurological functions relevant to ASD.

2. Results

2.1. Deep Phenotypic Analyses of MZ and DZ Twins: Influence of Zygosity and Diagnostic Concordance

A total of 284 pairs of twins represented in the Autism Genetic Resource Exchange (AGRE) were included in this study. The twins were sorted into subgroups based on validated zygosity (monozygotic versus dizygotic) as well as by diagnostic concordance (concordant or discordant) for ASD. Each individual's ADI-R scores for 88 items covering five ASD traits (spoken language, nonverbal communication, play skills, social interactions, and perseverative behaviors) were downloaded from AGRE and were used to establish trait severity distribution profiles for each subgroup of twins (Figure 1, see legend for nomenclature used for different twin subgroups). Among discordant twins who do not meet the ADI-R diagnostic criteria for autism (i.e., non-autistic co-twins), the trait distribution profiles show noticeably lower severity, as indicated by lower cumulative trait scores, among the DZ twins in comparison to the MZ twins. On the other hand, the discordant MZ and DZ twins who received an autism diagnosis exhibited similar severity profiles across each trait which closely tracked the severity profiles of both MZ and DZ twins who were concordant for autism diagnosis.

Boxplots of the cumulative trait scores for each trait exhibit the same pattern of severity where the non-autistic DZ twins have a significantly lower average severity for each trait in comparison to the non-autistic MZ twins, but all ASD-diagnosed twins exhibit similar average trait severity scores, regardless of zygosity or concordance (Figure 2). The comparisons of average severity scores for all ADI-R items that comprise each trait also reveal significant differences (p-values ≤ 0.05) between the non-autistic MZ and DZ twins for a majority of the items (Figure 3). Taken together, the significantly higher trait severity of non-autistic MZ twins in comparison to non-autistic DZ twins supports the notion that genetics is a strong determinant of the severity of virtually all autistic traits and behaviors, even in undiagnosed individuals. On the other hand, the almost identical severity profiles of the concordantly autistic but genetically different DZ co-twins suggest that shared environment may also contribute to trait severity. However, the specific relationships among genotype, environmental factors, and ASD phenotypes remain unknown.

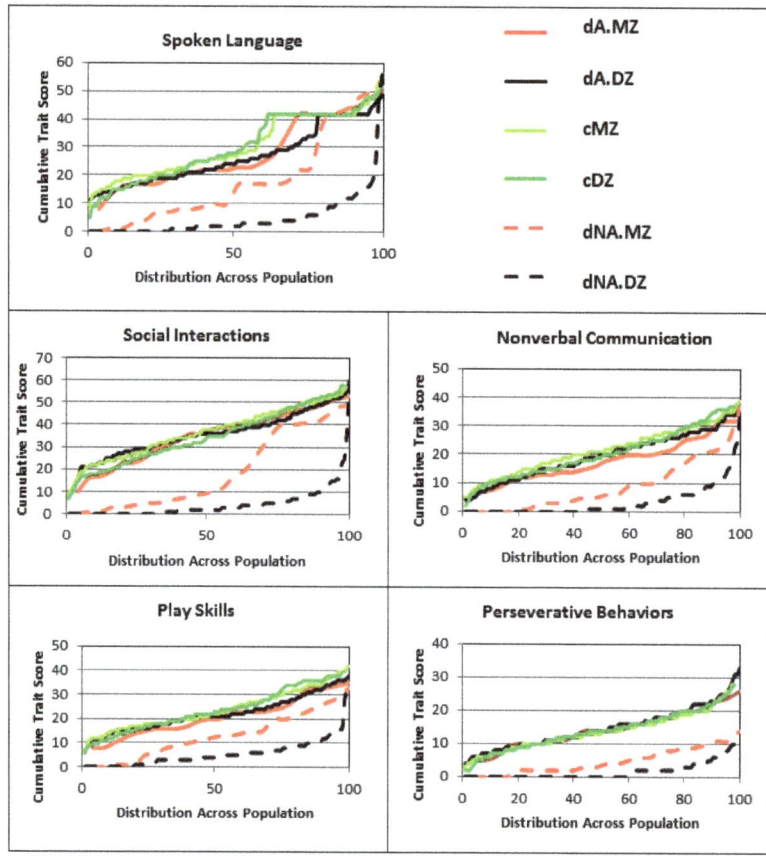

Figure 1. Phenotypic (trait) profiles based on cumulative ADI-R scores for spoken language, nonverbal communication, play skills, social skills/interactions, and perseverative behaviors. In order to better compare the distribution of traits in each twin subgroup, the total number of individuals comprising each group was normalized to 100. The concordant autistic monozygotic (MZ) and dizygotic (DZ) twin subgroups are identified as cMZ and cDZ, respectively, and the discordant autistic (dA) and non-autistic (dNA) MZ and DZ twin subgroups are referred to as dA.MZ, dA.DZ, dNA.MZ, and dNA.DZ, respectively.

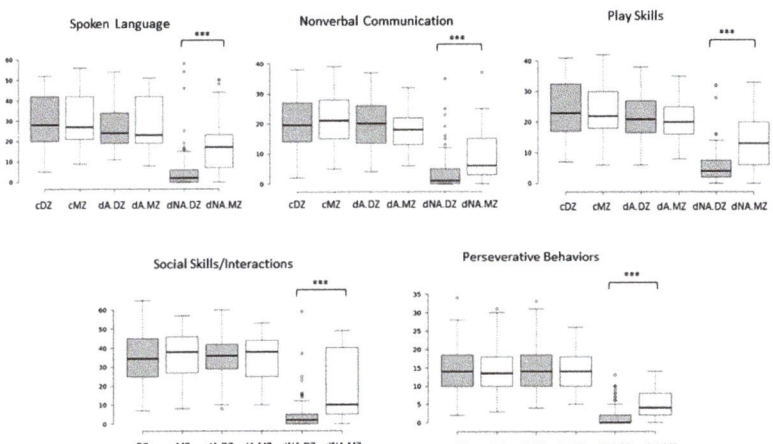

Figure 2. Boxplots showing range of trait scores of all twin groups. Student's *t*-test was used to show that there were significant differences between the trait scores for dNA.MZ and dNA.DZ twins. *** *p*-value ≤ 0.001.

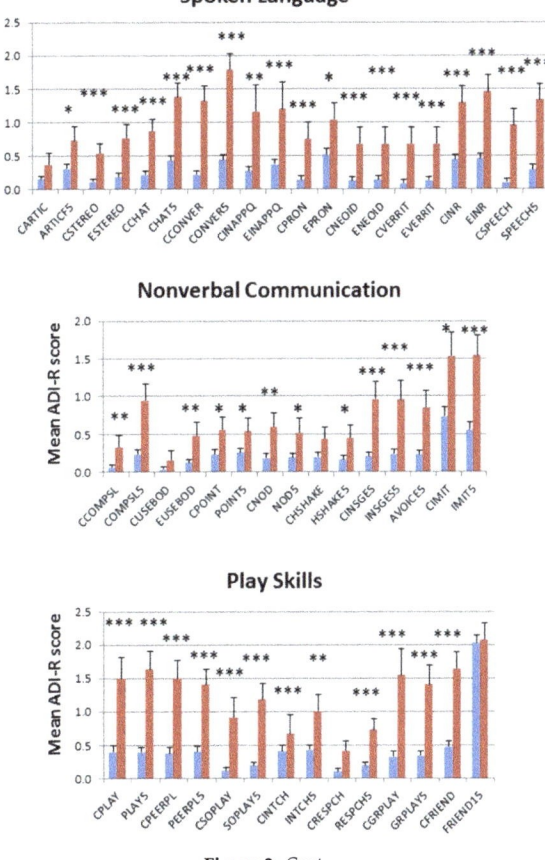

Figure 3. *Cont.*

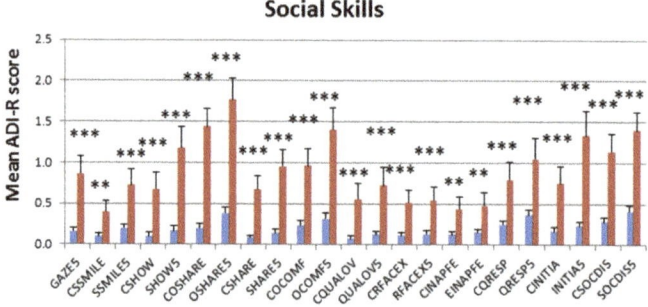

Figure 3. Comparison of average severity scores for dNA.MZ (red bars) and dNA.DZ (blue bars) twins across all ADI-R items (along horizontal axes) used to derive a cumulative trait score. * p-value ≤ 0.05, ** p-value ≤ 0.01, *** p-value ≤ 0.001.

2.2. Genotype–Phenotype Relationships Revealed by Quantitative Trait Association Analyses

Scheme 1 illustrates the overall design and workflow for the genetic analyses conducted in this study. Based upon the severity differences in multiple traits exhibited in each of the subgroups of twins, we conducted a series of quantitative trait association analyses to discover SNPs that may associate with the phenotypic differences in trait severity. Quantitative trait association analyses were conducted using the cumulative trait scores for each individual in each twin subgroup and their respective genotyping data derived from the study by Wang et al. (2009). QTNs with unadjusted p-values $\leq 1 \times 10^{-5}$ were selected for subsequent case-control association analyses. Results of the QTL analyses for each subgroup of twins are shown in Tables S1–S6 in Supplementary Materials. The combined sets of genes associated with the QTNs across all twin groups are shown in Table 1, with a Venn diagram showing the distribution of the overlapping genes among four of the five traits (Figure 4). Notably, there were no genes shared between those associated with perseverative behaviors and any of the other four traits. Hypergeometric distribution analyses of each set of QTN-associated genes indicated significant enrichment in genes from the SFARI database for all traits except non-verbal communication (Table 2).

Int. J. Mol. Sci. **2019**, *20*, 3804

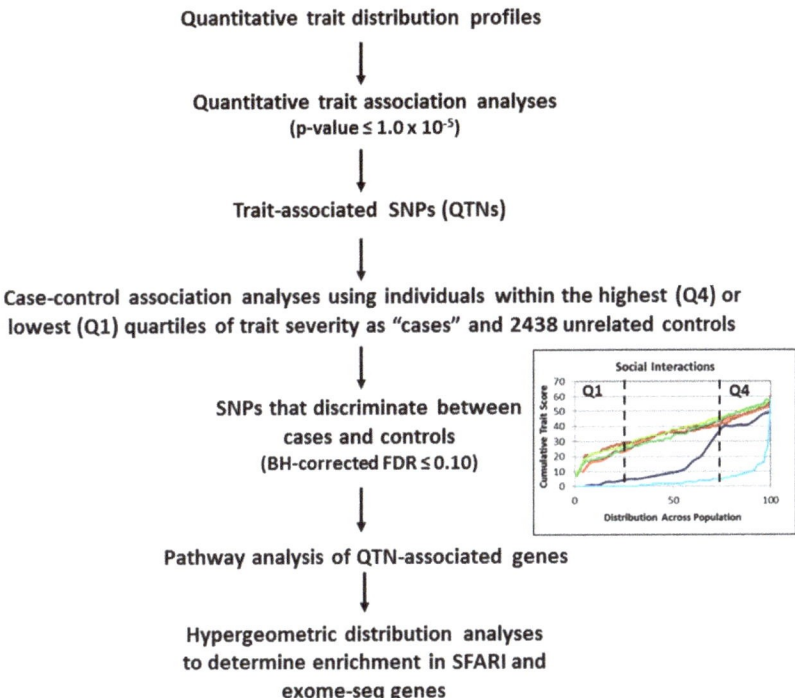

Scheme 1. Workflow for two-phase genetic analyses using both quantitative trait and case-control association analyses of individuals stratified according to severity of traits.

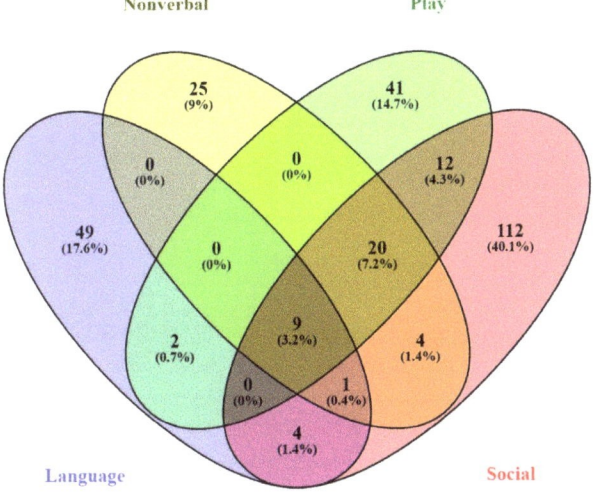

Figure 4. Venn diagram showing SNP-associated gene overlap among language, nonverbal communication, play skills, and social skills. There was no gene overlap between the genes associated with perseverative behaviors and those associated with any of the other four traits.

Table 1. Summary of genes associated with QTNs for each trait across all twin groups.

Spoken Language		Nonverbal Commun.		Play Skills				Social Skills				Pers. Behav.	
ADAM12	KLHL29	ABHD6	MGAT4C	ADAMTS8	KALRN	ABCC4		DCAF16	LHPP		RCOR1		APOLD1
ALOX12P1	L3MBTL4	ADAMTS8	MICA	ADPRHL1	KIRREL3	ABCD3		DCDC5	LMO1		REV1		BNIP3L
ANGPT1	LHFPL3	AGMO	MTCP1	AGMO	L3MBTL4	ACBD5		DGKH	LPPR4		RNASE8		C2orf88
BMP5	LHX4	AK097143	NCALD	AMPD3	LARGE	ADAMTS8		DLG2	LPPR5		RNF144B		CDH13
BMPR2	LRRFIP1	ANKRD44	NCAPG	ANKRD44	LCORL	ADARB1		DMRT2	LRIG3		RPTOR		CORO2A
C12orf42	LYPD6B	ANKS1B	NOP58	BEND4	LECT1	AGMO		DNAH9	LRRC4C		RUNX1		FAM136B
C3orf55	MGAT4C	BCAS3	NUP210P1	BMPR2	MARK3	AKAP6		DPF3	MAGI3		SGCZ		FHAD1
CCDC152	MGAT5	BMPR2	PAX3	C1orf143	MGAT4C	ALPK1		ELK3	MARK3		SHISA6		GABRR2
CCDC85A	NCALD	CADM1	PCDHGA1	CA10	MTCP1	AMPD2		ELOVL6	MCPH1		SLC16A9		GPC6
CCND3	NOP58	CCDC85A	PIEZO2	CCDC102B	MYH11	ANKRD32		EPHB1	MECOM		SLC44A1		GRAMD1C
CD101	NOS1AP	CCND3	PLCXD3	CCDC60	NCALD	ANKRD44		EPS15	MGAT4C		SLCO2B1		GRIP1
CDK5R1	NPAS3	CDH20	RARB	CCDC8	NCAPG	AOC1		EYS	MMP9		SPATA13		IL31RA
CHRM1	NRXN1	CEP95	RNF24	CCDC85A	NOP58	ARHGAP26		FAM210B	MTCP1		SPOP		KCNAB1
CHRNA7	NTM	CHL1	RYR2	CCND3	NRG2	ARL15		FAM89A	MYH11		SRD5A1		MAML2
CNTN1	OVCH2	CMKLR1	SKAP2	CHN2	PAG1	ASAP1		FAT4	MYO18B		SRGAP3		MRPS6
CNTN4	PAX3	COL20A1	SLC22A23	CHRM3	PARK2	ASXL3		FBXL7	NAALAD2		ST6GALNAC3		MTBP
CPM	PDE4B	CSMD1	SLC27A6	CLMP	PAX3	BC093087		FCER2	NCALD		STAC		MXRA5
CREM	PIEZO2	DCAF16	SPATA13	CMKLR1	PAX7	BMPR2		FHIT	NCAPG		STK11		OR2H2
CSMD1	PPIE	DLG2	STAC	CMTM7	PCDHGA1	BPIFB1		FRRS1L	NDRG2		STX8		PLCB1
DCTN5	SLC1A7	EPHB1	STK32B	COBLL1	PLCXD3	C10orf11		GCNT1	NOP58		SUPT3H		PLD6
DGKH	SLC30A8	EYS	THEG5	CPE	PSD3	C6orf106		GNE	OPA3		THEG5		PRICKLE1
DSCAM	SMEK1	FAT4	TMEM38A	CSMD1	RARB	C9orf171		GRID1	P4HA2		THSD4		PTPRD
DSCAML1	STX8	FLVCR1	TRIOBP	CTNND2	RPTOR	CA10		GRID2	PARK2		TMEM108		RAPGEF5
E2F7	SYT6	GCNT1	WBSCR17	DCAF16	SH3PXD2B	CASP6		GRM7	PARK3		TMEM135		RNLS
EP400	TCHP	IL1R2	WNK2	DFFA	SLC16A9	CASP8		HBS1L	PCDHGA1		TMEM245		SLC22A18
FAM49B	TLN2	ITIH5	ZNF207	DISC1	SLCO4A1	CCDC102B		HDAC11	PCSK5		TNS3		SORBS2
FMN1	TMEM192	KCNIP4		DLG2	SOX5	CCDC85A		HIST1H1D	PDE8A		TRDN		ST8SIA5
GOSR1	TNS3	L3MBTL4		DNAJC10	SPOP	CCND3		HIST1H2BF	PDGFC		TTC27		SYNPO2L
GPR139	TOP2B	LARGE		DPF3	STAC	CCSER1		HIST1H4E	PFKP		USP37		UNC13C
ID3	UNC5D	LCORL		E2F7	STEAP1B	CDH8		HIST1H4G	PIEZO2		WDSUB1		
JAZF1	WWC2	LDB2		EPHB1	STK38	CDK17		IGSF21	PITPNA		WNK2		
KIAA0947	YY1	LIM2		EYS	TECRL	CDK2		IKBKAP	PKD1L1		XYLT1		

Table 1. Cont.

Spoken Language	Nonverbal Commun.	Play Skills		Social Skills		Pers. Behav.
KIAA1549	LRRC4C	FAT4	THEG5	CEP95	ITGB3	PLCXD3	ZFP64
		FIP1L1	TMEM144	CMIP	KCND2	PLXDC1	ZNF142
		FZD4	TMEM161B	CMKLR1	KCNIP4	PREP	ZNF630
		GALNTL6	TNFSF12	CMYA5	KIAA0319	PRKCDBP	ZNF804B
		GCNT1	TP53	CNTN1	KIAA1377	PSD3	
		GPR56	TRDN	COLEC12	KIF13A	PTPRE	
		GREM1	VAV3	CR2	KLF12	PTPRK	
		HBS1L	WNK2	CSMD1	L3MBTL4	RABGAP1L	
		ID3	ZCCHC14	CTNNAL1	LARGE	RARB	
		ITSN1	ZNF385D	CTTNBP2	LCORL	RBFOX1	

Table 2. Hypergeometric distribution analyses of trait-associated genes and SFARI genes.

Hypergeometric Distribution Analyses of Enrichment of SFARI Genes Among ASD Trait-Associated Genes			
Trait	Number of Trait-Associated Genes	# Genes Represented within SFARI Gene	p-Value * for Enrichment
Language deficits	65	11	4.20×10^{-4}
Nonverbal communication	59	5	2.01×10^{-1}
Play skills	84	9	3.30×10^{-2}
Social skills	162	19	9.48×10^{-4}
Perseverative behaviors	29	5	1.68×10^{-2}

* For the hypergeometric distribution analyses, the total number of genes in the population was estimated to be 20,406, and the total number of ASD-associated genes in the SFARI gene database was 1079.

2.3. Case-Control Association Analyses Based on Individuals Stratified by Trait Severity for Each Subgroup of Twins

The SNPs used for case-control association analyses were limited to the trait-associated SNPs derived from QTL analyses involving the corresponding twin groups. Results of these case-control association analyses are presented in Tables S7–S12. Examination of these results for each set of twins reveals significant SNPs (corrected for multiple testing by Bonferroni and/or Benjamini–Hochberg methods) that differentiate between cases and controls. Moreover, for all SNPs that were found to be significantly associated with both the lowest quartile (Q1) and highest quartile (Q4) cases diagnosed with ASD, the minor allele frequencies (MAF) relative to that of controls were noticeably different, resulting in different odds ratios. That is, a specific trait-associated SNP that may be considered as predisposing to ASD in the Q4 subgroup with a high odds ratio (>1.0) was found to have a lower odds ratio (often <1.0) in the Q1 subgroup, further suggesting relevance to severity of that specific trait. Although a SNP may occasionally have a higher odds ratio in the Q1 than in the Q4 case group, the differences in MAFs still suggest that these subgroups based on trait severity are genetically distinct with respect to that genetic variant. Notably, the majority of significant SNPs in the non-autistic subgroups (dNA.MZ and dNA.DZ) were found in Q4, at the highest severity end of the trait distribution.

2.4. Enrichment of Known Autism Risk Genes from Case-Control Association Analyses

The SNP-associated genes derived from the case-control association analyses described above were compared to the complete set of autism risk genes that comprise the SFARI gene database. Table 3 shows that genes mapped to the trait-associated SNPs that are significant by case-control association analyses using individuals in both Q1 and Q4 as cases for each subgroup of twins are enriched among SFARI genes in three of the six twin groups (dNA.MZ, dNA.DZ, and cDZ). Together with the results shown in Table 2, these findings suggest that the experimental strategy of combining quantitative trait association analyses with case-control association analyses using cases stratified by trait severity is capable of identifying significant autism risk genes even with relatively small numbers of samples. Furthermore, the SNPs identified can be associated with severity of specific traits, thereby associating genotype with phenotype.

Table 3. Hypergeometric analyses of case-control associated genes and SFARI genes.

Case Groups (Combined Q1 and Q4) vs. Unaffected Controls	Number of Case-Associated Genes	# Genes Represented within SFARI Gene	Q-Value * for Enrichment
dA.MZ	13	0	1
dA.DZ	8	0	1
dNA.MZ	53	9	1.69×10^{-3}
dNA.DZ	19	4	1.59×10^{-2}
cMZ	29	2	4.58×10^{-1}
cDZ	23	4	3.10×10^{-2}

* For the hypergeometric distribution analyses, the total number of genes in the population was estimated to be 20,406; and the total number of ASD-associated genes in the SFARI gene database was 1079.

2.5. Functional Analysis of Genes Associated with QTNs from Quantitative Trait and Case-Control Association Analyses

Genes implicated by QTNs were analyzed using Ingenuity Pathway Analysis (IPA) software with a focus on identifying genes that impact nervous system development and function. Tables 4–8 show the neurological functions that are statistically enriched among genes implicated by QTNs associated with spoken language, nonverbal communication, play skills, social skills, and perseverative behaviors, respectively, for each subgroup of twins. Notably, many of the annotated functions are relevant to what is known about specific neuronal processes disrupted in ASD. Moreover, IPA analyses of genes associated with significant SNPs identified by case-control association analyses of both dNA.MZ and dNA.DZ subgroups in addition to the cDZ subgroup which are all enriched in SFARI genes also revealed significant over-representation of genes involved in neurological functions, behaviors, and disorders relevant to ASD, as shown in Tables 9–11, respectively.

Table 4. Neurological functions associated with genes implicated by language QTNs.

Functions Annotation	p-Value *	Genes
cell-cell adhesion of neurons	9.52×10^{-6}	CDK5R1, CNTN4, NRXN1
guidance of axons	9.66×10^{-6}	CDK5R1, CNTN1, CNTN4, LHX4, NRXN1, UNC5D
fasciculation of axons	8.24×10^{-5}	CDK5R1, CNTN1, CNTN4
abnormal morphology of brain	1.86×10^{-4}	CDK5R1, CHRM1, CHRNA7, CNTN1, ID3, LHX4, NPAS3, TOP2B
GABA-mediated receptor currents	6.98×10^{-4}	CHRNA7, NRXN1
abnormal morphology of granule cells	9.17×10^{-4}	CDK5R1, CNTN1
abnormal morphology of nervous system	1.48×10^{-3}	CDK5R1, CHRM1, CHRNA7, CNTN1, CNTN4, ID3, LHX4, NPAS3, TOP2B
stratification of cerebral cortex	1.75×10^{-3}	CDK5R1, TOP2B
formation of brain	2.52×10^{-3}	BMP5, CDK5R1, CNTN1, CREM, DSCAML1, NPAS3, TOP2B
memory	2.58×10^{-3}	CDK5R1, CHRM1, CHRNA7, CREM, NPAS3
abnormal morphology of molecular layer of cerebellum	2.63×10^{-3}	CDK5R1, CNTN1
formation of enteric ganglion	2.82×10^{-3}	PAX3
morphology of motor cortex	2.82×10^{-3}	CDK5R1
origination of axons	2.82×10^{-3}	CDK5R1
reorganization of molecular layer	2.82×10^{-3}	CDK5R1
sprouting of mossy fiber cells	2.82×10^{-3}	CDK5R1

* Fisher exact p-value which indicates the probability that the list of SNP-associated genes is not enriched for annotated function, using genes in IPA's Knowledgebase as the reference set of genes.

Table 5. Neurological functions associated with genes implicated by nonverbal QTNs.

Functions Annotation	p-Value *	Genes
organization of mossy fibers	2.60×10^{-3}	CHL1
formation of enteric ganglion	2.60×10^{-3}	PAX3
targeting of retinal ganglion cells	2.60×10^{-3}	EPHB1
cell-cell adhesion of astrocytes	2.60×10^{-3}	CADM1
maintenance of neural crest	5.18×10^{-3}	PAX3
survival of neural crest	5.18×10^{-3}	PAX3
innervation of forelimb	7.77×10^{-3}	BMPR2
differentiation of satellite cells	1.03×10^{-2}	PAX3
morphogenesis of optic nerve	1.29×10^{-2}	EPHB1
migration of pyramidal neurons	1.29×10^{-2}	CHL1
abnormal pruning of axons	1.29×10^{-2}	EPHB1
excitatory postsynaptic potential of neurons	1.39×10^{-2}	DLG2, RARB
formation of pyramidal neurons	1.55×10^{-2}	CHL1
synaptic depression of collateral synapses	1.80×10^{-2}	EPHB1
synaptic transmission of collateral synapses	1.80×10^{-2}	EPHB1
abnormal morphology of axons	2.29×10^{-2}	CHL1, EPHB1
development of retinal pigment epithelium	2.31×10^{-2}	RARB
abnormal morphology of optic tract	2.31×10^{-2}	EPHB1
abnormal morphology of hypoglossal nerve	2.82×10^{-2}	RARB
abnormal morphology of olfactory receptor neurons	3.32×10^{-2}	CHL1
abnormal morphology of mossy fibers	4.07×10^{-2}	CHL1
projection of axons	4.57×10^{-2}	CHL1
synaptic transmission of nervous tissue	4.74×10^{-2}	ANKS1B, EPHB1
abnormal morphology of neural arch	4.82×10^{-2}	RARB

* Fisher exact p-value which indicates the probability that the list of SNP-associated genes is not enriched for annotated function, using genes in IPA's Knowledgebase as the reference set of genes.

Table 6. Neurological functions associated with genes implicated by play skills QTNs.

Functions Annotation	p-Value *	Genes
formation of dendritic spines	6.97×10^{-4}	ITSN1, KALRN
short-term depression of calyx-type synapse	7.29×10^{-4}	ITSN1
neurotransmission of synapse	8.88×10^{-4}	CHRM3, PRKN
formation of tip of neurite-like extensions	1.46×10^{-3}	KALRN
elongation of dendritic spine neck	1.46×10^{-3}	ITSN1
long-term potentiation of Purkinje cells	1.46×10^{-3}	CHRM3
arrest in axonal transport of mitochondria	1.46×10^{-3}	PRKN
quantity of catecholaminergic neurons	1.46×10^{-3}	PRKN
length of neurons	2.18×10^{-3}	ITSN1, KALRN

Table 6. Cont.

Functions Annotation	p-Value *	Genes
excitation of striatal neurons	2.18×10^{-3}	PRKN
differentiation of satellite cells	2.91×10^{-3}	PAX7
replenishment of synaptic vesicles	2.91×10^{-3}	ITSN1
abnormal morphology of locus ceruleus	2.91×10^{-3}	PRKN
afterhyperpolarization of pyramidal neurons	4.36×10^{-3}	CHRM3
morphology of corticcal neurons	4.36×10^{-3}	KALRN
sensorimotor integration	5.09×10^{-3}	PRKN
abnormal morphology of substantia nigra	5.81×10^{-3}	PRKN
neurotransmission	6.89×10^{-3}	CHRM3,,KALRN, PRKN
morphogenesis of dendritic spines	7.26×10^{-3}	KALRN
retraction of dendrites	7.99×10^{-3}	KALRN
maturation of dendritic spines	8.71×10^{-3}	KALRN
length of axons	9.43×10^{-3}	KALRN
abnormal morphology of cerebral cortex	9.91×10^{-3}	KALRN,,PRKN
length of dendritic spines	1.38×10^{-2}	ITSN1
coordination	1.43×10^{-2}	KALRN, PRKN

* Fisher exact p-value which indicates the probability that the list of SNP-associated genes is not enriched for annotated function, using genes in IPA's Knowledgebase as the reference set of genes.

Table 7. Neurological functions associated with genes implicated by social skills QTNs.

Functions Annotation	p-Value *	Genes
abnormal morphology of thoracic vertebra	1.19×10^{-3}	DMRT2, FAT4, NDRG2
action potential of neurons	4.63×10^{-3}	DLG2, GRID2, KCND2, PARK7, RARB
abnormal morphology of Purkinje cells	4.78×10^{-3}	CNTN1, GRID2, PITPNA
innervation of climbing fiber	7.24×10^{-3}	GRID2
formation of enteric ganglion	7.24×10^{-3}	PAX3
development of climbing fiber	7.24×10^{-3}	GRID2
differentiation of branchial motor neurons	7.24×10^{-3}	RUNX1
targeting of retinal ganglion cells	7.24×10^{-3}	EPHB1
differentiation of visceral motor neurons	7.24×10^{-3}	RUNX1
abnormal morphology of Golgi interneurons	7.24×10^{-3}	CNTN1
proliferation of neuroglia	7.26×10^{-3}	CCND3, CDK2, CNTN1, MMP9, RUNX1
abnormal morphology of white matter	7.39×10^{-3}	PITPNA, SRGAP3
function of blood-brain barrier	9.99×10^{-3}	ABCC4, MMP9
abnormal morphology of lumbar vertebra	1.09×10^{-2}	DMRT2, FAT4
function of brain	1.12×10^{-2}	ABCC4, KCNIP4, MMP9
morphology of brain	1.18×10^{-2}	CASP6, CNTN1, EPHB1, GRID1, GRID2, MCPH1, MECOM, PARK7, PITPNA, SRGAP3
axonogenesis	1.31×10^{-2}	CASP6, EPHB1, GRID2, LRRC4C, PTPRE, STK11
arrest in cell cycle progression of oligodendrocyte precursor cells	1.44×10^{-2}	CDK2
abnormal morphology of superior ganglion of glossopharyngeal nerve	1.44×10^{-2}	MECOM
delay in initiation of pruning of axons	1.44×10^{-2}	CASP6
maintenance of neural crest	1.44×10^{-2}	PAX3
blood-cerebrospinal fluid barrier function	1.44×10^{-2}	ABCC4

* Fisher exact p-value which indicates the probability that the list of SNP-associated genes is not enriched for annotated function, using genes in IPA's Knowledgebase as the reference set of genes.

Table 8. Neurological functions associated with genes implicated by Perseverative behavior QTNs.

Diseases or Functions Annotation	p-Value *	Genes
paired-pulse facilitation of parallel fiber-Purkinje cell synapses	1.27×10^{-3}	UNC13C
early infantile epileptic encephalopathy type 12	1.27×10^{-3}	PLCB1
loss of hippocampal neurons	6.36×10^{-3}	PLCB1
epilepsy	1.27×10^{-2}	GABRR2, PLCB1, PRICKLE1
afterhyperpolarization of neurons	2.27×10^{-2}	KCNAB1
progressive myoclonic epilepsy	2.64×10^{-2}	PRICKLE1
status epilepticus	4.13×10^{-2}	GABRR2
density of synapse	4.61×10^{-2}	GRIP1
sedation	4.61×10^{-2}	GABRR2

* Fisher exact p-value which indicates the probability that the list of SNP-associated genes is not enriched for annotated function, using genes in IPA's Knowledgebase as the reference set of genes.

Table 9. Neurological functions implicated by QTN-associated genes in dNA.MZ.

Functions Annotation	p-value *	Genes
abnormal morphology of pyramidal neurons	5.59×10^{-5}	CHL1, CHRNA7, KALRN
GABA-mediated receptor currents	4.19×10^{-4}	CHRNA7, NRXN1
abnormal morphology of cerebral cortex	1.12×10^{-3}	CHL1, CHRNA7, KALRN, NPAS3
organization of mossy fibers	2.19×10^{-3}	CHL1
cell-cell adhesion of astrocytes	2.19×10^{-3}	CADM1
developmental process of synapse	2.35×10^{-3}	CADM1, CHRNA7, KALRN, NRXN1
formation of tip of neurite-like extensions	4.37×10^{-3}	KALRN
hyperexcitation of hippocampal neurons; short-term potentiation of hippocampus; nicotine-mediated receptor current	4.37×10^{-3}	CHRNA7
abnormal morphology of enlarged fourth cerebral ventricle	6.54×10^{-3}	NPAS3
miniature excitatory postsynaptic currents	7.15×10^{-3}	KALRN, NRXN1
abnormal morphology of lateral cerebral ventricle	7.64×10^{-3}	CHL1, NPAS3
differentiation of satellite cells	8.71×10^{-3}	PAX7
abnormal morphology of cingulate gyrus	8.71×10^{-3}	NPAS3
abnormal morphology of GABAergic neurons	8.71×10^{-3}	CHRNA7
migration of pyramidal neurons	1.09×10^{-2}	CHL1
pervasive developmental disorder	1.13×10^{-2}	BCAS3, PREP, SLC1A7
excitatory postsynaptic current	1.26×10^{-2}	KALRN, NRXN1
morphology of cortical neurons	1.30×10^{-2}	KALRN
formation of pyramidal neurons	1.30×10^{-2}	CHL1
maturatin of neurons	1.46×10^{-2}	KALRN, NRXN1
branching of axons	1.49×10^{-2}	KALRN, STK11
prepulse inhibition	1.56×10^{-2}	KALRN, NRXN1
abnormal morphology of enlarged third cerebral ventricle	1.74×10^{-2}	NPAS3
paired-pulse inhibition	1.74×10^{-2}	NRXN1
coordination	1.79×10^{-2}	CHRNA7, KALRN, NPAS3
abnormal morphology of cerebral aqueduct	1.95×10^{-2}	NPAS3
morphogenesis of dendritic spines	2.16×10^{-2}	KALRN
retraction of dendrites	2.38×10^{-2}	KALRN
activation of dopaminergic neurons	2.59×10^{-2}	CHRNA7
maturation of dendritic spines	2.59×10^{-2}	KALRN
abnormal morphology of olfactory receptor neurons	2.81×10^{-2}	CHL1
length of axons	2.81×10^{-2}	KALRN
spatial memory	2.88×10^{-2}	CHRNA7, KALRN, NPAS3
sleep disorders	3.06×10^{-2}	CHRNA7, PDE4B
neurotransmission	3.20×10^{-2}	ANKS1B, CHRNA7, KALRN, NRXN1
development of neurons	3.44×10^{-2}	CADM1, CHL1, CHRNA7, KALRN, NRXN1, STK11

* Fisher exact p-value which indicates the probability that the list of SNP-associated genes is not enriched for annotated function, using genes in IPA's Knowledgebase as the reference set of genes.

Table 10. Neurological functions implicated by QTN-associated genes in dNA.DZ.

Diseases or Functions Annotation	p-Value *	Genes
adhesion of cerebellar granule cell	8.65×10^{-4}	ADGRG1
migration of CA1 neuron	8.65×10^{-4}	DISC1
abnormal morphology of lumbar dorsal root ganglion	8.62×10^{-3}	GABBR1
abnormal morphology of somatic nervous system	1.03×10^{-2}	GABBR1
pervasive developmental disorder	1.44×10^{-2}	CORO2A, GABBR1
abnormal morphology of sciatic nerve	1.46×10^{-2}	GABBR1
positioning of neurons	1.55×10^{-2}	DISC1
development of olfactory cilia	1.80×10^{-2}	DISC1
progressive myoclonic epilepsy	1.80×10^{-2}	PRICKLE1
maturation of synapse	1.89×10^{-2}	DISC1
migration of neuronal progenitor cells	1.97×10^{-2}	ADGRG1
fragile X syndrome	2.48×10^{-2}	GABBR1
elongation of axons	2.73×10^{-2}	DISC1
migration of neurons	2.81×10^{-2}	ADGRG1, DISC1
abnormal morphology of myelin sheath	2.99×10^{-2}	GABBR1
differentiation of oligodendroccyte precursor cells	3.24×10^{-2}	DISC1
absense seizure	3.24×10^{-2}	GABBR1
passive avoidance learning	3.49×10^{-2}	GABBR1
inhibitory postsynaptic current	4.41×10^{-2}	GABBR1
electrophysiology of nervous system	4.74×10^{-2}	GABBR1

* Fisher exact p-value which indicates the probability that the list of SNP-associated genes is not enriched for annotated function, using genes in IPA's Knowledgebase as the reference set of genes.

Table 11. Neurological functions implicated by QTN-associated genes in cDZ.

Diseases or Functions Annotation	p-Value *	Genes
morphology of brain	1.51×10^{-3}	DSCAM, LHX4, PRKN, TOP2B
abnormal morphology of abducens nerve	1.73×10^{-3}	LHX4
arrest in axonal transport of mitochondria	1.73×10^{-3}	PRKN
quantity of catecholaminergic neurons	1.73×10^{-3}	PRKN
delay in specification of corticotroph cells	1.73×10^{-3}	LHX4
excitation of striatal neurons	2.59×10^{-3}	PRKN
startle response	2.60×10^{-3}	PLCB1, PRKN
development of granule cell layer	3.46×10^{-3}	CREM
function of central pattern generator	3.46×10^{-3}	DSCAM, LHX4, PRKN, TOP2B
development of cortical subplate	3.46×10^{-3}	TOP2B
abnormal morphology of locus ceruleus	3.46×10^{-3}	PRKN
morphogenesis of dendrites	3.67×10^{-3}	DSCAM, FMN1
loss of hippocampal neurons	4.32×10^{-3}	PLCB1, PRKN
development of central nervous system	5.75×10^{-3}	CREM, PLCB1, PRKN, TOP2B
abnormal morphology of amacrine cells	6.04×10^{-3}	DSCAM
sensorimotor integration	6.04×10^{-3}	PRKN
abnormal morphology of substantia nigra	6.90×10^{-3}	PRKN
abnormal morphology of neurons	7.53×10^{-3}	DSCAM, LHX4, PRKN
abnormal morphology of nervous system	8.50×10^{-3}	DSCAM, LHX4, PRKN, TOP2B
abnormal morphology of hypoglossal nerve	9.48×10^{-3}	LHX4
thickness of cerebral cortex	1.03×10^{-2}	DSCAM
quantity of gonadotropes	1.12×10^{-2}	LHX4
innervation of motor neurons	1.20×10^{-2}	TOP2B

Table 11. Cont.

Diseases or Functions Annotation	p-Value *	Genes
abnormal morphology of brain	1.22×10^{-2}	LHX4, PRKN, TOP2B
loss of neurons	1.27×10^{-2}	PLCB1, PRKN
curvature of vertebral column	1.80×10^{-2}	TOP2B
formation of brain	1.83×10^{-2}	CREM, PLCB1, TOP2B
stratification of cerebral cortex	1.89×10^{-2}	TOP2B
innervation of muscle	1.89×10^{-2}	TOP2B
abnormal morphology of adenohypophysis	1.97×10^{-2}	LHX4
quantity of nerve ending	2.14×10^{-2}	PRKN
guidance of motor axons	2.23×10^{-2}	LHX4
loss of dopaminergic neurons	2.23×10^{-2}	PRKN
abnormal morphology of spinal nerve	2.48×10^{-2}	LHX4
fasciculation of axons	2.56×10^{-2}	DSCAM
abnormal morphology of motor neurons	2.82×10^{-2}	LHX4
neuritogenesis	3.00×10^{-2}	DSCAM, FMN1, TOP2B
abnormal morphology of subventricular zone	3.07×10^{-2}	TOP2B
memory	3.36×10^{-2}	CREM, PLCB1
morphology of dendritic spines	3.57×10^{-2}	DSCAM
quantity of dendritic spines	3.99×10^{-2}	DSCAM
development of spinal cord	4.49×10^{-2}	TOP2B
abnormal morphology of olfactory bulb	4.57×10^{-2}	TOP2B
cell viability of cortical neurons	4.74×10^{-2}	PRKN
electrophysiology of nervous system	4.74×10^{-2}	PRKN

* Fisher exact p-value which indicates the probability that the list of SNP-associated genes is not enriched for annotated function, using genes in IPA's Knowledgebase as the reference set of genes.

2.6. Case-Control Association Analysis Using dNA.DZ Twins as Controls for dA.DZ Co-Twins

Given the differential diagnosis of discordant dizygotic twins with presumed genetic differences between the autistic and non-autistic co-twins, we conducted an exploratory case-control association analysis using the dNA.DZ twins ($n = 36$) as controls for the diagnosed dA.DZ co-twins ($n = 38$). Interestingly, over 140 genes were associated with a total of 390 SNPs that exhibited a nominal p-value ≤ 0.05 and odds ratio ≥ 3 (Table 12, complete case-control association data in Table S13). Hypergeometric distribution analyses showed that this set of genes was highly enriched for autism risk genes from the SFARI database ($q = 1.84 \times 10^{-7}$) and from an exome-sequencing study [23] ($q = 4.64 \times 10^{-8}$). Pathway analysis of this gene set using IPA revealed that netrin signaling (involving PRKG1, DCC, and PRKAG2) and axon guidance signaling (involving PRKCE, PDGFD, DCC, ROBO1, SLIT3, PRKAG2, NTNG1, PLCG2) were among the top 10 canonical pathways represented with Fisher's Exact p-values of 2.56×10^{-3} and 6.18×10^{-3}, respectively. Several of the above-mentioned genes (specifically, PRKCE, PRKAG2, and PLCG2) are also significantly over-represented in additional pathways potentially relevant to ASD, including melatonin signaling ($p = 1.18 \times 10^{-2}$) and synaptic long-term potentiation ($p = 4.45 \times 10^{-2}$). Functional analysis showed significant over-representation of many neurological processes commonly impacted by autism, notably neuritogenesis, axonogenesis, neuronal migration, and axon guidance (Table 13).

Table 12. Genes associated with SNPs identified by case-control association analyses using dA.DZ twins as cases and dNA.DZ twins as controls.

Case-control Association Analysis of dA.DZ vs. dNA.DZ					Overlap with SFARI	Overlap with Exome-seq [#]
(146 genes associated with SNPs with $p \leq 0.05$ and OR ≥ 3)					* Q = 1.84×10^{-7}	* Q = 4.64×10^{-8}
ABCA13	DCC	KCTD16	PCSK6	RPH3AL	ABCA13	ABCA13 OR1J2
ACVRL1	DKK3	KIAA0232	PDCD4	SCOC	CACNA1A	ALDH3B2 PCM1
ALDH3B2	DMD	KIAA1407	PDE3A	SEC16B	CACNA2D3	ALMS1 PCSK6
ALMS1	DNAH5	KLHDC7A	PDE9A	SETBP1	CNTN4	ARHGAP28 PDCD4
ANO4	DST	KLHL1	PDGFD	SFMBT2	CSMD1	ATP8B4 PDE9A
ARHGAP28	ESRRB	KSR2	PDXK	SLC12A2	CTNND2	C20orf96 PDGFD
ATP8B4	EXOSC1	LDLRAD3	PDZD2	SLC22A23	DMD	CACNA1A PDZD2
ATXN3	FAM216A	LIN52	PEX13	SLC25A21	DST	CACNA2D3 PKNOX2
BBIP1	FAM89A	LPHN3	PGAM1P5	SLC39A11	ESRRB	CDK14 PLCG2
C20orf96	FAT4	LRP11	PIP5K1B	SLC5A12	FER	CSMD1 PRKAG2
CACNA1A	FER	LRP1B	PIP5K1C	SLIT3	FHIT	CSMD3 PRKCE
CACNA2D3	FERMT1	MAL2	PKNOX2	SMC6	GABRB1	CTNND2 PRPF4B
CACNG2	FHIT	MARCH1	PLCG2	SNX9	GRIP1	DCC PSD3
CARD6	FLIP1L	MAST4	POU2F3	SORCS2	MCPH1	DMD RBMS3
CCDC102B	FREM1	MCPH1	PPARGC1A	SYT9	NELL1	DNAH5 RHBDF2
CCDC111	GABRB1	MIPEP	PRKAG2	TBCE	NTNG1	DST RNF213
CCDC176	GALC	MPP7	PRKCE	TMEM182	NXPH1	ESRRB ROBO1
CCDC3	GAS7	MYO15B	PRKG1	TMTC2	PSD3	FAT4 RPH3AL
CD36	GNN	MYOM3	PRPF4B	TRIP11	RBMS3	FERMT1 SCOC
CDK14	GPR124	NCOR2	PSD3	TTC7A	ROBO1	GALC SEC16B
CDKAL1	GPR125	NELL1	QRTRTD1	TUBGCP5	SETBP1	HEG1 SETBP1
CLYBL	GRIP1	NMNAT2	RABGAP1L	VIT	SLC39A11	KIAA0232 SLC22A23
CMSS1	HAL	NRDE2	RASGEF1B	XRCC4	SLIT3	KIAA1407 SLC39A11
CNOT10	HEG1	NTNG1	RBMS3	YIPF5	SNTG2	LRP11 SMC6
CNTN4	HSPA12A	NXPH1	RCN1	ZDDGGC16	TUBGCP5	LRP1B TMTC2
CSMD1	HVCN1	OAS2	RGS17			MCPH1 TRIP11
CSMD3	IFT81	OR1J2	RHBDF2			MYOM3 TTC7A
CTNND2	IRS1	OR8U8	RNF180			NCOR2 TUBGCP5
CWC27	KCNIP4	PALLD	RNF213			NELL1 YIPF5
CYMP	KCNN3	PCM1	ROBO1			NTNG1

* Q indicates probability of enrichment in SFARI or exome-seq genes from hypergeometric distribution analysis.
[#] Exome-seq genes were downloaded from study by Iossifov et al. [23].

Table 13. Neurological functions of SNP-associated genes from dA.DZ vs. dNA.DZ case-control association analysis.

Function Annotation	p-Value *	Genes
development of neurons	5.50×10^{-6}	ADGRL3, CACNA1A, CACNG2, CNTN4, CTNND2, DCC, DMD, FER, GAS7, KLHL1, NTNG1, PALLD, PCM1, PIP5K1B, PIP5K1C, PRKCE, PRKG1, ROBO1, SLC12A2, SLIT3, TBCE
neuritogenesis	3.57×10^{-5}	CACNA1A, CNTN4, CTNND2, DCC, FER, GAS7, KLHL1, NTNG1, PALLD, PIP5K1B, PIP5K1C, PRKCE, PRKG1, ROBO1, SLIT3, TBCE
axonogenesis	2.58×10^{-4}	CACNA1A, CNTN4, DCC, NTNG1, PIP5K1C, PRKG1, ROBO1, TBCE
migration of neurons	6.40×10^{-4}	ADGRL3, DCC, PCM1, PEX13, PIP5K1C, PRKG1, ROBO1, SLC12A2
development of sensory projections	7.83×10^{-4}	ROBO1, SLIT3
pathfinding of neurons	2.02×10^{-3}	DCC, ROBO1
morphology of nervous system	2.62×10^{-3}	ADGRA2, BBIP1, CACNA1A, CNTN4, DCC, KLHL1, MCPH1, NCOR2, PALLD, PCSK6, PEX13, PPARGC1A, ROBO1, SLC12A2, XRCC4

Table 13. Cont.

Function Annotation	p-Value *	Genes
guidance of axons	4.61×10^{-3}	CNTN4, DCC, PRKG1, ROBO1, SLIT3
abnormal morphology of forebrain	4.80×10^{-3}	ADGRA2, BBIP1, DCC, NCOR2, PPARGC1A, ROBO1
formation of dendrites	4.83×10^{-3}	CACNA1A, GAS7, KLHL1, PRKG1, ROBO1
developmental process of synapse	5.28×10^{-3}	ADGRL3, CACNA1A, CACNG2, DCC, DMD, SLC12A2
quantity of oxytocin neurons	6.19×10^{-3}	DCC
synaptic transmission of stellate cells	6.19×10^{-3}	CACNG2
guidance of corticocortical axons	1.23×10^{-2}	ROBO1
quantity of vasopressin neurons	1.23×10^{-2}	DCC
activation of Purkinje cells	1.23×10^{-2}	CACNA1A
afterhyperpolarization of dopaminergic neurons	1.23×10^{-2}	KCNN3
size of hippocampal commissure	1.23×10^{-2}	ROBO1
startle response	1.74×10^{-2}	CACNA2D3, CSMD1, PPARGC1A
inhibition of presympathetic neurons	1.85×10^{-2}	SLC12A2
fragmentation of myelin sheath	1.85×10^{-2}	GALC
maturation of cerebellum	1.85×10^{-2}	CACNA1A
turnover of synaptic vesicles	1.85×10^{-2}	CACNA1A
density of synapse	2.20×10^{-2}	CTNND2, GRIP1
morphogenesis of neurites	2.43×10^{-2}	CACNA1A, CNTN4, CTNND2, FER, GAS7, PALLD, PRKG1, ROBO1

* Fisher exact p-value which indicates the probability that the list of SNP-associated genes is not enriched for annotated function, using genes in IPA's Knowledgebase as the reference set of genes.

3. Discussion

The goals of this study were to: (1) examine the influence of genetics on specific behaviors and traits of ASD; (2) identify SNPs (i.e., QTNs) that associate with a particular ASD trait; (3) determine if trait QTNs can discriminate between cases and controls, where the cases are individuals at the extremes of phenotypic severity across five autistic traits; and (4) to identify pathways and functions implicated by the genes associated with the QTNs. To accomplish these goals, we developed a novel approach which utilized MZ and DZ twins who are either concordant or discordant for diagnosis of autism to reveal differences in phenotypic severity among and within the subgroups of twins defined by diagnostic status and by zygosity. Then, we used the phenotypic (trait) profiles of each subgroup of twins to perform quantitative trait association analyses to identify SNPs that may be functionally associated with the respective ASD trait (i.e., QTNs). Case-control association analyses were then performed with the QTNs for five autistic behavioral traits using the six different subgroups of twins at the extreme ends (i.e., lowest and highest quartiles) of the respective quantitative trait distribution curves as cases and a large group of unrelated controls. We show here that this novel combination of experimental strategies allowed us to identify significant SNPs that could distinguish individuals with autism from controls. Genes harboring these SNPs are significantly enriched for autism risk genes annotated by SFARI Gene.

3.1. Severity of Autistic Traits Are Strongly Influenced by Genetics

Numerous studies using both monozygotic and dizygotic twins have sought to determine the role of genetics versus environment with varying results, as described earlier. The quantitative trait distribution profiles generated in this study demonstrate significant differences in severity between clinically discordant non-autistic MZ and DZ co-twins, with the profiles of the MZ twins being significantly more severe than DZ twins across all traits, while the profiles of all diagnosed twins are virtually indistinguishable from each other, regardless of zygosity (Figures 1 and 2). These differences in trait severity between the non-autistic MZ and DZ twins are seen even at the most fundamental level, that is, at the level of specific ADI-R items which comprise each trait, demonstrating the strong influence of genetics on a broad spectrum of ASD-associated behaviors and characteristics (Figure 3). In other words, a non-autistic identical twin exhibits a significantly higher severity of autistic traits in comparison to an undiagnosed non-identical twin who shares only a part of his/her autistic co-twin's genes.

3.2. Quantitative Trait Association Analyses Reveal SNPs that Associate with a Specific ASD Trait

QTL association analyses allowed us to discover SNPs that may be functionally relevant to autism traits. The genes associated with trait QTNs (Table 1) are over-represented in a number of neurological functions related to autism. The neurological functions associated with each set of trait genes are shown in Tables 4–8. SNPs associated with spoken language implicate genes involved in cell–cell adhesion of neurons, axon guidance and fasciculation, GABA-mediated receptor currents, and morphology of different brain regions, including the cerebral cortex, cerebellum, and corpus callosum, which are all impacted in ASD (Table 4). Another set of SNPs associated with nonverbal communication implicate genes that play a role in cell–cell adhesion of astrocytes, organization and morphology of mossy fibers, axon pruning, migration of pyramidal neurons, and synaptic transmission of collateral synapses (Table 5). SNPs associated with play skills highlight genes involved in dendritic spine formation, synaptic transmission, and long-term potentiation of Purkinje cells (Table 6). Purkinje cell morphology, neurotransmission, axonogenesis, and differentiation of motor neurons are functions over-represented among genes associated with social QTNs (Table 7). QTNs associated with perseverative behaviors point to genes involved in epileptic encephalopathy, loss of hippocampal neurons, and certain higher level functions such as social transmission of food preference, mating, spatial learning, and motor learning (Table 8). Interestingly, the genes associated with the QTNs for perseverative behaviors do not overlap with those associated with any of the other traits, while there is an overlap of 20 genes harboring QTNs for nonverbal, play and social skills (Figure 4), suggesting interrelated proficiencies involving the latter functions. These studies thus help to link genotype to genes and phenotypes and reveal some of the biological processes that may underlie specific ASD traits. The relevance of the above-described neurological functions to ASD further suggested that some of these QTNs may be able to distinguish cases from controls.

3.3. Trait-Associated QTNs Can Discriminate between Cases and Controls

Case-control association analyses using individuals at the extremes of phenotypic (i.e., trait) severity (Q1 and Q4) as cases enabled the identification of significant trait QTNs that were demonstrated to discriminate between cases and controls. This approach allowed reduction in the phenotypic heterogeneity of the individuals within each subgroup of twins for genetic analyses. In fact, genetic differences between the first and fourth quartiles of trait severity for all twin subgroups are quite clear. Notably, for SNPs associated with both Q1 and Q4 subgroups, the odds ratios for the two extreme groups are distinctly different and often in opposite directions (that is, greater or less than 1) relative to unrelated controls (Tables S7–S12), thereby supporting the associative nature of the specific SNP with that particular trait. Thus, the genetic heterogeneity of cases with respect to these trait-associated SNPs reflects the phenotypic heterogeneity of individuals at the extreme ends of the trait distribution profiles. In addition, hypergeometric distribution analyses of the genes derived from case-control analyses of twin subgroups show significant enrichment in SFARI autism risk genes in three of the twin subgroups (dNA.MZ, dNA.DZ, and cDZ) (Table 3). The over-representation of SFARI-annotated autism risk genes among those revealed here through case-control analyses indicates that the reduction in heterogeneity of cases at the extremes of the trait spectrum allows the detection of significant genetic variants differentiating cases and controls with relatively few samples, while also implicating novel ASD-associated genes that may be replicated by future studies. Although there is precedence for the use of individuals at the extremes of autistic traits for phenotype analyses [24–27], no other study

3.4. Genetic Differences between Discordant DZ Twins Strongly Associate with Autism Risk Genes

The availability of genome-wide genotype data for both autistic and non-autistic DZ co-twins in our study prompted us to examine the feasibility of performing a case-control analysis in which the group of non-autistic DZ twins was used as a control for the group of autistic co-twins. Although none of the 3400 SNPs with raw p-values ≤ 0.05 remained significant after correction for multiple testing, there were 390 SNPs with nominal p-values ≤ 0.05 and odds ratios ≥ 3 (ranging from 3 to 11) (Table S13). Hypergeometric distribution analysis of the 146 SNP-associated protein-coding genes showed significant enrichment in ASD-risk genes annotated by SFARI Gene as well as in genes revealed by exome sequencing [23]. Table 13 shows that this set of genes is highly enriched for ASD-associated neuronal functions including development, migration and pathfinding of neurons, neuritogenesis, axonogenesis, and guidance of axons, as well as synaptic development and transmission.

While the use of discordant non-autistic DZ twins as a control group for their autistic co-twins in case-control association analyses may seem unconventional, there is precedence for family-based genetic studies in which concordant MZ twin pairs were compared against their parents by whole genome and exome sequencing, with each study revealing novel and rare variants in the probands [28,29]. The use of both concordant and discordant MZ and DZ twins to investigate the contribution of pre-and post-zygotic de novo CNVs to ASD and other neurodevelopmental disorders [30] further illustrates the value of using diagnostic concordance and discordance in dissecting the complex genetic underpinnings of ASD.

3.5. Advantages and Limitations of Study Design

An advantage of quantitative trait association analysis is that it allows the identification of SNPs that may potentially be more functionally related to the condition, thus reducing the number of SNPs to be considered for further case-control association analyses. A possible disadvantage is that this procedure may exclude some ASD-relevant but not trait-associated SNPs from case-control analyses. Another limitation is that we did not separately analyze male and female twins due to the relatively small and variable number of females in the different subgroups of twins, and thus cannot eliminate sex as a confounding factor. However, a prior analysis of affected males and females from the AGRE repository using cluster analyses of ADI-R scores as described previously [17] showed no obvious sex differences in subphenotypes [31].

Because of the extreme heterogeneity of ASD, there has been increasing attempts to stratify or subgroup individuals with ASD by specific phenotypes to obtain more homogeneous sample groups for large-scale genetics analyses. While some autism studies have been conducted using individuals at the top 5% of an autistic trait [24,25,27,32], no other study has performed genetic case-control association analyses on subgroups of twins stratified by trait severity in this manner. Although the use of both MZ and DZ twins at the extremes of trait severity reduces the genetic heterogeneity of 'cases' when compared against a large group of unrelated controls, sample sizes at these extremes are a limitation of this study. Another limitation is that there is no empirical validation of the significant SNPs identified by case-control analyses as this was purely an in silico study, and we did not have access to the twins' biological samples for follow-up genotype analyses. On the other hand, the identification of some significant SNPs (with different odds ratios) for samples in the first and fourth quartiles of trait severity in case-control analyses replicates the association of those SNPs with ASD in distinct subgroups of individuals. Despite these limitations, case-control analyses revealed a number of significant trait-associated SNPs that implicate genes that converge on certain neurological functions associated with ASD, suggesting that disruption of those functions or pathways may play a role in the manifestation of that specific trait in ASD. Notably, multiple genes are associated with each of the five traits reflecting the multi-genic nature of ASD, even at these fundamental levels. However, no information is available on the functional significance of the specific SNPs with respect to gene regulation or to protein function and expression, and many SNPs are in noncoding regions which require further exploration.

Case-control association analyses using clinically discordant DZ twins as both cases and controls, while underpowered, identified a large number of nominally significant SNPs associated with genes that are significantly enriched in autism risk genes. While this study shows that reduction of genetic heterogeneity by stratification of cases according to trait severity or by use of discordant DZ twins as cases and controls increases the ability to identify common genetic variants associated with ASD, future studies with greater numbers of individuals in each subgroup are required to replicate these findings.

4. Summary

We present here a novel experimental design using MZ and DZ twins, either concordant or discordant for ASD, which evaluates the role of genetics in contributing to the severity of autistic traits and identifies significant SNPs that can distinguish cases from unaffected controls by capitalizing on the extreme phenotypic differences exhibited especially by discordant MZ and DZ twins. Although prior studies have consistently indicated that genetics is a major contributor to the overall diagnosis of ASD, deep phenotypic profiling shows that almost all ASD traits are significantly more severe in non-autistic MZ twins than in non-autistic DZ twins, suggesting a dominant influence of genotype on ASD phenotypes probed by the majority of items on the ADI-R diagnostic instrument [16]. At the same time, the similarity of trait-severity profiles among all autistic subgroups suggests that the ADI-R, often considered the gold-standard instrument for autism diagnostics, captures the essential components of ASD across the ASD population.

Quantitative trait association analyses using ASD trait profiles reveal SNPs (QTNs) associated with genes that provide meaningful insight into neurological functions and pathways commonly associated with ASD, thus linking genotype to phenotype (i.e., specific traits) as well as to underlying molecular pathology. Moreover, reducing phenotypic heterogeneity by using individuals at the extremes of trait severity for case-control association analyses with the trait-associated QTNs resulted in the identification of SNPs that significantly discriminate both affected and non-autistic co-twins from a large group of unrelated controls. These results suggest an underlying genetic liability towards autistic traits, even in the undiagnosed individuals (i.e., non-autistic co-twins). Genes implicated by the QTNs that survive correction for multiple testing in case-control association analyses are statistically enriched in ASD-associated genes revealed by significant overlap with those in the SFARI Gene database. Finally, case-control association analysis using dA.DZ twins as cases and their discordant non-autistic co-twins (dNA.DZ) as 'controls' also reveals a large number of neurologically relevant genes that are significantly over-represented in both SFARI Gene and exome sequencing datasets.

5. Materials and Methods

5.1. ASD Subphenotype Analysis and Generation of Trait Severity Distribution Profiles

Detailed demographic information of the 284 pairs of twins included in this study is shown in Table S14. Of these sets of twins, 88 monozygotic (MZ) pairs were concordant for diagnosis of ASD, while 25 MZ pairs were discordant. Among the dizygotic (DZ) twins, 56 pairs were concordantly autistic, while 115 pairs were discordant for diagnosis. As mentioned earlier, we label the concordant autistic MZ and DZ twin subgroups as cMZ and cDZ, respectively, and the discordant autistic (dA) and non-autistic (dNA) MZ and DZ twin subgroups as dA.MZ, dA.DZ, dNA.MZ, and dNA.DZ, respectively. ADI-R diagnostic scoresheets for all sets of twins were downloaded from the AGRE repository. It should be noted that ADI-R scoresheets were available for both the autistic and non-autistic (discordant) co-twins in order to establish concordance. Raw scores for 88 items from the ADI-R scoresheet which related to five ASD traits (spoken language, nonverbal communication, play skills, social skills, and perservative behaviors) were extracted from each individual's scoresheet, and the ADI-R scores were then adjusted according to previously described methods [17]. The specific items related to each trait are shown in Table S15. The average score for each ADI-R item, as well as the cumulative score for a specific trait, was calculated for each of the six twin subgroups. Quantitative trait distribution profiles for each twin subgroup were created by graphing each individual's cumulative score for each trait. To account for differences in the number of individuals in the different subgroups of twins, the total number of individuals in each subgroup was normalized to 100 to facilitate graphical comparisons between trait severity distribution profiles based on zygosity as well as on diagnostic concordance or discordance. The student's two-sample t-test in the StatPac statistical software package (https://statpac.com/index.htm) was used to determine significance of differences in severity scores of overall ASD traits and specific ADI-R items based on p-values ≤ 0.05.

5.2. Source of Genetic Data

Genome-wide genotype data for the twins and 2438 unaffected (non-autistic) controls were derived from a previously published genome-wide association study (GWAS) by Wang et al. [33], with data previously cleaned by Jennifer K. Lowe in the laboratory of Daniel H. Geschwind, M.D., Ph.D. at UCLA. Briefly, genotyping data were generated on Illumina HumanHap550 BeadChip arrays with over 550,000 SNP markers. Quality control procedures required DNA samples to have ≥ 0.95 call rate with minor allele frequency ≥ 0.05, and p-values testing significant deviation from Hardy–Weinberg equilibrium that were ≥ 0.001. Only subjects of European ancestry were genotyped and thus, only Caucasian twins could be included in the genetic association analyses, eliminating concerns about population stratification as a confounding factor. This publicly available dataset contained the genotypes for 74.3% of MZ twins (85 pairs) and ~85.4% of DZ twins (146 pairs) in this study. Controls were comprised of 2438 unrelated non-autistic individuals of European ancestry for whom genome-wide genotyping data was also available from the same GWAS study [33]. The workflow for the genetic association analyses performed on the twin data is shown in Scheme 1 for clarity.

5.3. Quantitative Trait Loci (QTL) Association Analyses

PLINK 1.07 software [34] was used to perform all genetic association analyses. Quantitative trait association analyses utilized the cumulative trait scores and the respective genotype data from the above-mentioned dataset for each individual within a specific twin subgroup as previously described [19]. Single nucleotide polymorphisms (SNPs) with unadjusted p-value $\leq 1.0 \times 10^{-5}$ were identified as QTNs which were subsequently used in case-control association analyses as described below. The overlap of trait-associated genes implicated by the SNPs was determined using Venny 2.1.0, an online software package for creating Venn diagrams [35].

5.4. Case-Control Association Analyses

To reduce ASD heterogeneity for genetic analyses, only cases at the extremes of a defined ASD trait were used in separate case-control association analyses. These individuals exhibited cumulative trait severity scores within the first or fourth quartiles. The first quartile (Q1) was comprised of twins who exhibited the least severe phenotype for that trait and the fourth quartile (Q4) was comprised of twins who exhibited the highest severity for that trait. Cumulative trait scores at Q1 and Q4 for each subgroup of twins were determined using Tyers Box Plot software [36] (see Scheme 1 and Figure 2). Individuals with cumulative scores less than or equal to that determined by Q1 and greater than or equal to that determined by Q4 were used in case-control association analyses against 2438 unrelated controls from the study of Wang et al. [33], focusing on the SNPs discovered by QTL analysis. Discordant non-autistic twins for whom genome-wide genotyping data were available were also stratified and analyzed in the same way. Because only one individual of a pair of MZ twins was included in the original genome-wide genotyping analysis [33], the genotype data of each dA.MZ twin was used for his or her respective dNA.MZ co-twin in case-control analyses. SNPs were considered significant if the adjusted Benjamini–Hochberg FDR was ≤ 0.10.

5.5. SNP Annotation and Functional Analyses of Associated Genes

Significant SNPs were annotated using SNPper [37] and/or SNPnexus [38]. Both are web-based applications that allow downloading of information on SNPs according to user-defined criteria, such as chromosomal position, band, alleles, closest gene, role (e.g., coding exon, promoter, intron, 3'-UTR), amino acid change, and position. The SNP-associated genes were analyzed using Ingenuity Pathway Analysis (IPA) software (QIAGEN, Redwood City, CA) with a focus on genes involved in neurological functions and pathways. Significance for enrichment of genes associated with a particular pathway or function included in IPA's Knowledgebase was determined by right-tailed Fisher's exact test (p-value ≤ 0.05).

5.6. Hypergeometric Distribution Analyses for Gene Enrichment

SNP-associated genes were then compared to a list of known autism risk genes in the SFARI Gene database [39] and/or a list of ASD-associated genes identified by an exome sequencing study [23]. Hypergeometric distribution probabilities for over-representation of overlapped genes within the SFARI dataset or among ASD genes identified by exome sequencing were calculated using the CASIO Keisan Online Calculator (http://keisan.casio.com/exec/system/1180573201), with significance determined by an upper cumulative q-value ≤ 0.05.

6. Conclusions

Deep phenotyping analysis of monozygotic and dizygotic twins concordant or discordant for diagnosis of ASD indicates that the identical genotype of non-autistic MZ twins with their respective affected co-twins strongly influences the severity of autistic traits in comparison to the trait severity expressed by non-autistic DZ twins. Quantitative trait association analyses using trait distribution profiles and genotype data for the respective twin groups identify SNPs linked to traits. Case-control association analyses using these QTNs and individuals at the extremes of trait distribution profiles reveal significant SNPs associated with genes that are functionally significant to the known pathobiology of ASD. Finally, we suggest that more effective treatment strategies may be derived by associating specific phenotypes with genotype-implicated genes and related functional deficits manifested by a given subgroup of individuals.

Supplementary Materials: Supplementary materials can be found at http://www.mdpi.com/1422-0067/20/15/3804/s1, Table S1: All trait QTNs for cMZ twins, Table S2: All trait QTNs for dA.MZ twins, Table S3: All trait QTNs for dNA.MZ twins, Table S4: All trait QTNs for cDZ twins, Table S5: All trait QTNs for dA.DZ twins, Table S6: All trait QTNs for dNA.DZ twins, Table S7: Case-control by quartile analysis of cMZ twins, Table S8: Case-control by quartile analysis of dA.MZ twins, Table S9: Case-control by quartile analysis of dNA.MZ twins, Table S10: Case-control by quartile analysis of cDZ twins, Table S11: Case-control by quartile analysis of dA.DZ twins, Table S12: Case-control by quartile analysis of dNA.DZ twins, Table S13: Case-control analysis using dA.DZ as cases and dNA.DZ as controls, Table S14: Demographic information for all twins from AGRE repository, Table S15: ADI-R items used for quantitative trait severity profiles and analyses.

Author Contributions: Conceptualization, V.W.H.; Phenotype analysis, C.A.D.; Genetic analyses, V.W.H.; SNP annotation and hypergeometric analyses, J.J.D. and V.W.H.; Original draft preparation, V.W.H. and C.A.D.; Review and editing, C.A.D., J.J.D., and V.W.H.; Supervision, V.W.H.

Acknowledgments: This research received no external funding. This study was an in silico reanalysis of existing genome-wide genotyping data. The authors are grateful to Zohreh Talebizadeh (Children's Mercy Hospital, Kansas City, MO, USA) and Olivia Veatch (Univ. of Pennsylvania, Philadelphia, PA, USA) for helpful discussion and comments on a draft of the manuscript.

Conflicts of Interest: The authors declare no conflict of interest.

References

1. American Psychiatric Association. *Diagnostic and Statistical Manual of Mental Disorders (DSM-5)*; American Psychiatric Publishing: Washington, DC, USA, 2013.
2. Masi, A.; DeMayo, M.M.; Glozier, N.; Guastella, A.J. An overview of autism spectrum disorder, heterogeneity and treatment options. *Neurosci. Bull.* **2017**, *33*, 183–193. [CrossRef] [PubMed]
3. Bailey, A.; Le Couteur, A.; Gottesman, I.; Bolton, P. Autism as a strongly genetic disorder: Evidence from a british twin study. *Psychol. Med.* **1995**, *25*, 63–77. [CrossRef] [PubMed]
4. Ronald, A.; Hoekstra, R.A. Autism spectrum disorders and autistic traits: A decade of new twin studies. *Am. J. Med. Genet. Part B Neuropsychiatr. Genet.* **2011**, *156*, 255–274. [CrossRef] [PubMed]
5. Trouton, A.; Spinath, F.M.; Plomin, R. Twins Early Development Study (TEDS): A multivariate, longitudinal genetic investigation of language, cognition and behavior problems in childhood. *Twin Res.* **2002**, *5*, 444–448. [CrossRef] [PubMed]
6. Mevel, K.; Fransson, P.; Bölte, S. Multimodal brain imaging in autism spectrum disorder and the promise of twin research. *Autism* **2015**, *19*, 527–541. [CrossRef]
7. Frans, E.M.; Sandin, S.; Reichenberg, A.; Långström, N.; Lichtenstein, P.; McGrath, J.J.; Hultman, C.M. Autism risk across generations: A population-based study of advancing grandpaternal and paternal age. *JAMA Psychiatry* **2013**, *70*, 516–521. [CrossRef]
8. Bölte, S.; Willfors, C.; Berggren, S.; Norberg, J.; Poltrago, L.; Mevel, K.; Coco, C.; Fransson, P.; Borg, J.; Sitnikov, R.; et al. The roots of autism and ADHD twin study in Sweden (RATSS). *Twin Res. Hum. Genet.* **2014**, *17*, 164–176. [CrossRef]
9. Hallmayer, J.; Cleveland, S.; Torres, A.; Phillips, J.; Cohen, B.; Torigoe, T.; Miller, J.; Fedele, A.; Collins, J.; Smith, K.; et al. Genetic heritability and shared environmental factors among twin pairs with autism. *Arch. Gen. Psychiatry* **2011**, *68*, 1095–1102. [CrossRef]
10. Gaugler, T.; Klei, L.; Sanders, S.J.; Bodea, C.A.; Goldberg, A.P.; Lee, A.B.; Mahajan, M.; Manaa, D.; Pawitan, Y.; Reichert, J.; et al. Most genetic risk for autism resides with common variation. *Nat. Genet.* **2014**, *46*, 881–885. [CrossRef]
11. Tick, B.; Bolton, P.; Happé, F.; Rutter, M.; Rijsdijk, F. Heritability of autism spectrum disorders: A meta-analysis of twin studies. *J. Child Psychol. Psychiatry Allied Discip.* **2016**, *57*, 585–595. [CrossRef]
12. Colvert, E.; Tick, B.; McEwen, F.; Stewart, C.; Curran, S.R.; Woodhouse, E.; Gillan, N.; Hallett, V.; Lietz, S.; Garnett, T.; et al. Heritability of autism spectrum disorder in a UK population-based twin sample. *JAMA Psychiatry* **2015**, *72*, 415–423. [CrossRef] [PubMed]
13. Taylor, M.J.; Gustafsson, P.; Larsson, H.; Gillberg, C.; Lundström, S.; Lichstenstein, P. Examining the association between autistic traits and atypical sensory reactivity: A twin study. *J. Am. Acad. Child Adolesc. Psychiatry* **2018**, *57*, 96–102. [CrossRef] [PubMed]
14. Lewis, G.J.; Shakeshaft, N.G.; Plomin, R. Face identity recognition and the social difficulties component of the autism-like phenotype: Evidence for phenotypic and genetic links. *J. Autism Dev. Disord.* **2018**, *48*, 2758–2765. [CrossRef] [PubMed]
15. Isaksson, J.; Van't Westeinde, A.; Cauvet, É.; Kuja-Halkola, R.; Lundin, K.; Neufeld, J.; Willfors, C.; Bolte, S. Social cognition in autism and other neurodevelopmental disorders: A co-twin control study. *J. Autism Dev. Disord.* **2019**, *49*, 2838–2848. [CrossRef] [PubMed]
16. Lord, C.; Rutter, M.; Couteur, A.L. Autism diagnostic interview-revised: A revised version of a diagnostic interview for caregivers of individuals with possible pervasive developmental disorders. *J. Autism Dev. Disord.* **1994**, *24*, 659–685. [CrossRef] [PubMed]
17. Hu, V.W.; Steinberg, M.E. Novel clustering of items from the autism diagnostic interview-revised to define phenotypes within autism spectrum disorders. *Autism Res.* **2009**, *2*, 67–77. [CrossRef] [PubMed]
18. Hu, V.W.; Sarachana, T.; Kim, K.S.; Nguyen, A.; Kulkarni, S.; Steinberg, M.E.; Luu, T.; Lai, Y.; Lee, N.H. Gene expression profiling differentiates autism case-controls and phenotypic variants of autism spectrum disorders: Evidence for Circadian rhythm dysfunction in severe autism. *Autism Res.* **2009**, *2*, 78–97. [CrossRef]
19. Hu, V.W.; Addington, A.; Hyman, A. Novel autism subtype-dependent genetic variants are revealed by quantitative trait and subphenotype association analyses of published GWAS data. *PLoS ONE* **2011**, *6*, e19067. [CrossRef]

20. Talebizadeh, Z.; Arking, D.E.; Hu, V.W. A novel stratification method in linkage studies to address inter and intra family heterogeneity in autism. *PLoS ONE* **2013**, *8*, e67569. [CrossRef]
21. Veatch, O.J.; Pendergast, J.S.; Allen, M.J.; Leu, R.M.; Johnson, C.H.; Elsea, S.H.; Malow, B.A. Genetic variation in melatonin pathway enzymes in children with autism spectrum disorder and comorbid sleep onset delay. *J. Autism Dev. Disord.* **2014**, *45*, 100–110. [CrossRef]
22. Talebizadeh, Z.; Shah, A.; DiTacchio, L. The potential role of a retrotransposed gene and a long noncoding RNA in regulating an X-linked chromatin gene (KDM5C): Novel epigenetic mechanism in autism. *Autism Res.* **2019**, *12*, 1007–1021. [CrossRef]
23. Iossifov, I.; O'Roak, B.J.; Sanders, S.J.; Ronemus, M.; Krumm, N.; Levy, D.; Stessman, H.A.; Witherspoon, K.T.; Vives, L.; Patterson, K.E.; et al. The contribution of de novo coding mutations to autism spectrum disorder. *Nature* **2014**, *515*, 216–221. [CrossRef]
24. Ronald, A.; Happé, F.; Price, T.S.; Baron-Cohen, S.; Plomin, R. Phenotypic and genetic overlap between autistic traits at the extremes of the general population. *J. Am. Acad. Child Adolesc. Psychiatry* **2006**, *45*, 1206–1214. [CrossRef]
25. Robinson, E.B.; Koenen, K.C.; McCormick, M.C.; Munir, K.; Hallett, V.; Happé, F.; Plomin, R.; Ronald, A. Evidence that autistic traits show the same etiology in the general population and at the quantitative extremes (5%, 2.5%, and 1%). *Arch. Gen. Psychiatry* **2011**, *68*, 1113–1121. [CrossRef]
26. Frazier, T.W.; Thompson, L.; Youngstrom, E.A.; Law, P.; Hardan, A.Y.; Eng, C.; Morris, N. A twin study of heritable and shared environmental contributions to autism. *J. Autism Dev. Disord.* **2014**, *44*, 2013–2025. [CrossRef]
27. Veatch, O.J.; Sutcliffe, J.S.; Warren, Z.E.; Keenan, B.T.; Potter, M.H.; Malow, B.A. Shorter sleep duration is associated with social impairment and comorbidities in ASD. *Autism Res.* **2017**, *10*, 1221–1238. [CrossRef]
28. McKenna, B.; Koomar, T.; Vervier, K.; Kremsreiter, J.; Michaelson, J.J. Whole-genome sequencing in a family with twin boys with autism and intellectual disability suggests multimodal polygenic risk. *Cold Spring Harbor Mol. Case Stud.* **2018**, *4*, a003285. [CrossRef]
29. Egawa, J.; Watanabe, Y.; Sugimoto, A.; Nunokawa, A.; Shibuya, M.; Igeta, H.; Inoue, E.; Hoya, S.; Orime, N.; Hayashi, T.; et al. Whole-exome sequencing in a family with a monozygotic twin pair concordant for autism spectrum disorder and a follow-up study. *Psychiatry Res.* **2015**, *229*, 599–601. [CrossRef]
30. Stamouli, S.; Anderlid, B.-M.; Willfors, C.; Thiruvahindrapuram, B.; Wei, J.; Berggren, S.; Nordgren, A.; Scherer, S.W.; Lichtenstein, P.; Tammimies, K.; et al. Copy number variation analysis of 100 twin pairs enriched for neurodevelopmental disorders. *Twin Res. Hum. Genet.* **2018**, *21*, 1–11. [CrossRef]
31. Hu, V.W. Cluster Analyses of Females with Autism According to ADI-R Severity Scores. Unpublished.
32. Robinson, E.B.; Koenen, K.C.; McCormick, M.C.; Munir, K.; Hallett, V.; Happé, F.; Plomin, R.; Ronald, A. A multivariate twin study of autistic traits in 12-year-olds: Testing the fractionable autism triad hypothesis. *Behav. Genet.* **2012**, *42*, 245–255. [CrossRef]
33. Wang, K.; Zhang, H.; Ma, D.; Bucan, M.; Glessner, J.T.; Abrahams, B.S.; Salyakina, D.; Imielinski, M.; Bradfield, J.P.; Sleiman, P.M.A.; et al. Common genetic variants on 5p14.1 associate with autism spectrum disorders. *Nature* **2009**, *459*, 528–533. [CrossRef]
34. Purcell, S.; Neale, B.; Todd-Brown, K.; Thomas, L.; Ferreira, M.A.R.; Bender, D.; Maller, J.; Sklar, P.; De Bakker, P.I.W.; Daly, M.J.; et al. PLINK: A tool set for whole-genome association and population-based linkage analyses. *Am. J. Hum. Genet.* **2007**, *81*, 559–575. [CrossRef]
35. Oliveros, J.C.; Venny. An Interactive Tool for Comparing Lists with Venn's Diagrams. 2007. Available online: http://bioinfogp.cnb.csic.es/tools/venny/index.html (accessed on 17 June 2019).
36. Spitzer, M.; Wildenhain, J.; Rappsilber, J.; Tyers, M. BoxPlotR: A web tool for generation of box plots. *Nat. Methods* **2014**, *11*, 121–122. [CrossRef]
37. Riva, A.; Kohane, I.S. SNPper: Retrieval and analysis of human SNPs. *Bioinformatics* **2002**, *18*, 1681–1685. [CrossRef]

38. Dayem Ullah, A.Z.; Oscanoa, J.; Wang, J.; Nagano, A.; Lemoine, N.R.; Chelala, C. SNPnexus: Assessing the functional relevance of genetic variation to facilitate the promise of precision medicine. *Nucleic Acids Res.* **2018**, *46*, W109–W113. [CrossRef]
39. Basu, S.N.; Kollu, R.; Banerjee-Basu, S. AutDB: A gene reference resource for autism research. *Nucleic Acids Res.* **2009**, *37*, D832–D836. [CrossRef]

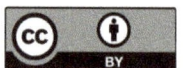

© 2019 by the authors. Licensee MDPI, Basel, Switzerland. This article is an open access article distributed under the terms and conditions of the Creative Commons Attribution (CC BY) license (http://creativecommons.org/licenses/by/4.0/).

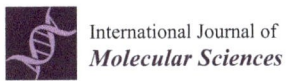

Case Report

Significantly Elevated *FMR1* mRNA and Mosaicism for Methylated Premutation and Full Mutation Alleles in Two Brothers with Autism Features Referred for Fragile X Testing

Michael Field [1,†], Tracy Dudding-Byth [1,2,†], Marta Arpone [3,4], Emma K. Baker [3,4,5], Solange M. Aliaga [3,4], Carolyn Rogers [1], Chriselle Hickerton [3], David Francis [6], Dean G. Phelan [6], Elizabeth E. Palmer [1], David J. Amor [3,4], Howard Slater [3,4,6], Lesley Bretherton [3,4,7,8], Ling Ling [3] and David E. Godler [3,4,*]

1. Genetics of Learning Disability Service, Hunter Genetics, Waratah, NSW 2298, Australia
2. Grow-up Well WPriority Research Centre, University of Newcastle, Newcastle, NSW 2308, Australia
3. Diagnosis and Development, Murdoch Children's Research Institute, Royal Children's Hospital, Parkville, VIC 3052, Australia
4. Department of Paediatrics, Faculty of Medicine, Dentistry and Health Sciences, University of Melbourne, Parkville, VIC 3052, Australia
5. School of Psychology and Public Health, La Trobe University, Bundoora, VIC 3086, Australia
6. Victorian Clinical Genetics Services, Murdoch Children's Research Institute, Royal Children's Hospital, Parkville, VIC 3052, Australia
7. Psychology Service, The Royal Children's Hospital, Parkville, VIC 3052, Australia
8. Melbourne School of Psychological Sciences, University of Melbourne, Parkville, VIC 3052, Australia
* Correspondence: david.godler@mcri.edu.au
† These authors contributed equally to the work.

Received: 2 July 2019; Accepted: 7 August 2019; Published: 11 August 2019

Abstract: Although fragile X syndrome (FXS) is caused by a hypermethylated full mutation (FM) expansion with ≥200 cytosine-guanine-guanine (CGG) repeats, and a decrease in *FMR1* mRNA and its protein (FMRP), incomplete silencing has been associated with more severe autism features in FXS males. This study reports on brothers (B1 and B2), aged 5 and 2 years, with autistic features and language delay, but a higher non-verbal IQ in comparison to typical FXS. CGG sizing using AmplideX PCR only identified premutation (PM: 55–199 CGGs) alleles in blood. Similarly, follow-up in B1 only revealed PM alleles in saliva and skin fibroblasts; whereas, an FM expansion was detected in both saliva and buccal DNA of B2. While Southern blot analysis of blood detected an unmethylated FM, methylation analysis with a more sensitive methodology showed that B1 had partially methylated PM alleles in blood and fibroblasts, which were completely unmethylated in buccal and saliva cells. In contrast, B2 was partially methylated in all tested tissues. Moreover, both brothers had *FMR1* mRNA ~5 fold higher values than those of controls, FXS and PM cohorts. In conclusion, the presence of unmethylated FM and/or PM in both brothers may lead to an overexpression of toxic expanded mRNA in some cells, which may contribute to neurodevelopmental problems, including elevated autism features.

Keywords: fragile X syndrome; autism; RNA toxicity; DNA methylation; mosaicism; pediatrics; MS-QMA; AmplideX

1. Introduction

Fragile X syndrome (FXS) is a leading single-gene cause of inherited intellectual disability (ID), with a prevalence of up to 1 in 4000 [1]. The vast majority (~90%) of males affected by FXS, and ~50% of females, show autism spectrum disorder (ASD) features, including speech perseveration, compulsions, echolalia, repetitive behaviors, poor eye contact, and deficits in social communication [2–5]. Many of these features are shared with idiopathic ASD [6]. The primary molecular cause of FXS is abnormal regulation of the fragile X mental retardation 1 (*FMR1*) gene due to the presence of ≥200 cytosine-guanine-guanine (CGG) repeats, termed full mutation (FM), within the *FMR1* promoter (reviewed in Kraan et al. [7]). These FM alleles are thought to silence *FMR1* transcription [8–12] through epigenetic changes at the *FMR1* promoter, including increased DNA methylation. Loss of *FMR1* mRNA in turn leads to depletion of the fragile X mental retardation protein (FMRP) [13–16], which is the primary cause of FXS symptomology, as FMRP has a critical function in synaptic plasticity and normal brain development [17–21].

In contrast, smaller CGG alleles (55–199 repeats), termed premutation (PM), usually have an unmethylated *FMR1* promoter, but abnormally increased levels of expanded PM mRNA [22,23]. In some PM carriers, the transcription of *FMR1* mRNA from expanded alleles has been associated with "RNA gain of function" toxicity, implicated in late onset disorders such as Fragile X-associated Tremor/Ataxia Syndrome (FXTAS) [22,23]. Other factors proposed to contribute to PM-related disorders are expanded repeat associated non-AUG translation, and increased transcription of *ASFMR1/FMR4* originating from the same locus as *FMR1* (reviewed in Kraan et al. [7]). In FXS, these mechanisms have not been comprehensively studied, but may explain significant variability in the type and severity of the FXS phenotype, beyond FMRP deficiency. This is consistent with our recent study suggesting that, in the majority (60%) of FXS males, FM mRNA can still be detected, and that this incomplete silencing in males <19 years of age is associated with more severe autism features, but not more severe ID [6]. This led us to propose that FXS can be stratified based on complete and incomplete silencing, with the two reciprocal mechanisms of RNA toxicity and FMRP deficiency contributing to overlapping aspects of FXS, namely the ID and autism phenotype in each individual that has incomplete silencing. This is particularly important as mosaicism for active and inactive expanded alleles may be more common than previously reported (10% to 40%) [5,11,15,24–29], based on the detection of *FMR1* mRNA in more than 60% of FM males [6]. The difference of >20% in the reported prevalence of mosaicism in FXS by Southern blot analysis as opposed to incomplete *FMR1* silencing detected by real-time PCR [6], is likely due to the limited analytical sensitivity of methylation-sensitive Southern blot analysis (the 'gold standard' FXS diagnostic test used in earlier studies) that does not detect mosaic alleles in less than 20% of cells [26]. Extreme examples of low level methylation mosaicism found in <20% of cells have previously been described in rare adult individuals with unmethylated FM (UFM) alleles that typically have mild ID (but are at risk of premutation phenotypes such as FXTAS) [30].

This study, for the first time, describes two brothers with UFM alleles detected by Southern blot analysis in a pediatric setting. Based on non-verbal intellectual functioning assessments, the brothers are 'higher functioning' compared to typical FXS, but have autism features ranging from mild to severe. The detailed clinical and molecular follow-up is described. This includes the detection of low-level mosaicism for methylated PM and FM alleles in different tissues. The CGG sizing and *FMR1* mRNA analysis of the two brothers are also compared with family members ascertained through cascade testing, typical FXS, age-matched children with PM, and typically developing (TD) controls.

2. Results

2.1. Medical History

B1 was born at term after an uncomplicated pregnancy and delivery. His parents became concerned with his development from an early age. He had extreme shyness, disliked new social circumstances, avoided some physical contact, and had limited eye contact. He was difficult to settle and he was often irritable and upset. His early motor milestones were normal, but language was significantly delayed. A clinical evaluation with the Griffiths Mental Developmental Scales, Extended Revised led to a diagnosis of mild global developmental delay, with significant difficulties with language and play skills.

Fragile X testing by Southern blot analysis of DNA extracted from blood and microarray analysis were performed at the age of 3 years. Southern blot analysis detected an abnormal 1.42 kb pfxa3 fragment equivalent to approximately 170 CGG repeats expansion. No pathogenic copy number variants (ISCA 60K) were identified through a chromosomal microarray. The results of psychometric testing (Stanford-Binet Intelligence Scales 5th Edition) [31] at the age of 4.5 years were consistent with a mild ID, with relative strengths in nonverbal abilities. The Adaptive Behavioural Assessment System (ABAS-II) results indicated a mild deficit in everyday functioning. He was treated with fluoxetine, which improved his social anxiety. After B1's fragile X genetic testing, cascade testing was carried out for other family members. The mother of both brothers was found to have a 74 CGG expanded allele; the maternal half-sister, maternal aunt, and maternal grandfather were also all identified as having a PM allele (Figure 1A).

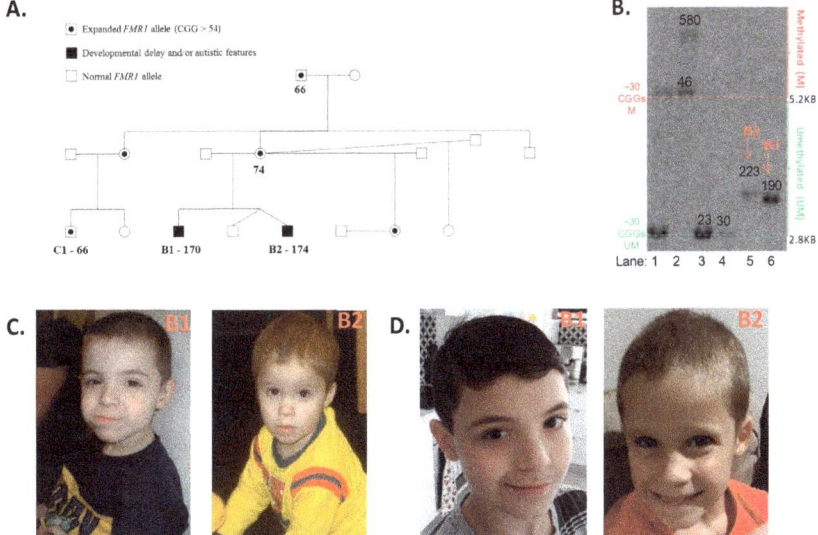

Figure 1. (**A**) Family pedigree, with expansion sizes from AmplideX testing. None of the individuals had manifested symptoms consistent with fragile X syndrome or fragile X-associated disorders, such as Fragile X-associated Tremor/Ataxia Syndrome (FXTAS) or Fragile X-associated Primary Ovarian Insufficiency (FXPOI). The brothers' have two half-sisters, one of which was identified as carrying a premutation (PM) allele and the other as carrying a normal fragile X mental retardation 1 (*FMR1*) allele. B1's cousin (C1) was identified at 1 year and 11 months of age as carrying an *FMR1* PM allele of 66 CGG repeats. (**B**) Methylation-sensitive Southern blot analysis of the *NruI* restriction site within the *FMR1* CpG island in blood. The DNA samples from the two brothers in question are located in lanes 5 and 6. B2 has a 223 CGG unmethylated allele, while B1 has a 190 CGG repeat unmethylated allele. A typical female (CGG < 44) is in lane 1, while typical males (CGG < 44) are in lanes 3 and 4; and a full mutation (FM) female with a 100% methylated 580 CGG allele is in lane 2. The numbers superimposed on the blot indicate CGG sizing. The lower limit of detection for the Southern blot analysis of FM alleles on a normal allele background is 20%. (**C**) Photos of B1 and B2 at the ages of 5 and 2 years, respectively; written informed consent was obtained from the mother of the brothers to include these images in the publication (**D**) Photos of B1 and B2 at the ages of 10 and 7 years, respectively; written informed consent was obtained from the mother of the brothers to include these images in the publication. Note: Comparator DNA used of methylation-sensitive Southern blot analysis in (**B**) were also sized using standard CGG sizing PCR.

B2 is the younger brother of B1, who is a dizygous twin. The twins were conceived before the *FMR1* CGG expansion was identified in B1. B2 and his twin brother were delivered at term by elective caesarean section, in good condition after a pregnancy complicated by gestational hypertension. The twins were admitted for two days in the newborn nursery for blood sugar instability and required intravenous fluids. However, there were no ongoing neonatal concerns and the boys were discharged home on day four of life. There were no concerns about B2's development in the first year of life; he fed and slept well and all his motor milestones were in the normal range. He had surgery for left cryptorchidism, but his medical history was otherwise unremarkable. B2's mother became concerned about his development and behaviour around two years of age. Although B2 did not have typical craniofacial features of fragile X syndrome, he had a slightly longer face than his twin brother, which was visible at the time of assessment (Figure 1C) and also more recently (Figure 1D). He was normocephalic, had a normal tone and power, with a normal gait, and did not have joint hypermobility. At 9 months of age, fragile X PCR with AmplideX commercial kit was performed on their DNA extracted from blood, which identified a normal triplet repeat size (29 CGG repeats) in one of the twins, but a 174 PM CGG repeats expansion in B2.

2.2. Extended FMR1 CGG Testing

Extended *FMR1* testing was initiated to test the hypothesis that the neurodevelopmental phenotypes in B1 and B2 were due to the presence of FM alleles in tissues other than blood. For these extended studies, B1 and B2 were recruited into the FREE FX study at 5.6 and 2.7 years of age, respectively, but were not included in previous FREE FX study publications due to uncertainty about molecular diagnosis [6].

In blood, methylation-sensitive Southern blot analysis demonstrated the presence of unmethylated alleles of 190 CGGs in B1 and 223 CGGs in B2 (Figure 1B). These results are consistent with those previously reported for rare 'high functioning' FXS males with fully unmethylated FM alleles [32–34]. AmplideX testing of blood at the time of the FREE FX study assessments showed an allele of 168 CGGs in B1, while for B2, there were three alleles detected of 165, 185, and 199 CGGs (Figure 2B). AmplideX CGG sizing analysis in tissues other than blood showed that for B1, CGG sizing in saliva was consistent with that in blood. However, in fibroblasts, the sizing was different, with mosaicism for 140 CGG and 156 CGG alleles detected. In contrast, for B2, all alleles in the PM range were consistent between the tissues tested. However, for B2, in buccal epithelial cells (BEC) and saliva, FM alleles were also detected, which were not identified in blood. Subsequently, B2 received a molecular diagnosis of FXS that was not initially given by standard testing of blood.

The variability in CGG sizing between tissues was also investigated in both brothers using FastFraX 5′ and 3′ melting curve analysis (MCA) assays, using samples from C1 (cousin, as reference) [35]. Surprisingly, there was no amplification by the 3′ MCA assay in B1 and B2, while amplification occurred by 3′ MCA for C1, with the 5′ MCA performed on the same samples from B1, B2, and C1 displaying amplification, as expected (Supplemental Figure S1). This suggested that one of the primer sites for the 3′ MCA assay had a de novo sequence change of unknown significance in all tissues tested in both brothers that prevented primer binding and amplification, but not in their cousin. As a follow-up, sanger sequencing of the 3′ MCA *FMR1* exon 1 binding site inclusive of the ATG translation start site, and surrounding regions, was performed. However, no sequence variants were detected in both brothers compared to controls (Supplemental Figures S3 and S4). This suggested that a de novo sequence change was present for the binding site of the primer anchored at the 3′ end of the CGG repeat, rather than the primer overlapping with the ATG site within the exon 1.

2.3. FMR1 Methylation and Gene Expression Analyses

Methylation analysis using Methylation-Specific Quantitative Melt Analysis (MS-QMA) identified methylated alleles in both brothers in multiple tissues (Figure 3A,B) that were not present in 17 control males and 14 PM males co-run with these samples. However, the methylated peaks of ~5% in both brothers did overlap with those found in 41 FM only males and 18 typical PM/FM mosaics also co-run with the B1 and B2 samples (Supplemental Figure S2). The levels observed in both brothers were also consistent with those of the spiking reference sample, which contained 6% methylated FM and 94% unmethylated normal size male DNA (Figure 3C). Presence of the unmethylated expanded alleles in the majority of cells was consistent with *FMR1* mRNA analyses in blood for both brothers (Figure 4), where the levels in both brothers were ~5 fold higher than the levels observed in male and female controls. Interestingly, of the 13 PM male reference samples (most children or adolescents), only one had analogous *FMR1* mRNA levels. None of the FM only or PM/FM mosaic males had mRNA levels remotely close to those observed in the brothers, with the C1 PM (66 CGGs) cousin having mRNA levels just above the control range.

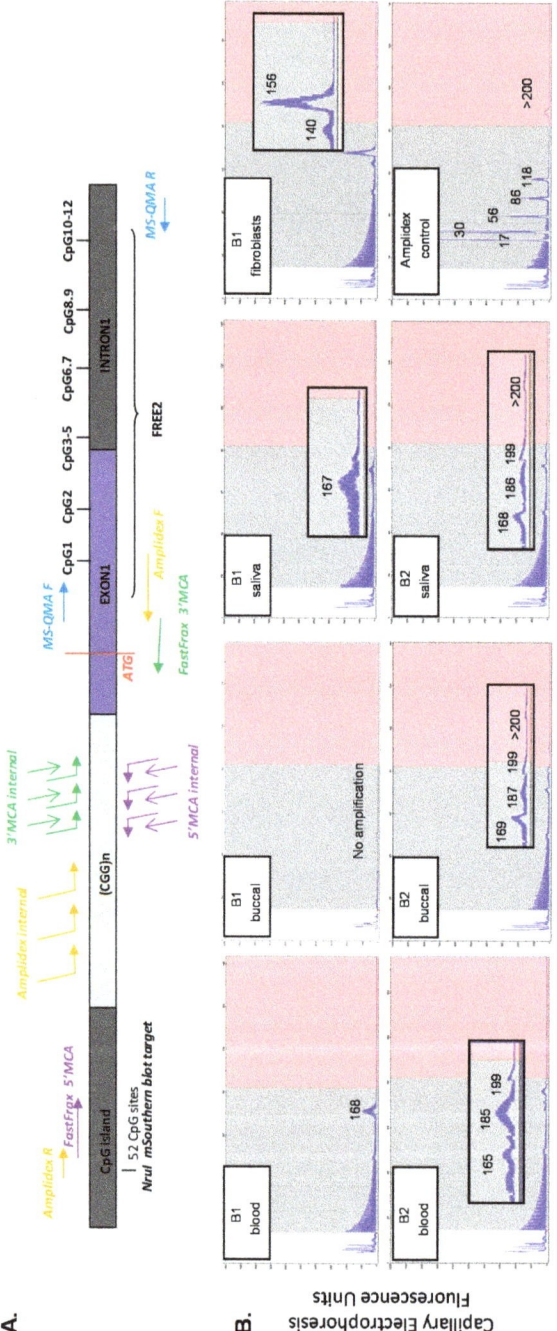

Figure 2. (**A**) Organization of the fragile X mental retardation 1 (*FMR1*) 5' region, including the cytosine-guanine-guanine (CGG) expansion and primer binding site locations for AmplideX CGG sizing PCR, FastFraX High-Resolution Melt Analysis, and Methylation-Specific Quantitative Melt Analysis (MS-QMA), in relation to Fragile X-Related Epigenetic Element 2 (FREE2); the *FMR1* CpG island and methylation sensitive restriction site *NruI* analysed using routine fragile X Southern blot testing; and two *HpaII* sites targeted by AmplideX methylation PCR. Note: The *FMR1* translation start site is indicated in red overlapping with FastFraX 3' melting curve analysis (MCA) primer. (**B**) AmplideX triplet-repeat primed long range PCR results for B1 and B2, for blood, buccal, saliva, and fibroblast DNA. Note: a reference sample co-run with the samples in question is included as the AmplideX sizing control in (**B**).

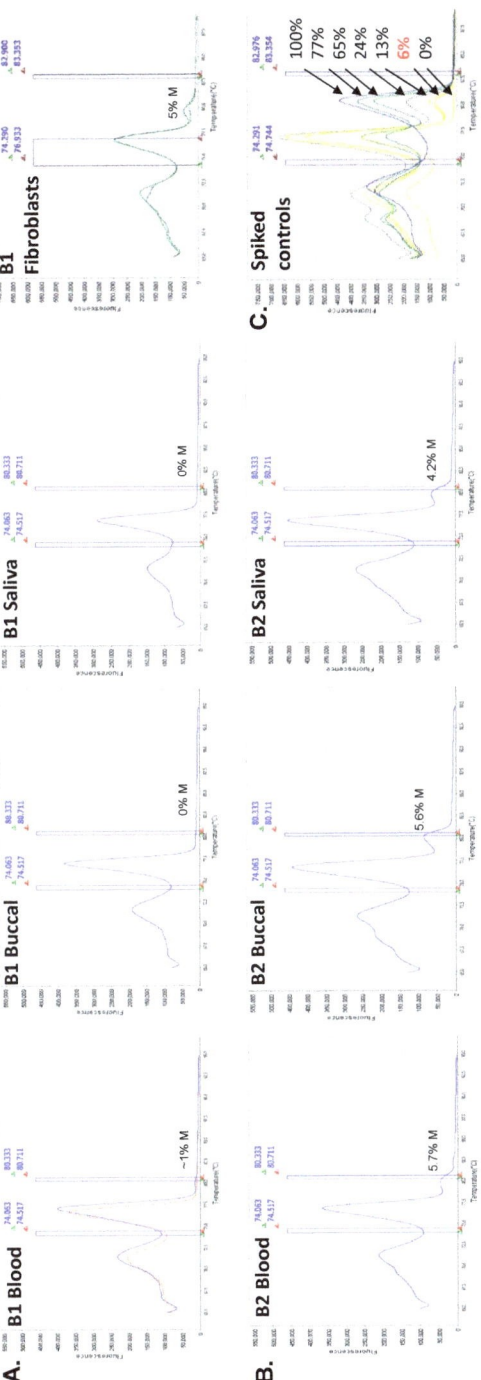

Figure 3. Derivative curve high-resolution melt profiles and mean methylation output ratios of CpG sites located within the Fragile X-Related Epigenetic Element 2 (FREE2) region assessed using Methylation-Specific Quantitative Melt Analysis (MS-QMA) between different tissues for (**A**) B1 and (**B**) B2. (**C**) DNA samples from lymphoblasts of a fragile X syndrome (FXS) male with the fragile X mental retardation 1 (*FMR1*) promoter 100% methylated spiked with DNA from a typically developing control (cytosine-guanine-guanine (CGG) < 44) with the *FMR1* promoter 0% methylated. These samples were mixed at different ratios for the MS-QMA methylation reference curve, with the expected % of methylation indicated on the plot for each derivative curve profile.

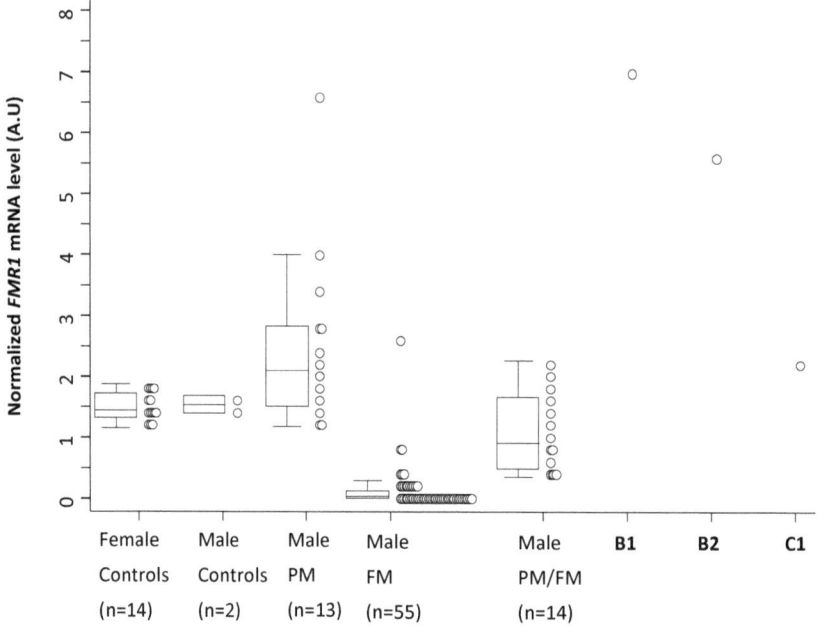

Figure 4. Comparison of fragile X mental retardation 1 (*FMR1*) mRNA levels in blood in the probands, control, premutation (PM), full mutation (FM) only, and PM/FM mosaic reference cohorts. Note: Control reference ranges included in blood of females (age 22 to 54 years; cytosine-guanine-guanine (CGG) < 44) and males (age 7.7–8.1 years) typically developing (TD) controls; males with PM alleles (3.4 to 23.6 years); and males with FM only alleles and PM/FM mosaic alleles (1.89 to 43.17 years). Control children had no family history of developmental delay and their mothers had CGG size < 44.

2.4. Neurodevelopmental Outcomes at the Time of Recruitment

In B1, the cognitive assessment as part of the FREE FX study highlighted receptive language difficulties, which greatly influenced his performance in the IQ test. He showed significant variability in his cognitive abilities. His verbal skills were a cognitive weakness, reflected in his verbal IQ (VIQ) score of 72 falling in the borderline range. His overall nonverbal problem-solving skills were in the low average range, with a performance IQ (PIQ) score of 84. His processing speed index (PSI) score was 71, which fell in the borderline range. His overall intellectual functioning, as reflected in the Full Scale IQ (FSIQ), was 77. Based on the Autism Diagnostic Observation Schedule Second Edition (ADOS-2) assessment, B1 met the cut-off for autism spectrum, with an overall ADOS-2 calibrated severity score (CSS) of 4. His Social Affect (SA) CSS was 3 (non-spectrum range), whilst his Restricted and Repetitive Behavior (RRB) CSS was 6 (autism range). B1's scores on the Child Behavior Checklist (CBCL) were in the normal range for the Total Problem and Externalizing problem scales, but fell in the borderline range for the Internalizing problems scale. Moreover, the Pervasive Developmental Problems subscale score fell in the clinical range and the Withdrawn subscale score fell in the borderline range. At the time of the research assessment, B1 was enrolled in a small mainstream primary school with additional learning support. He was reported to play alongside other children and although still shy, he did not have any major challenging behaviours. He had no seizures and was taking 2 mg/day of sertraline.

During assessment, as part of the FREE FX study, B2 predominantly used non-word vocalizations and jabbering; although on a number of occasions, he used single words and word approximations. Moreover, his formal developmental assessment with the Mullen Scales of Early Learning (MSEL) showed that his receptive and expressive language skills were respectively similar to that expected of an infant aged 10 and 17 months old, a marked discrepancy from his chronological age (31 months). He did not obtain a valid score (T ≥ 20) on the receptive language subdomain of the MSEL; a further indication of the significant impairment in this area. B2's ratio VIQ [36] was 44. In contrast, his performance in tasks assessing visual reception and fine motor skills was much better, obtaining age equivalents of 25 and 20 months, respectively, and a ratio non-verbal IQ (NVIQ) of 73. His overall MSEL Early Learning Composite score (using a default minimum T score of 20 for his Receptive Language domain) was 56, more than three standard deviations below the mean score (mean = 100; SD = 15) of similar aged peers, indicating a significant developmental delay. B2's difficulties with social communication, his engagement in sensory seeking and repetitive behaviours, and restricted interests observed during the ADOS-2 assessment led to an ADOS-2 classification of autism, with an overall ADOS CSS of 7. His SA CSS score of 5 fell in the autism spectrum range, whereas his RRB CSS of 10 fell in the autism range, the highest severity level for this domain for children with ASD of his age and verbal abilities. B2's CBCL Total, Internalizing, and Externalizing problem scales scores were all in the normal range. However, his score in the Withdrawn and Pervasive Developmental Problems subscales fell in the clinical range. His mother reported significant concerns regarding his very limited speech and social anxiety.

3. Discussion

This study describes two young brothers with expanded *FMR1* alleles, who were 'higher functioning' based on intellectual functioning assessments compared to a typical FXS cohort reported in previous studies [6]. Specifically, B1 had a PIQ score three standard deviations above the mean of the FREE FX typical FXS male cohort, while B2 had a non-verbal (NVIQ) score that was nearly two standard deviations above the same mean. Regarding VIQ, B1's score was 1 SD greater than the FXS group mean, while B2 fell within 1 SD of the typical FXS cases on this measure. B2's greater difficulties with expressive and receptive language skills may be closely linked to his more severe autism phenotype. In contrast, B1 presented mild autism features, though still met the ADOS-2 cut-off for autism spectrum. Based on methylation-sensitive Southern blot analysis of blood DNA, both brothers have been described as having UFM alleles approaching 200 CGGs in blood. Previous studies have described adults with similar Southern blot profiles, explaining their higher intellectual functioning through the *FMR1* promoter being completely unmethylated and expressing *FMR1* FM mRNA and FMRP [32–34]. These adult males with unmethylated alleles (FM and PM/FM mosaic) and incomplete silencing of *FMR1* mRNA from expanded FM alleles are at risk of FXTAS, based on clinical assessments and magnetic resonance imaging (MRI) features [30,37,38]. In these studies, it was hypothesized that expression of the UFM RNA is a contributor to the neurodegenerative features observed in some adults, through the same RNA toxicity mechanism as in PM-related disorders. However, the interplay between intellectual functioning and autism severity in the pediatric setting has not previously been characterized in individuals with UFM alleles.

In this study, additional molecular analyses with more sensitive techniques, such as MS-QMA and AmplideX PCR, indicate that a small proportion of cells in blood and other tissues have methylated PM and FM alleles that were not detected by Southern blot analysis. These findings are partly consistent with a previous study examining tissue heterogeneity in *FMR1* methylation and CGG size post-mortem, in a 79-year-old 'high-functioning' male with unmethylated PM and FM alleles detected in blood by Southern blot analysis [34]. In this male, a complete unmethylated PM/FM allele smear was found in blood by Southern blot analysis; however, in multiple other tissues, including the parietal lobe, methylated FM alleles were detected. Together, this suggests that the detection of methylated alleles varies with the tissue tested and the analytical sensitivity of the technique used. With the addition of more sensitive technologies to complement Southern blot analysis, the UFM classification in some of these cases is likely to be replaced with the term 'low-level methylation mosaicism'. Moreover, these males with low-level somatic mosaicism may not be as uncommon as previously thought. One reason for this may be that these unmethylated alleles are somatically unstable, with a significant proportion of these cases that have retraction down to a normal repeat size currently not being detected by standard testing [26].

It is also important to note that based on CGG sizing and methylation analysis of multiple tissues, B1 was found to have multiple methylated alleles in the PM range in a small proportion of cells (e.g., 170 CGG repeats in blood, but 140 and 156 CGG alleles in fibroblasts). This is consistent with an earlier study [26] that also reported a male with a methylated PM allele of 110 CGG repeats, in the absence of an FM, with a FSIQ value of 46. Together, this suggests that as part of somatic retraction below an FM allele size, some alleles may remain methylated in a proportion of cells, and may not be fully functional, with this proportion and CGG sizing differing between tissues. For the two brothers, however, the RNA toxicity, rather than FMRP deficiency, is likely to be the primary factor contributing to the autism phenotype. This is consistent with FM RNA levels being ~5 fold greater than in the reference sample of typically developing controls, PM/FM mosaic and FM only males affected with FXS, and the PM cousin (C1) with 66 CGGs. This is also consistent with our earlier study showing that FM males with incomplete silencing of *FMR1* had more severe autism features compared to the FM group where *FMR1* mRNA could not be detected [6].

This study also detected a potential sequence variant in the *FMR1* promoter overlapping with the 3′ MCA FastFraX primer binding site at the 3′ end of the CGG repeat. While the functional and clinical significance of this potential variant is uncertain, it did not inhibit *FMR1* transcription in both brothers. Similarly, previous studies have reported a sequence variant located next to the CGG repeat in FXS individuals displaying somatic retractions [30]. The loss of primer binding sites that may be associated with somatic retraction is an important limitation of all standard and long-range PCR-based methods, including AmplideX and FastFraX, as it may lead to expanded alleles being missed or not amplified, as demonstrated by the 3′ MCA assay for both brothers in this study, and for AmplideX previously [30].

In summary, the study reports two brothers with low-level methylation mosaicism not detected by standard testing in blood, who may be mistaken for males with rare UFM alleles, when based alone on Southern blot analysis of blood DNA. Moreover, in both brothers, *FMR1* mRNA levels were increased ~5-fold compared to typical developing controls, and significantly above the levels reported from PM, FM only, and PM/FM mosaic male cohorts from a previous study [6]. The abnormally elevated levels of *FMR1* mRNA in the two brothers may have led to *FMR1* mRNA-related cellular "toxicity". It is plausible that an FXS patho-mechanism exists whereby active unmethylated FM and/or PM alleles lead to the expression of toxic expanded mRNA in some cells, in conjunction with possible reduced *FMR1* mRNA and FMRP levels in other cells with *FMR1* methylation detected by MS-QMA. A combination of these two mechanisms in different cells may contribute to the brothers' neurodevelopmental problems, including the elevated ASD symptoms. This hypothesis is also in line with the findings reported by Baker et al. [6] showing that males with FM-only CGG expansions (aged < 19 years), who expressed FM *FMR1* mRNA, had significantly more severe ASD symptoms measured with the ADOS-2 compared to males with FM-only alleles who had completely silenced *FMR1*. The main limitations of this study are that the FMRP levels in blood and direct sequencing of the 3′ MCA binding site, anchored at the 5′ end of the CGG repeat, suspected to be modified in both brothers, have not been tested and performed. Future studies will address these limitations to shed light on the effect of the potential 3′ MCA variant (to be confirmed through DNA sequencing) on FMRP structure and function, and possibly further explain the phenotype presented by these two young children.

4. Materials and Methods

4.1. Ethics Approval and Consent

All aspects of this study have received ethical approval by The Royal Children's Hospital Human Research Ethics Committee (Single Site Reference numbers: HREC 34227, HREC 33066—Multi site HREC Reference Number: HREC/13/RCHM/24, approved on 24 May 2013).

4.2. Recruitment and Assessments

Affected family members include two brothers, B1, age 5.6 years, and B2, age 2.7 years, and their cousin C1, age 3.4 years. All were recruited through their clinical geneticist into the FREE FX study [6]. As part of the FREE FX study, the brothers' neurodevelopmental outcomes were evaluated through a medical and developmental history questionnaire prepared ad hoc for this study, the ADOS-2 (Module 2 for B1 and Module 1 for B2) [39], the Wechsler Preschool and Primary Scale of Intelligence–Third Edition (WPPSI-III) (Australian) (B1) [40], MSEL (B2) [41], and CBCL [42]. Both brothers' and their cousin's buccal epithelial cells, saliva, and venous blood samples were collected at the time of their participation in the study. A skin biopsy for genetic testing on fibroblasts was performed on B1, as part of his clinical care. Molecular data for positive and negative control cohorts used as reference data in this study were analysed previously [6,43,44] and from a newly recruited control and PM participants as part of the FREE FX study.

4.3. Sample Processing

Up to four BEC samples were collected per participant using the Master Amp Buccal Swab Brush kit (Epicentre Technologies, Madison, WI, USA), as previously described [45]. A single saliva sample was collected for each participant using the Oragene® DNA Self-Collection Kit (DNA Genotek, Global) and was processed as per the manufacturer's instructions. As part of a clinical genetic follow-up, and not as part of his involvement in the FREE FX study, a skin biopsy was performed for B1 to obtain fibroblasts. The DNA extracts were evaluated using a NanoDrop 2000 spectrophotometer (Thermo Fisher Scientific, Foster City, CA, USA). Ten ml of venous blood, from B1 and B2 and from two control male participants (aged 7.6 and 8.1 years, respectively), was used for peripheral blood mononuclear cell (PBMC) isolation using Ficoll gradient separation [46]. Isolated PBMCs were used for RNA extraction (RNeasy kit; Qiagen Inc., Hilden Germany) for gene expression analyses [46]. Total RNA extraction, purification, and reverse transcription were performed as previously described [47].

4.4. Methylation Specific-Quantitative Melt Analysis (MS-QMA)

DNA samples were extracted from BEC, saliva, venous blood, and fibroblasts, and transferred into 96-well plates to be treated with sodium bisulphite. An EZ DNA Methylation-Gold™ kit (Zymo research, Irvine, CA, USA) was used to bisulphite convert each sample in two separate reactions, with each conversion analysed in duplicate reactions. FREE2 DNA methylation analysis was performed using MS-QMA, as previously described [43]. Specifically, ninety-six samples were bisulfite converted at a time (3 controls and 93 unknown samples per plate) and were serially diluted four times post-conversion. These included positive and negative control cohorts used as reference data in this study, as well as samples in question from B1, B2, and C1. The bisulfite converted DNA was then transferred into a 384 well format for real-time PCR analysis utilizing MeltDoctor™ high-resolution melt reagents in 10 μL reactions, as per the manufacturer's instructions (Life technologies, Foster City, CA, USA). A unique primer set was used for real-time PCR that targets specific CpG sites within the Fragile X-Related Epigenetic Element 2 (FREE2) region, at the *FMR1* exon1/intron 1 boundary [43]. The annealing temperature for the thermal cycling protocol was 650 °C for 40 cycles. The ViiA™ 7 Real-Time PCR System (Life technologies, Foster City, CA, USA) was then used to quantify the DNA concentration of the unknown samples using the relative standard curve method post bisulfite conversion, by measuring the rate of dye incorporation into double stranded DNA. To progress to the next stage of the MS-QMA analysis, the unknown samples had to be within this dynamic linear range.

The products from a methylated and unmethylated FREE2 sequence were then separated into single strands in the temperature range of 74 and 82 °C as part of the high-resolution melt step that followed the real-time PCR in a close tube format. The HRM Software Module for ViiA™ 7 System was then used to plot the rate of PCR product separation to single strands, with the difference in fluorescence converted to Aligned Fluorescence Units (AFU).

The AFU conversion to the methylation percentage was performed at 78 °C, and all of the above quality control steps, were analysed simultaneously for 384 reactions at a time using Q-MAX software (Curve Tomorrow, Melbourne, Australia), developed to automate the process.

This software utilizes a custom-designed computer algorithm to simultaneously perform multiple quality control checks to determine DNA concentrations and quality post-bisulfite conversion using raw RT-PCR and high-resolution melt data for all dilutions from each bisulfite reaction. The high-resolution melt data for those sample dilutions outside the QC ranges were discarded from the quantitative methylation analysis by Q-MAX software, and were not used for the final aggregate methylation ratio calculation. The high-resolution melt profiles discarded from quantitative assessments by Q-MAX, however, were used for visual assessments for the presence or absence of abnormal methylation compared to control melt curves (Figure 3). Males were considered to have positive MS-QMA results if they had >2% methylation derived through Q-MAX and/or one of more high-resolution melt curve profiles that had derivative high-resolution melt plots with the presence of a peak originating from methylated alleles, at the same melting temperature as in FXS male controls (Figure 3).

4.5. Methylation Analysis and CGG Sizing Using Southern Blot and AmplideX PCR

Methylation-sensitive Southern blot analysis of the *NruI* restriction site within the *FMR1* CpG island was performed for the two brothers' venous blood DNA samples, using a fully validated methylation-sensitive Southern blot procedure with appropriate normal and abnormal controls, as described previously [48]. The *FMR1* CGG repeat size was assessed using a fully validated PCR assay with a precision of +/− one triplet repeat across the normal and grey zone ranges, performed using a fragment analyser (MegaBACE, GE Healthcare, Chicago, Illinois, IL, USA), with the upper limit of detection of 170 repeats, as described previously [49]. CGG sizing using both brothers' BEC, saliva, venous blood, and fibroblast (only B2) DNA was also performed using the AmplideX®™ *FMR1* PCR Kit as per the manufacturer's instructions [50] (Asuragen, Austin, TX, USA). The *FMR1* CGG size in DNA extracted from venous blood from the two brothers was further investigated by Southern blot testing at the Victorian Clinical Genetics Services (VCGS) (without the use of methylation sensitive restriction enzymes), as described previously [48].

4.6. Melting Curve Analysis (MCA) to Determine the Presence of Expanded FMR1 Alleles

Five prime and 3′ MCA high-resolution melt analyses were also undertaken in the BEC, saliva, and venous blood DNA of both brothers, in the fibroblasts DNA of B1, and in the venous blood DNA of C1, as per the manufacturer's instructions for the FastFraX commerical kit (Biofactory, Singapore) [35]. Specifically, 5′ and 3′ PCR reactions were performed for each sample, with each assay having one of the primers anchored at one end of the CGG repeat. Each assay contained 5 units of HotStarTaq DNA polymerase (Qiagen), 2.5× Q-Solution (Qiagen), 1× of the supplied PCR buffer (Qiagen), 0.1× SYBR Green I nucleic acid dye (Roche Applied Science, Upper Bavaria, Germany), and 50 ng genomic DNA. The 5′ PCR used a deoxynucleoside triphosphate mix consisting of 0.2 mmol/L each of dATP, dTTP, and dCTP, and 0.1 mmol/L each of 7-deaza-2′-dGTP (7-deaza-dGTP) and dGTP (Roche Molecular Diagnostics, Upper Bavaria, Germany). The 3′-PCR used a deoxynucleoside triphosphate mix consisting of 0.2 mmol/L each of dATP, dTTP, dCTP, and dGTP, and primer sequences and concentrations as previously described [35], with primer locations indicated in Figure 2A. The 5′ and 3′-PCR reactions were performed separately under identical thermocycling conditions in a ViiA™ 7 Real-Time PCR System (Life technologies, Foster City, CA). An initial denaturation step at 95 °C for 15 min was followed by 40 cycles of 99 °C for 2 min, 65 °C for 2 min, and 72 °C for 3 min, and then a final extension step at 72 °C for 10 min. PCR amplicons were then melted (after completion of the PCR program), consisting of denaturation at 95 °C for 1 min, a temperature-hold step at 60 °C for 1 min, and a temperature ramp from 60 °C to 95 °C at a rate of 0.01 °C/s. Reference male samples were co-run with the samples in question, including an FM (530 CGG), a PM (170 CGG), and a normal size (NS) control (30 CGG). Positive and negative calls were made based on the presence or absence of the difference in the profile fluorescence at the melting temperature threshold (85 °C for 5′ MCA; 90 °C for 3′MCA) compared to male reference samples.

4.7. Sanger Sequencing

Sanger sequencing of the 3′ MCA *FMR1* exon 1 binding site inclusive of the ATG translation start site, and surrounding regions was performed at the Australian Genome Research Facility Ltd in blood of B1 and B2, and compared to 2 reference samples from typically developing controls co-run with these samples. The data was re-analysed at the Victorian Clinical Genetics Services (VCGS), using Mutation Surveyor®V4.0.9 software (SoftGenetics®, State College, PA, USA) to detect and report SNPs as previously described [51].

4.8. FMR1 mRNA Analysis

Gene expression analyses were performed using reverse transcription real-time quantitative PCR (RT-PCR) on a ViiaTM 7 System (Life Technologies, Global), with the relative standard curve method as described in Kraan et al. [52]. The mean 5′and 3′ *FMR1* mRNA levels were normalized to the mean of *EIF4A2* and *SDHA* mRNA levels used as internal controls, expressed in arbitrary units (a.u) [52]. The summary measure used for mRNA expression levels for each participant was calculated by averaging the four arbitrary unit outputs originating from the two separate cDNA reactions, with each of these analysed in two separate RT-PCR reactions, performed for each RNA sample [52,53].

Supplementary Materials: The following are available online at http://www.mdpi.com/1422-0067/20/16/3907/s1.

Author Contributions: Conceptualization: M.F., T.D.-B., D.J.A., and D.E.G.; data curation: M.A., E.K.B., S.M.A., D.G.P., and L.L.; formal analysis: M.F., T.D.-B., M.A., E.K.B., E.E.P., and L.B.; funding acquisition: M.F., H.S., D.J.A., and D.E.G.; investigation: M.F., T.D.-B., M.A., S.M.A., C.R., C.H., D.F., E.E.P., L.L., D.G.P., and D.E.G.; resources: M.A., H.S., and D.E.G.; supervision: M.F., H.S., L.B., and D.E.G.; visualization: D.E.G.; writing—original draft preparation: M.F., T.D.-B., M.A., E.K.B., D.J.A., and D.E.G.; All authors have reviewed and provided corrections, and have agreed to be co-authors on the submitted version of the paper.

Funding: This work was funded by The Victorian Government's Operational Infrastructure Support Program, Murdoch Children's Research Institute, Royal Children's Hospital Foundation, Martin & E.H. Flack Trust, Pierce Armstrong Trust, Financial Markets Foundation for Children (Australia) (FMFC; grant number: 2017-361), and the National Health and Medical Research Council (NHMRC; project grant numbers: 1049299 and 1103389). D.E.G. was supported by the Next Generation Clinical Researchers Program—Career Development Fellowship Funded by the Medical Research Future Fund (grant number 1141334). M.A. was supported by the International Postgraduate Research Scholarship (IPRS) and the Research Training Program Fee offset scholarship funded by the Australian Government and awarded by the University of Melbourne, and in part by the Diagnosis and Development group of the Murdoch Children's Research Institute.

Acknowledgments: We sincerely thank the family described in this study and all participants and their parents/guardians for their contribution, support and generosity, which have been greatly appreciated. We also thank Annabel May Marsh for assisting with participants' psychological assessments.

Conflicts of Interest: David E. Godler is named as an inventor on patent applications (PCT/AU2010/000169 and PCT/AU2014/00004) related to the technology described in this article. The other authors declare that the research was conducted in the absence of any commercial or financial relationships that could be construed as a potential conflict of interest.

References

1. Vissers, L.E.; Gilissen, C.; Veltman, J.A. Genetic studies in intellectual disability and related disorders. *Nat. Rev. Genet.* **2016**, *17*, 9–18. [CrossRef] [PubMed]
2. Clifford, S.; Dissanayake, C.; Bui, Q.M.; Huggins, R.; Taylor, A.K.; Loesch, D.Z. Autism spectrum phenotype in males and females with fragile X full mutation and premutation. *J. Autism Dev. Disord.* **2007**, *37*, 738–747. [CrossRef] [PubMed]
3. Hall, S.S.; Lightbody, A.A.; Reiss, A.L. Compulsive, self-injurious, and autistic behavior in children and adolescents with fragile X syndrome. *Am. J. Ment. Retard.* **2008**, *113*, 44–53. [CrossRef]
4. Mazzocco, M.M.; Kates, W.R.; Baumgardner, T.L.; Freund, L.S.; Reiss, A.L. Autistic behaviors among girls with fragile X syndrome. *J. Autism Dev. Disord.* **1997**, *27*, 415–435. [CrossRef] [PubMed]

5. Merenstein, S.A.; Sobesky, W.E.; Taylor, A.K.; Riddle, J.E.; Tran, H.X.; Hagerman, R.J. Molecular-clinical correlations in males with an expanded *FMR1* mutation. *Am. J. Med. Genet.* **1996**, *64*, 388–394. [CrossRef]
6. Baker, E.K.; Arpone, M.; Aliaga, S.M.; Bretherton, L.; Kraan, C.M.; Bui, M.; Slater, H.R.; Ling, L.; Francis, D.; Hunter, M.F.; et al. Incomplete silencing of full mutation alleles in males with fragile X syndrome is associated with autistic features. *Mol. Autism.* **2019**, *10*, 21. [CrossRef] [PubMed]
7. Kraan, C.M.; Godler, D.E.; Amor, D.J. Epigenetics of fragile X syndrome and fragile X-related disorders. *Dev. Med. Child Neurol.* **2018**. [CrossRef] [PubMed]
8. Heitz, D.; Rousseau, F.; Devys, D.; Saccone, S.; Abderrahim, H.; Le Paslier, D.; Cohen, D.; Vincent, A.; Toniolo, D.; Della Valle, G.; et al. Isolation of sequences that span the fragile X and identification of a fragile X-related CpG island. *Science* **1991**, *251*, 1236–1239. [CrossRef] [PubMed]
9. Oberle, I.; Rousseau, F.; Heitz, D.; Kretz, C.; Devys, D.; Hanauer, A.; Boue, J.; Bertheas, M.F.; Mandel, J.L. Instability of a 550-base pair DNA segment and abnormal methylation in fragile X syndrome. *Science* **1991**, *252*, 1097–1102. [CrossRef]
10. Pieretti, M.; Zhang, F.P.; Fu, Y.H.; Warren, S.T.; Oostra, B.A.; Caskey, C.T.; Nelson, D.L. Absence of expression of the FMR-1 gene in fragile X syndrome. *Cell* **1991**, *66*, 817–822. [CrossRef]
11. Rousseau, F.; Heitz, D.; Biancalana, V.; Blumenfeld, S.; Kretz, C.; Boué, J.; Tommerup, N.; Hagen, C.V.D.; DeLozier-Blanchet, C.; Croquette, M.-F.; et al. Direct diagnosis by DNA analysis of the fragile X syndrome of mental retardation. *N. Engl. J. Med.* **1991**, *325*, 1673–1681. [CrossRef] [PubMed]
12. Sutcliffe, J.S.; Nelson, D.L.; Zhang, F.; Pieretti, M.; Caskey, C.T.; Saxe, D.; Warren, S.T. DNA methylation represses FMR-1 transcription in fragile X syndrome. *Hum. Mol. Genet.* **1992**, *1*, 397–400. [CrossRef] [PubMed]
13. Devys, D.; Lutz, Y.; Rouyer, N.; Bellocq, J.-P.; Mandel, J.-L. The FMR–1 protein is cytoplasmic, most abundant in neurons and appears normal in carriers of a fragile X premutation. *Nat. Genet.* **1993**, *4*, 335–340. [CrossRef] [PubMed]
14. Feng, Y.; Zhang, F.; Lokey, L.; Chastain, J.; Lakkis, L.; Eberhart, D.; Warren, S. Translational suppression by trinucleotide repeat expansion at *FMR1*. *Science* **1995**, *268*, 731–734. [CrossRef] [PubMed]
15. Pretto, D.; Yrigollen, C.M.; Tang, H.T.; Williamson, J.; Espinal, G.; Iwahashi, C.K.; Durbin-Johnson, B.; Hagerman, R.J.; Hagerman, P.J.; Tassone, F. Clinical and molecular implications of mosaicism in *FMR1* full mutations. *Front. Genet.* **2014**, *5*, 318. [CrossRef] [PubMed]
16. Willemsen, R.; Smits, A.; Mohkamsing, S.; van Beerendonk, H.; de Haan, A.; de Vries, B.; van den Ouweland, A.; Sistermans, E.; Galjaard, H.; Oostra, B.A. Rapid antibody test for diagnosing fragile X syndrome: A validation of the technique. *Hum. Genet.* **1997**, *99*, 308–311. [CrossRef] [PubMed]
17. Gothelf, D.; Furfaro Joyce, A.; Hoeft, F.; Eckert Mark, A.; Hall Scott, S.; O'Hara, R.; Erba Heather, W.; Ringel, J.; Hayashi Kiralee, M.; Patnaik, S.; et al. Neuroanatomy of fragile X syndrome is associated with aberrant behavior and the fragile X mental retardation protein (FMRP). *Ann. Neurol.* **2007**, *63*, 40–51. [CrossRef]
18. Irwin, S.A.; Galvez, R.; Greenough, W.T. Dendritic spine structural anomalies in fragile-X mental retardation syndrome. *Cereb Cortex* **2000**, *10*, 1038–1044. [CrossRef]
19. Jeanne, W.I.; Greenough, W.T. Synaptic synthesis of the fragile X protein: Possible involvement in synapse maturation and elimination. *Am. J. Med. Genet.* **1999**, *83*, 248–252.
20. Pfeiffer, B.E.; Huber, K.M. The state of synapses in fragile X syndrome. *Neuroscientist* **2009**, *15*, 549–567. [CrossRef]
21. Sidorov, M.S.; Auerbach, B.D.; Bear, M.F. Fragile X mental retardation protein and synaptic plasticity. *Mol. Brain* **2013**, *6*, 15. [CrossRef] [PubMed]
22. Rodriguez-Revenga, L.; Madrigal, I.; Badenas, C.; Xuncla, M.; Jimenez, L.; Mila, M. Premature ovarian failure and fragile X female premutation carriers: No evidence for a skewed X-chromosome inactivation pattern. *Menopause* **2009**, *16*, 944–949. [CrossRef] [PubMed]
23. Sherman, S.L. Premature ovarian failure in the fragile X syndrome. *Am. J. Med. Genet.* **2000**, *97*, 189–194. [CrossRef]
24. Nolin, S.L.; Glicksman, A.; Houck, G.E., Jr.; Brown, W.T.; Dobkin, C.S. Mosaicism in fragile X affected males. *Am. J. Med. Genet.* **1994**, *51*, 509–512. [CrossRef] [PubMed]

25. Rousseau, F.; Heitz, D.; Tarleton, J.; MacPherson, J.; Malmgren, H.; Dahl, N.; Barnicoat, A.; Mathew, C.; Mornet, E.; Tejada, I.; et al. A multicenter study on genotype-phenotype correlations in the fragile X syndrome, using direct diagnosis with probe StB12.3: The first 2,253 cases. *Am. J. Hum. Genet.* **1994**, *55*, 225–237.

26. Aliaga, S.M.; Slater, H.R.; Francis, D.; Du Sart, D.; Li, X.; Amor, D.J.; Alliende, A.M.; Santa Maria, L.; Faundes, V.; Morales, P.; et al. Identification of Males with Cryptic Fragile X Alleles by Methylation-Specific Quantitative Melt Analysis. *Clin. Chem.* **2016**, *62*, 343–352. [CrossRef] [PubMed]

27. Bonarrigo, F.A.; Russo, S.; Vizziello, P.; Menni, F.; Cogliati, F.; Giorgini, V.; Monti, F.; Milani, D. Think about it: *FMR1* gene mosaicism. *J. Child Neurol.* **2014**, *29*, NP74–NP77. [CrossRef]

28. Jiraanont, P.; Kumar, M.; Tang, H.-T.; Espinal, G.; Hagerman, P.J.; Hagerman, R.J.; Chutabhakdikul, N.; Tassone, F. Size and methylation mosaicism in males with fragile X syndrome. *Expert Rev. Mol. Diagn.* **2017**, *17*, 1023–1032. [CrossRef]

29. Orrico, A.; Galli, L.; Dotti, M.T.; Plewnia, K.; Censini, S.; Federico, A. Mosaicism for full mutation and normal-sized allele of the *FMR1* gene: A new case. *Am. J. Med. Genet.* **1998**, *78*, 341–344. [CrossRef]

30. Hwang, T.Y.; Aliaga, S.; Arpone, M.V.; Francis, D.; Li, X.; Chong, B.; Slater, H.R.; Rogers, C.; Bretherton, L.; Hunter, M.; et al. Partially Methylated Alleles, Microdeletion and Tissue Mosaicism in a Fragile X Male with Tremor and Ataxia at 30 Years of Age: A Case Report. *Am. J. Med. Genet.* **2016**, *170*, 3327–3332. [CrossRef]

31. Roid, G.H. *Stanford-Binet Intelligence Scales-Fifth Edition (SB5) Examiner's Manual*; Riverside Publishing: Itasca, IL, USA, 2003.

32. Hagerman, R.J.; Hull, C.E.; Safanda, J.F.; Carpenter, I.; Staley, L.W.; O'Connor, R.A.; Seydel, C.; Mazzocco, M.M.; Snow, K.; Thibodeau, S.N.; et al. High functioning fragile X males: Demonstration of an unmethylated fully expanded FMR-1 mutation associated with protein expression. *Am. J. Med. Genet.* **1994**, *51*, 298–308. [CrossRef] [PubMed]

33. Basuta, K.; Schneider, A.; Gane, L.; Polussa, J.; Woodruff, B.; Pretto, D.; Hagerman, R.; Tassone, F. High functioning male with fragile X syndrome and fragile X-associated tremor/ataxia syndrome. *Am. J. Med. Genet. A* **2015**, *167*, 2154–2161. [CrossRef] [PubMed]

34. Taylor, A.K.; Tassone, F.; Dyer, P.N.; Hersch, S.M.; Harris, J.B.; Greenough, W.T.; Hagerman, R.J. Tissue heterogeneity of the *FMR1* mutation in a high-functioning male with fragile X syndrome. *Am. J. Med. Genet.* **1999**, *84*, 233–239. [CrossRef]

35. Teo, C.R.; Law, H.Y.; Lee, C.G.; Chong, S.S. Screening for CGG repeat expansion in the *FMR1* gene by melting curve analysis of combined 5′ and 3′ direct triplet-primed PCRs. *Clin. Chem.* **2012**, *58*, 568–579. [CrossRef] [PubMed]

36. Bishop, S.L.; Guthrie, W.; Coffing, M.; Lord, C. Convergent validity of the Mullen Scales of Early Learning and the differential ability scales in children with autism spectrum disorders. *Am. J. Intellect. Dev. Disabil.* **2011**, *116*, 331–343. [CrossRef]

37. Santa Maria, L.; Pugin, A.; Alliende, M.; Aliaga, S.; Curotto, B.; Aravena, T.; Tang, H.T.; Mendoza-Morales, G.; Hagerman, R.; Tassone, F. FXTAS in an unmethylated mosaic male with fragile X syndrome from Chile. *Clin. Genet.* **2013**. [CrossRef] [PubMed]

38. Hwang, Y.T.; Dudding, T.; Aliaga, S.M.; Arpone, M.; Francis, D.; Li, X.; Slater, H.R.; Rogers, C.; Bretherton, L.; du Sart, D.; et al. Molecular Inconsistencies in a Fragile X Male with Early Onset Ataxia. *Genes* **2016**, *7*, 68. [CrossRef]

39. Lord, C.; Rutter, M.; DiLavore, P.; Risi, S.; Gotham, K.; Bishop, S. *Autism Diagnostic Observation Schedule, Second Edition: ADOS-2*; Western Psychological Services: Torrance, CA, USA, 2012.

40. Wechsler, D. *Wechsler Preschool & Primary Scale of Intelligence–Third Edition Australian Standardised Edition (WPPSI-III Australian)*; Pearson Clinical and Talent Assessment Australia and New Zealand: Sydney, NSW, Australia, 2004.

41. Mullen, E.M. *Mullen Scales of Early Learning: AGS Edition (MSEL:AGS)*; American Guidance Services, Inc.: Circle Pines, MN, USA, 1995.

42. Achenbach, T.M.; Rescorla, L.A. *Manual for the ASEBA Preschool Forms & Profiles*; University of Vermont, Research Center for Children, Youth, & Families: Burlington, VT, USA, 2000.

43. Inaba, Y.; Schwartz, C.E.; Bui, Q.M.; Li, X.; Skinner, C.; Field, M.; Wotton, T.; Hagerman, R.J.; Francis, D.; Amor, D.J.; et al. Early Detection of Fragile X Syndrome: Applications of a Novel Approach for Improved Quantitative Methylation Analysis in Venous Blood and Newborn Blood Spots. *Clin. Chem.* **2014**. [CrossRef]

44. Godler, D.E.; Inaba, Y.; Schwartz, C.E.; Bui, Q.M.; Shi, E.Z.; Li, X.; Herlihy, A.S.; Skinner, C.; Hagerman, R.J.; Francis, D.; et al. Detection of skewed X-chromosome inactivation in Fragile X syndrome and X chromosome aneuploidy using quantitative melt analysis. *Expert Rev. Mol. Med.* **2015**, *17*, e13. [CrossRef]
45. Arpone, M.; Baker, E.K.; Bretherton, L.; Bui, M.; Li, X.; Whitaker, S.; Dissanayake, C.; Cohen, J.; Hickerton, C.; Rogers, C.; et al. Intragenic DNA methylation in buccal epithelial cells and intellectual functioning in a paediatric cohort of males with fragile X. *Sci. Rep.* **2018**, *8*, 3644. [CrossRef]
46. Loesch, D.Z.; Godler, D.E.; Evans, A.; Bui, Q.M.; Gehling, F.; Kotschet, K.E.; Trost, N.; Storey, E.; Stimpson, P.; Kinsella, G.; et al. Evidence for the toxicity of bidirectional transcripts and mitochondrial dysfunction in blood associated with small CGG expansions in the *FMR1* gene in patients with parkinsonism. *Genet. Med.* **2011**, *13*, 392–399. [CrossRef]
47. Godler, D.E.; Loesch, D.Z.; Huggins, R.; Gordon, L.; Slater, H.R.; Gehling, F.; Burgess, T.; Choo, K.H. Improved methodology for assessment of mRNA levels in blood of patients with *FMR1* related disorders. *BMC Clin. Pathol.* **2009**, *9*, 5. [CrossRef]
48. Francis, D.; Burgess, T.; Mitchell, J.; Slater, H. Identification of small FRAXA premutations. *Mol. Diagn.* **2000**, *5*, 221–225. [CrossRef]
49. Khaniani, M.S.; Kalitsis, P.; Burgess, T.; Slater, H.R. An improved Diagnostic PCR Assay for identification of Cryptic Heterozygosity for CGG Triplet Repeat Alleles in the Fragile X Gene (*FMR1*). *Mol. Cytogenet.* **2008**, *1*, 5. [CrossRef]
50. Chen, L.; Hadd, A.G.; Sah, S.; Houghton, J.F.; Filipovic-Sadic, S.; Zhang, W.; Hagerman, P.J.; Tassone, F.; Latham, G.J. High-resolution methylation polymerase chain reaction for fragile X analysis: Evidence for novel *FMR1* methylation patterns undetected in Southern blot analyses. *Genet. Med.* **2011**, *13*, 528–538. [CrossRef]
51. Weckx, S.; Del-Favero, J.; Rademakers, R.; Claes, L.; Cruts, M.; De Jonghe, P.; Van Broeckhoven, C.; De Rijk, P. novoSNP, a novel computational tool for sequence variation discovery. *Genome Res.* **2005**, *15*, 436–442. [CrossRef]
52. Kraan, C.M.; Cornish, K.M.; Bui, Q.M.; Li, X.; Slater, H.R.; Godler, D.E. β-glucuronidase mRNA levels are correlated with gait and working memory in premutation females: Understanding the role of FMR1 premutation alleles. *Sci. Rep.* **2016**, *6*, 29366.
53. Kraan, C.M.; Cornish, K.M.; Bui, Q.M.; Li, X.; Slater, H.R.; Godler, D.E. beta-glucuronidase use as a single internal control gene may confound analysis in *FMR1* mRNA toxicity studies. *PLoS ONE* **2018**, *13*, e0192151. [CrossRef]

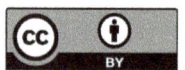

© 2019 by the authors. Licensee MDPI, Basel, Switzerland. This article is an open access article distributed under the terms and conditions of the Creative Commons Attribution (CC BY) license (http://creativecommons.org/licenses/by/4.0/).

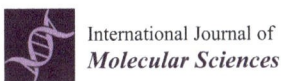

Article

Associations between Monocyte and T Cell Cytokine Profiles in Autism Spectrum Disorders: Effects of Dysregulated Innate Immune Responses on Adaptive Responses to Recall Antigens in a Subset of ASD Children

Harumi Jyonouchi [1,2,*] and Lee Geng [1]

1 Department of Pediatrics, Saint Peter's University Hospital (SPUH), New Brunswick, NJ 08901, USA; lgeng@saintpetersuh.com
2 Department of Pediatrics, Rutgers-Robert Wood Johnson medical school, New Brunswick, NJ 08901, USA
* Correspondence: hjyonouchi@saintpetersuh.com; Tel.: +732-339-7780; Fax: +732-937-9428

Received: 26 July 2019; Accepted: 23 September 2019; Published: 24 September 2019

Abstract: Changes in monocyte cytokine production with toll like receptor (TLR) agonists in subjects with autism spectrum disorders (ASD) were best reflected by the IL-1β/IL-10 ratios in our previous research. The IL-1β/IL-10 based subgrouping (low, normal, and high) of ASD samples revealed marked differences in microRNA expression, and mitochondrial respiration. However, it is unknown whether the IL-1β/IL-10 ratio based subgrouping is associated with changes in T cell cytokine profiles or monocyte cytokine profiles with non-TLR agonists. In ASD ($n = 152$) and non-ASD ($n = 41$) subjects, cytokine production by peripheral blood monocytes (PBMo) with TLR agonists and β-glucan, an inflammasome agonist, and T cell cytokine production by peripheral blood mononuclear cells (PBMCs) with recall antigens (Ags) (food and candida Ags) were concurrently measured. Changes in monocyte cytokine profiles were observed with β-glucan in the IL-1β/IL-10 ratio based ASD subgroups, along with changes in T cell cytokine production and ASD subgroup-specific correlations between T cell and monocyte cytokine production. Non-ASD controls revealed considerably less of such correlations. Altered innate immune responses in a subset of ASD children are not restricted to TLR pathways and correlated with changes in T cell cytokine production. Altered trained immunity may play a role in the above described changes.

Keywords: ASD; cytokine; monocyte; β-glucan; T cell cytokine; trained immunity; maternal immune activation

1. Introduction

Autism spectrum disorder (ASD) is a behaviorally defined syndrome and the effects of genetic and environmental factors that form its pathogenesis, likely vary in individuals with ASD diagnosis. However, recent research is increasingly supporting the role of immune mediated inflammation in its pathogenesis [1–3]. In fact, one of the most extensively studied animal models of ASD is generated by inducing sterile inflammation in pregnant rodents through intraperitoneal injection of stimulants of innate immunity, such as endotoxin [4]. This model which is called maternal immune activation (MIA) has been shown to create lasting neurodevelopmental and behavioral changes in offspring, as well as lasting effects on T cell functions [4–6]. Perinatal stresses causing immune activation such as maternal infection, during pregnancy, has also been implicated with pathogenesis of ASD and other neuropsychiatric conditions [7,8]. In our clinic, we have also observed that some ASD subjects reveal fluctuating behavioral symptoms and even repeated loss of once acquired cognitive activity following each immune insult. In addition, our previous research indicated an association between fluctuating behavioral symptoms and dysregulated innate immune responses [9,10].

The MIA model relies on the induction of sterile immune activation through non-specific stimulants of innate immunity. However, the lack of antigen (Ag)-specific immune memory in innate immunity, as opposed to adaptive immunity, has made the lasting effects of puzzling. Although neuronal damage caused by innate immune activation in mothers could cause lasting effects in neuronal development, if this is the case, such neurodevelopmental changes will remain static, as seen in patients with cerebral palsy. However, we observed that ASD subjects reveal fluctuating behavioral symptoms following immune insults (mainly microbial infection) repeatedly affect behavioral symptoms along with a high frequency of co-morbid conditions. That is, these ASD subjects develop multi-system inflammation not restricted to the brain (inflammatory subtype) [11]. In addition, direct damage to the brain by MIA would not explain MIA's lasting effects on T cell functions [6].

The recent discovery of innate immune memory (IIM) may explain many aspects of the lasting effects of MIA. Reprogramming of innate immunity via metabolic and epigenetic changes following initial innate immune stimulus, was first realized as a part of the non-specific effects of vaccinations such as Bacillus Calmette–Guérin (BCG) [12]. Such effects of IIM were termed as trained immunity (TI). It has been shown that TI causes hyper-responsiveness of innate immunity against second stimuli, which can be totally different from the 1st stimuli, since TI is established through metabolic and subsequent epigenetic modulation of innate immune cells [12–15]. On the other hand, the 1st innate immune stimuli can also cause subsequent hypo-responsiveness of innate immunity (tolerance) as shown in endotoxin tolerance [16]. Innate immune tolerance is also thought to be induced by metabolic and epigenetic regulation [17,18]. Induction of innate immune memory appears to be associated with dose, kinds of stimuli, and other environmental and genetic factors [19].

We have previously reported that some ASD subjects reveal changes in monocyte activation status at the level of cytokine production, expression of microRNA (miRNAs), and mitochondrial respiration [20,21]. Our research has also revealed that the above-described changes are closely associated with production of monocyte cytokines as well as the ratio of IL-1β/IL-10 [20,21]. In these studies, we used a panel of agonists of toll like receptors (TLRs) for stimulating peripheral blood monocytes (PBMo), main innate immune cells in the peripheral blood. It was found that subgrouping of ASD subjects based on IL-1β/IL-10 ratios help identify ASD subjects who have dysregulated innate immune responses; high or low ratio ASD subgroup reveal marked differences in miRNA expression and mitochondrial respiration [20,21]. These findings support the presence of maladapted TI in these ASD children.

In the animal model of TI, with β-glucan derived from *Candida albicans* used as an initial stimulus, the IL-1β family was reported to have a major role in the development of TI [22]. Additionally, β-glucan tends to induce TI, but not tolerance, while endotoxin tends to induce tolerance when given at a low dose [23]. β-glucan is a representative dectin-1 agonist, which stimulates canonical inflammasomes of innate immune cells, leading to cleavage of proinflammatory cytokines, especially IL-1β and IL-18. Inflammasome mediated pathways are different from TLR mediated pathways, but often they exert converging effects on activation of innate immunity [24,25]. It is also noted that miRNAs have important regulatory roles in inflammasome priming and activation [25]. Thus, it can be hypothesized that TI suspected in ASD children will include multiple pathways of innate immunity, including both TLRs and inflammasome mediated pathways.

We also noted that in the low IL-1β/IL-10 ratio ASD subgroup, there is a higher frequency of non-IgE mediated food allergy (NFA) as compared to the normal ratio ASD subgroups [21]. NFA is thought to be associated with cellular immune reactivity to common food proteins, and we have previously reported that ASD children reveal increased T cell cytokine production (TNF-α, IFN-γ, and IL-12) against cow's milk proteins at a high frequency. Given these findings, it may be hypothesized that exaggerated innate immune responses due to maladapted TI could result in the alternation of adaptive immune responses, resulting in unwanted T cell responses to benign environmental Ags, such as food proteins, and self-Ags.

This study was formulated to examine the above described hypothesis by assessing whether changes in the monocyte cytokine production are detected under β-glucan stimulated cultures in IL-1β/IL-10 based ASD subgroups, and whether T cell cytokine production in response to luminal antigens differ among IL-1β/IL-10 based ASD subgroups. This study determined monocyte cytokine profiles in responses to β glucan, in comparison with their responses to TLR agonists, and T cell cytokine profiles in response to food and candida proteins in ASD ($n = 152$) and control non-ASD ($n = 41$) subjects. Samples from ASD subjects were subdivided into the IL-1β/IL-10 based subgroups (high, normal, and low) as reported previously [20]. The results obtained support our hypotheses described above.

2. Results

2.1. Clinical Characteristics in the IL-1β/IL-10 Based ASD Subgroups

A summary of clinical characteristics of the ASD subgroups are shown in Table 1. There are no statistical differences in gender frequency and clinical characteristics (ASD severity, cognitive development, sleep, GI symptoms, history of non-IgE mediated food allergy (NFA), seizure disorders, specific antibody deficiency, AR, and asthma) by Chi-Square test ($p > 0.05$) (Table 1). Ages in the ASD subgroups did not differ ($p > 0.05$ by Kruskal–Wallis test). History of NFA tended to be higher in the low IL-1β/IL-10 ratio group than the normal ratio ASD subgroup, but this was not statistically significant ($p = 0.1286$ by Fisher's exact test).

Table 1. Demographics and clinical features in the IL-1β/IL-10 based autism spectrum disorder (ASD) subgroups.

	IL-1β/IL-10 Ratio Based ASD Subgroups		
	High ($n = 65$)	Normal ($n = 51$)	Low ($n = 36$)
Age (year) median (range)	9.9 (2.5–26.3)	8.5 (2.2–24.5)	11.4 (2.6–22.4)
Age (year) Mean ± SD [1]	11.3 ± 5.8	10.6 ± 6.1	12.1 ± 5.6
Gender (M:F)	52:13 (80.0%:20.0%)	46:5 (80.4%:19.6%)	32:4 (88.9%:11.1%)
Ethnicity	AA 5, Asian 17, W 40, Mixed 5	AA 2, Asian 12, W 35, mixed 2	AA 4, Asian 5, W 27,
Clinical Characteristics [2]			
ASD severity			
Severe	39/65 (60.0%)	31/51 (60.8%)	20/36 (55.6%)
Moderate	13/65 (20.0%)	9/51 (17.6%)	9/36 (25.0%)
Mild	13/65 (20.0%)	11/51 (21.6%)	7/36 (19.4%)
Cognitive development (<1st %)	39/65 (60.0%)	38/51 (74.5%)	25/36 (69.4%)
Disturbed sleep	21/65 (32.3%)	16/51 (33.3%)	12/36 (33.3%)
GI symptoms	46/65 (70.8%)	36/51 (70.6%)	29/36 (80.6%)
History of NFA	30/65 (46.2%)	22/51 (43.1%)	22/36 (61.1%)
Seizure disorders	7/65 (10.8%)	8/51 (8.3%)	3/36 (8.3%)
Specific antibody deficiency	11/65 (16.9%)	7/51 (13.75)	8/36 (22.2%)
Allergic rhinitis	15/65 (23.1%)	10/51 (19.6%)	5/36 (13.9%)
Asthma	8/65 (12.3%)	4/51 (7.8%)	4/36 (11.1%)

[1] Abbreviations used: AA, African Americans; ADHD, attention deficit hyperactivity disorder; AEDs, anti-epileptic drugs; F, female; GI, gastrointestinal; M, male; NFA, non-IgE mediated food allergy; SD, standard deviations; SSRIs, selective serotonin receptor inhibitors; W, Caucasians. [2] No significant differences in frequency of clinical characteristics in the IL-1β/IL-10 ratio based ASD subgroup by Chi-Square test ($p > 0.05$).

We also assessed the frequency of prescription medication use in the IL-1β/IL-10 ratio based ASD subgroups. Table 2 summarizes frequency of intake of prescription medications at the time of sample obtainment. For ASD subjects who had samples taken at multiple time points, the medications taken at each time-point was assessed. There was no difference in the frequency of medication intake between the ASD subgroups ($p > 0.05$ by Chi-Square test). Co-variance analysis rejected the effects of the above described clinical characteristics and prescription medication use on IL-1β/IL-10 ratios under all the culture conditions tested in this study.

Table 2. Frequency of medication use in the IL-1β/IL-10 based ASD subgroups.

	IL-1β/IL-10 Ratio Based ASD Subgroups (Sample Numbers)		
	High (n = 70) [1]	Normal (n = 74)	Low (n = 43)
	Medication Use [2]		
Neuroleptics	6/70 (8.6%)	12/74 (15.7%)	6/43 (14.6 %)
ADHD medications	11/70 (15.7%)	6/74 (8.1%)	8/43 (18.6%)
AEDs	12/70 (17.1%)	13/74 (17.6%)	6/43 (14.6 %)
SSRIs	13/70 (18.5%)	11/74 (14.9%)	8/43 (18.6%)

[1] Frequency of medication use at the time of sample obtainment. It should be noted that samples were obtained at 2–4 time points in a total of 25 ASD subjects. Frequency of medication use did not significantly differ in the IL-1β/IL-10 based ASD subgroups by Chi-Square test ($p > 0.05$). [2] Medications on which study subjects were on when blood samples were obtained.

2.2. Changes in Monocyte Cytokine Production in Response to Candida Heat Extract (β-Glucan) the IL-1β/IL-10 Based ASD Subgroups

Since TLR agonists were used to generate IL-1β/IL-10 ratios for subgrouping ASD samples previously, we also assessed the effects of β-glucan, a ligand to dectin 1 which activates innate immunity through inflammasome. We used candida heat extract as a source of β-glucan. One of the reasons that we used β-glucan is that this is widely used for TI induction [12]. Under β-glucan stimulated cultures, significant changes in IL-1β/IL-10 ratios and in the production of IL-1β, IL-10, TNF-α, sTNFRII, and CC-chemokine-ligand-2 (CCL2) were observed (Table 3). There is a tendency of high production of inflammatory cytokines (IL-1β and TNF-α) in the high ratio ASD subgroup, while the low ratio ASD subgroup revealed higher levels of counter-regulatory cytokines (IL-10, sTNFRII, and TGFβ) and CCL2, chemokine under the β-glucan stimulated cultures (Table 3). Therefore, differences were the most apparent between the high vs. low ratio ASD subgroups (Table 3). Such changes were not observed in the production of IL-6, IL-12, IL-23, and CCL7. The changes in monocyte cytokine profiles were more evident with stimulus of β-glucan as compared to monocyte cytokine production without stimuli (Table 3).

We were able to obtain samples at 2–4 different time points in 22 ASD subjects to test longitudinal changes in each subject. With the use of repeated measures of analysis of variance, significant variability was observed in IL-1β/IL-10 ratios under the cultures without stimulus and β-glucan stimulated cultures (F-ratio 5.0 and 3.88, with $p < 0.01$ and $p < 0.02$, respectively).

Table 3. Changes in IL-1β/IL-10 ratios and monocyte production in the IL-1β/IL-10 based ASD subgroups under β-glucan stimulated culture conditions.

Cytokines Produced	IL-1β/IL-10 Ratio Based ASD Subgroups			Non-ASD Controls (n = 41)	p-Value [4]
	High (n = 70) [1]	Normal (n = 74)	Low (n = 43)		
Without Stimuli (Medium Only) [6]					
IL-1β/IL-10	1.44 ± 1.9 [2,6]	0.71 ± 0.48	0.42 ± 0.29	1.02 ± 2.06	0.00000
IL-1β	208.8 ± 233.1 [3]	201.2 ± 236.9	101.6 ± 93.9 [6]	260.8 ± 317.5 [5]	0.00612
IL-10	212.3 ± 170.9	248.6 ± 211.7	299.2 ± 271.7	436.4 ± 837.0 [5]	0.09448
TNF-α	76.2 ± 136.0 [6]	42.9 ± 116.8	15.7 ± 26.0	81.9 ± 121.1	0.00006
sTNFRII	301.1 ± 167.9	370.5 ± 187.2	340.8 ± 169.8	331.3 ± 200.8	0.19151
TGFβ	577.4 ± 321.0 [6]	370.5 ± 187.2	691.3 ± 328.8	650.6 ± 328.9	0.00703
CCL2	18,423 ± 7617	18,519 ± 6259	17,637 ± 8364	18,554 ± 7775	0.90492
With β-Glucan					
IL-1β/IL-10	15.4 ± 20.6 [6]	4.1 ± 2.1	2.7 ± 1.7	4.5 ± 3.1	0.00000
IL-1β	2355.1 ± 1077.5 [6]	2266.6 ± 1083.6	1541.8 ± 776.9 [6]	1812.3 ± 1028.3	0.00008
IL-10	266.4 ± 205.7 [6]	670.7 ± 394.8	806.5 ± 469.4	517.7 ± 395.8	0.00000
TNF-α	1456.6 ± 1125.3 [6]	1096.7 ± 967.0	740.1 ± 484.4 [6]	1138.6 ± 876.1	0.00761
sTNFRII	426.7 ± 227.1 [6]	722.2 ± 464.5	825.1 ± 518.9	595.8 ± 567.9	0.00000
TGFβ	439.6 ± 298.0 [6]	588.4 ± 298.3	598.3 ± 259.3	560.8 ± 298.5	0.00312
CCL2	4640 ± 3741 [6]	7308 ± 5596	10001 ± 7502 [6]	6807 ± 6568	0.00000

[1] Total sample numbers in the group; [2] The results are expressed as mean values ± SD. [3] Cytokine concentrations are shown as pg/mL; [4] p values by one-way ANOVA with α = 0.2 (Terry–Hoeffding test). Comparisons between groups by ANOVA with α = 0.05. [5] Values from non-ASD controls differed from ASD subgroups. [6] Differed from other ASD subgroups by ANOVA (α = 0.05).

2.3. Changes in T Cell Cytokine Production in the IL-1β/IL-10 Based ASD Subgroups

We then tested whether T cell cytokine production differs among the study groups, including non-ASD controls. Numerically significant differences were found between the study groups in the production of IFN-γ (medium only and in response to candida), TNF-α (in all the culture conditions), and IL-10 (in response to β-LG and gliadin), as shown in Table 4. When the whole ASD samples were compared with non-ASD controls, no significant differences were observed ($p > 0.05$). These changes are mainly due to higher production of TNF-α and IL-10 in the high IL-1β/IL-10 ratio ASD subgroup as compared to other study groups (Table 4). On the other hand, IFN-γ production was lower in the high ratio ASD subgroup, as compared to the normal and low ratio ASD subgroups in the cultures without stimuli or with candida protein (Table 4). In addition, the low ratio subgroup revealed lower IL-10 production in response to gliadin than other study groups (Table 4).

When we assessed the variability of the production T cell cytokines, no significant time-dependent variations were found under all culture conditions, except for IFN-γ production under soy-protein stimulated cultures (F-ratio 4.93, $p < 0.01$).

Table 4. T cell cytokine production by peripheral blood mononuclear cells (PBMCs) in response to β-LG, gliadin, or candida Ag in the IL-1β/IL-10 based ASD subgroups.

Cytokines	IL-1β/IL-10 Ratio Based ASD Subgroups			Non-ASD Controls (n = 41)	p-Value [3]
	High (n = 70) [1]	Normal (n = 74)	Low (n = 43)		
IFN-γ					
medium only	54.5 ± 155.5 [2]	65.1 ± 183.9	71.1 ± 134.6	28.7 ± 39.5	0.3431
β-lactoglobulin	152.4 ± 229.9	112.7 ± 181.6	178.6 ± 291.7	77.8 ± 122.9	0.3486
gliadin	107.4 ± 179.3	94.2 ± 192.6	114.3 ± 212.7	43.5 ± 56.1	0.2129
Candida	189.4 ± 290.9	278.9 ± 442.7	265.0 ± 351.3	172.3 ± 342.1 [4]	0.0119
TNF-α					
medium only	31.2 ± 136.9	25.2 ± 130.1	61.7 ± 177.5	0.9 ± 2.4	0.0309
β-lactoglobulin	230.7 ± 219.2 [5]	137.3 ± 201.0	108.8 ± 191.2	154.0 ± 196.8	0.00043
gliadin	220.9 ± 219.4 [5]	125.1 ± 193.0	90.5 ± 173.4	112.9 ± 159.0	0.00002
Candida	64.6 ± 219.2	38.3 ± 139.2	58.8 ± 183.3	28.7 ± 85.5	0.01695
IL-10					
medium only	60.4 ± 161.3	38.5 ± 98.3	80.6 ± 164.1	30.5 ± 63.3	0.107
β-lactoglobulin	1358.5 ± 523.7 [5]	1146.4 ± 495.1	1044.3 ± 526.6	1119.2 ± 423.1	0.0073
gliadin	808.3 ± 371.0 [5]	760.4 ± 446.8	572.1 ± 387.7 [5]	742.5 ± 374.7	0.0063
Candida	66.6 ± 91.0	41.5 ± 60.0	60.4 ± 90.1	93.6 ± 152.0 [4]	0.9926

[1] Total sample numbers in each study group. [2] The results are expressed as mean values ± SD. Cytokine concentrations are shown as pg/mL; [3] p values by one-way ANOVA with α = 0.2 (Terry–Hoeffding test). Comparisons between groups by ANOVA with α = 0.05. [4] Values from non-ASD controls differed from ASD subgroups. [5] Differed from other ASD subgroups by ANOVA (α = 0.05).

2.4. Associations between T Cell Cytokine Production by Peripheral Blood Mononuclear Cells (PBMCs) and Monocyte Cytokine Production

Since we observed differences in the production of IFN-γ, TNF-α, and IL-10 by peripheral blood mononuclear cells (PBMCs) under cultures stimulated with β-LG, gliadin, and candida, we assessed whether production of these cytokines revealed any correlation with the cytokines produced by PBMo in response to TLR agonists and/or β-glucan.

When IFN-γ production by PBMCs were compared with monocyte cytokine profiles, we observed significant correlations between IFN-γ levels produced by PBMCs and levels of monocyte cytokines produced by PBMo in the ASD subgroups (Table 5). Interestingly, correlations markedly differed among the ASD subgroups, while the non-ASD controls revealed little correlations. Such correlations were most notable between IL-6 and CCL2 production by PBMo and IFN-γ production by PBMCs in response to candida proteins in the normal ratio ASD subgroup (Table 5).

Table 5. Correlations between IFN-γ production by PBMCs and monocyte cytokine production.

Correlation Coefficient	IL-1β/IL-10 Ratio Based ASD Subgroups			Non-ASD Controls (n = 41)
	High (n = 70) [1]	Normal (n = 74)	Low (n = 43)	
	In Response to β-Lactoglobulin			
IL-1β/IL-10 ratio				
No stimulant [3]	–	–	0.3236 (p < 0.05)	–
LPS	–	0.3084 (p < 0.02) [2]	–	–
CL097	–	−0.2662 (p < 0.05)	–	–
IL-1β				
No stimulant	0.2668 (p < 0.05)	—	0.3941 (p < 0.02)	–
LPS	0.3141 (p < 0.02)	0.3663 (p < 0.005)	–	–
CL097	—	−0.2714 (p < 0.05)	0.3912 (p < 0.02)	–
IL-10				
No stimulant	0.332 (p < 0.01)	–	0.3258 (p < 0.05)	–
Zymosan	–	0.2439 (p < 0.05)	–	–
CL097	–	–	–	−0.3586 (p < 0.05)

Table 5. Cont.

Correlation Coefficient	IL-1β/IL-10 Ratio Based ASD Subgroups			Non-ASD Controls ($n = 41$)
	High ($n = 70$) [1]	Normal ($n = 74$)	Low ($n = 43$)	
IL-6				
No stimulant	0.2917 ($p < 0.05$)	0.2744 ($p < 0.05$)	–	0.3351 ($p < 0.05$)
LPS	–	0.3216 ($p < 0.01$)	–	–
sTNFRII				
No stimulant	−0.2524 ($p < 0.05$)	–	–	–
β-glucan	−0.3615 ($p < 0.005$)	–	–	–
CCL2				
No stimulant	–	0.2928 ($p < 0.02$)	–	–
β-glucan	–	0.2511 ($p < 0.05$)	–	–
In Response to Gliadin				
IL-1β/IL-10 ratio				
No stimulant	–	–	0.3772 ($p < 0.02$)	–
LPS	–	0.3843 ($p < 0.005$)	–	–
IL-1β				
No stimulant	0.2713 ($p < 0.05$)	–	0.4462 ($p < 0.005$)	–
LPS	–	0.481 ($p < 0.0001$)	–	–
IL-10				
No stimulant	0.2748 ($p < 0.05$)	–	–	–
LPS	–	0.3413 ($p < 0.005$)	–	–
TNF-α				
No stimulant	0.3398 ($p < 0.01$)	–	–	–
Zymosan	–	–	–	−0.326 ($p < 0.05$)
IL-6				
No stimulant	0.2621 ($p < 0.05$)	0.2426 ($p < 0.05$)	–	–
LPS	–	0.396 ($p < 0.001$)	–	–
Zymosan	–	0.3036 ($p < 0.02$)	–	–
sTNFRII				
Zymosan	−0.3397 ($p < 0.01$)	–	–	–
β-glucan	−0.4695 ($p < 0.0001$)	–	–	–
In Response to Candida Protein				
IL-1β/IL-10 ratio				
No stimulant	–	−0.324 ($p < 0.01$)	–	–
IL-1β				
No stimulant	–	0.2607 ($p < 0.05$)	–	–
Zymosan	–	−0.2677 $p < 0.05$)	–	–
IL-10				
No stimulant	–	0.2567 ($p < 0.05$)	–	–
IL-6				
No stimulant	–	0.379 ($p < 0.001$)	–	–
Zymosan	–	0.2932 ($p < 0.02$)	–	–
β-glucan	–	0.2507 ($p < 0.05$)	–	–
sTNFRII				
No stimulant	–	–	–	−0.3515 ($p < 0.05$)
LPS	–	–	–	−0.346 ($p < 0.05$)
Zymosan	–	–	–	−0.3768 ($p < 0.05$)
CCL2				
No stimulant	–	0.3071 ($p < 0.01$)	–	–
Zymosan	–	0.2385 ($p < 0.05$)	–	–
CL097	–	0.3292 ($p < 0.005$)	–	–
β-glucan	–	0.277 ($p < 0.05$)	–	−0.4391 ($p < 0.01$)

[1] Total sample numbers in each study group; [2] Correlation coefficient by Spearman test with p value shown in ( ) when p value is at least $p < 0.05$. [3] Culture conditions monocyte cytokines produced under.

As for TNF-α production, production of TNF-α by PBMCs in response to β-LG and gliadin and that by PBMo revealed a significant correlation with TNF-α production by PBMo in response to TLR agonists and β-glucan (Table 6). Such correlations were most notable in the high ratio ASD subgroup. However, such correlations were also noted in the low ratio and non-ASD subgroups as well, but to a lesser extent (Table 6). On the other hand, few correlations were found in the normal ratio ASD subgroups (Table 6). It should be noted that PBMCs from the normal ratio ASD subgroup produced equivalent amounts of TNF-α, as compared to both the low ratio ASD subgroup and the non-ASD controls (Table 4), making it unlikely that the lack of correlations in the normal ASD subgroup is associated with low TNF-α production. The high and low ratio ASD subgroups revealed positive associations between TNF-α production by PBMCs in response to candida protein, and production of IL-1β, IL-6, IL-10, and sTNFRII by PBMo.

Table 6. Correlations between TNF-α production by PBMCs and monocyte cytokine production.

Correlation Coefficient	IL-1β/IL-10 Ratio Based ASD Subgroups			Non-ASD Controls ($n = 41$)
	High ($n = 70$) [1]	Normal ($n = 74$)	Low ($n = 43$)	
	In Response to β-Lactoglobulin			
IL-1β/IL-10 ratio				
LPS [3]	–	–	–	0.3541 ($p < 0.05$)
CL097	–	−0.2744 ($p < 0.05$) [2]	0.3916 ($p < 0.02$)	–
IL-1β				
LPS	0.2858 ($p < 0.05$)	–	–	0.3411 ($p < 0.05$)
CL097	0.4575 ($p < 0.0005$)	–	0.4069 ($p < 0.02$)	0.5101 ($p < 0.005$)
IL-10				
No stimulant	0.3339 ($p < 0.01$)	–	–	–
LPS	0.2858 ($p < 0.05$)	–	–	–
CL097	–	0.253 ($p < 0.05$)	–	–
TNF-α				
No stimulant	0.4883 ($p < 0.0001$)	–	–	0.569 ($p < 0.0002$)
LPS	0.6857 ($p < 0.0001$)	–	–	0.5103 ($p < 0.002$)
Zymosan	0.4558 ($p < 0.0005$)	–	–	0.3469 ($p < 0.05$)
CL097	0.5481 ($p < 0.0001$)	–	0.3364 ($p < 0.05$)	0.4643 ($p < 0.005$)
β-glucan	0.5469 ($p < 0.0001$)	–	–	–
IL-6				
No stimulant	0.3887 ($p < 0.02$)	–	–	–
LPS	0.2776 ($p < 0.05$)	–	0.3197 ($p < 0.05$)	0.4241 ($p < 0.01$)
sTNFRII				
LPS	–	–	–	−0.4695 ($p < 0.005$)
Zymosan	–	–	–	−0.3532 ($p < 0.05$)
CL097	–	0.2632 ($p < 0.05$)	−0.3166 ($p < 0.05$)	−0.4571 ($p < 0.005$)
β-glucan	–	–	–	–
CCL2				
β-glucan	–	–	–	−0.4411 ($p < 0.01$)
	In Response to Gliadin			
IL-1β/IL-10 ratio				
LPS	–	0.2515 ($p < 0.05$)	–	–
CL097	–	−0.3013 ($p < 0.02$)	0.3561 ($p < 0.05$)	–
IL-1β				
LPS	0.3098 ($p < 0.02$)	0.2441 ($p < 0.05$)	–	–
CL097	0.2944 ($p < 0.02$)	–	0.4395 ($p < 0.005$)	–
β-glucan	–	0.2633 ($p < 0.05$)	–	–

Table 6. Cont.

Correlation Coefficient	IL-1β/IL-10 Ratio Based ASD Subgroups			Non-ASD Controls (n = 41)
	High (n = 70) [1]	Normal (n = 74)	Low (n = 43)	
IL-10				
No stimulant	0.2823 ($p < 0.05$)	–	–	–
LPS	0.3098 ($p < 0.02$)	–	–	–
CL097	02917 ($p < 0.02$)	–	0.3642 ($p < 0.02$)	–
TNF-α				
No stimulant	0.5168 ($p < 0.0001$)	–	0.5156 ($p < 0.001$)	0.4179 ($p < 0.01$)
LPS	0.6777 ($p < 0.0001$)	–	0.3462 ($p < 0.02$)	0.452 ($p < 0.005$)
Zymosan	0.4567 ($p < 0.0001$)	–	–	–
CL97	0.4268 ($p < 0.0005$)	–	0.4201 ($p < 0.01$)	0.5626 ($p < 0.001$)
β-glucan	0.4778 ($p < 0.0001$)	–	–	–
IL-6				
CL097	0.2612 ($p < 0.05$)	–	0.3937 ($p < 0.02$)	0.3695 ($p < 0.05$)
β-glucan	–	–	–	0.3939 ($p < 0.02$)
sTNFRII				
CL097	–	0.2481 ($p < 0.05$)	–	–
CCL2				
β-glucan	−0.2509 ($p < 0.05$)	–	–	−0.327 ($p < 0.05$)
In Response to Candida Protein				
IL-1β/IL-10 ratio				
No stimulant	−0.3303 ($p < 0.01$)	–	–	–
CL097	–	–	0.5351 ($p < 0.005$)	–
IL-1β				
Zymosan	–	–	−0.4518 ($p < 0.005$)	0.3507 ($p < 0.05$)
CL097	0.4228 ($p < 0.0005$)	–	0.5832 ($p < 0.0001$)	–
β-glucan	–	–	−0.3169 ($p < 0.05$)	–
IL-10				
CL097	0.2486 ($p < 0.05$)	–	0.4879 ($p < 0.001$)	–
sTNFRII				
CL097	0.4237 ($p < 0.0005$)	–	0.5626 ($p < 0.0001$)	–
β-glucan	0.2814 ($p < 0.02$)	–	–	–
IL-6				
CL097	0.3848 ($p < 0.005$)	–	0.5636 ($p < 0.0001$)	–
CCL2				
CL097	–	–	–	−0.3362 ($p < 0.05$)

[1] Total sample numbers in each study group; [2] Correlation coefficient by Spearman test with p value shown in ( ) when p value is at least $p < 0.05$. [3] Culture conditions monocyte cytokines produced under.

When we examined correlations between IL-10 production by PBMCs and monocyte cytokine production, we found different correlating patterns between the ASD subgroups in response to β-LG and gliadin, while the non-ASD controls revealed little correlations (Table 7). In response to candida protein, only the high ratio ASD subgroup revealed positive correlations between IL-10 production by PBMCs and monocyte cytokine production (Table 7). Non-ASD controls revealed positive correlations between IL-10 production by PBMCs and sTNFRII production by PBMo, and negative correlations between IL-10 production by PBMCs and CCL2 production by PBMo.

Table 7. Correlation between IL-10 production by PBMCs and monocyte cytokine production.

Correlation Coefficient	IL-1β/IL-10 Ratio Based ASD Subgroups			Non-ASD Controls ($n = 41$)
	High ($n = 70$) [1]	Normal ($n = 74$)	Low ($n = 43$)	
In Response to β-Lactoglobulin				
IL-1β/IL-10 ratio				
Zymosan [3]	−0.3281 ($p < 0.01$) [2]	–	−0.3223 ($p < 0.05$)	–
CL097	–	–	0.3407 ($p < 0.05$)	–
IL-1β				
LPS	0.4682 ($p < 0.0001$)	0.3497 ($p < 0.005$)	–	–
CL097	0.3247 ($p < 0.02$)	–	0.4745 ($p < 0.005$)	–
IL-10				
No stimulant	0.4606 ($p < 0.0005$)	–	–	–
LPS	0.3998 ($p < 0.005$)	0.5026 ($p < 0.0001$)	0.3545 ($p < 0.05$)	0.5166 ($p < 0.005$)
Zymosan	0.2924 ($p < 0.05$)	–	–	–
CL097	–	–	0.3848 ($p < 0.02$)	–
TNF-α				
No stimulant	0.3132 ($p < 0.02$)	–	–	–
LPS	0.5669 ($p < 0.0001$)	0.3322 ($p < 0.01$)	–	–
CL097	0.3086 ($p < 0.02$)	–	0.4028 ($p < 0.02$)	–
IL-6				
LPS	–	0.2552 ($p < 0.05$)	–	–
CL097	–	–	0.4028 ($p < 0.02$)	–
In Response to Gliadin				
IL-1β/IL-10 ratio				
LPS	–	0.2504 ($p < 0.05$)	–	–
Zymosan	−0.252 ($p < 0.05$)	−0.2656 ($p < 0.05$)	–	–
CL097	–	–	0.3138 ($p < 0.05$)	–
IL-1β				
LPS	0.3834 ($p < 0.005$)	0.3866 ($p < 0.005$)	–	–
CL097	–	–	0.4537 ($p < 0.005$)	–
β-glucan	–	0.2576 ($p < 0.05$)	–	–
IL-10				
No stimulant	0.3233 ($p < 0.01$)	0.2398 ($p < 0.05$)	–	–
LPS	–	0.4354 ($p < 0.0005$)	0.3524 ($p < 0.05$)	–
Zymosan	0.3459 ($p < 0.005$)	–	–	–
CL097	–	–	0.3962 ($p < 0.02$)	–
β-glucan	0.2745 ($p < 0.05$)	–	–	–
TNF-α				
No stimulant	–	–	0.3378 ($p < 0.05$)	–
LPS	0.3368 ($p < 0.01$)	–	–.	–
Zymosan	0.285 ($p < 0.05$)	–	–	–
CL97	–	–	0.3422 ($p < 0.05$)	–
IL-6				
CL097	–	–	0.3235 ($p < 0.05$)	–
β-glucan	–	–	–	0.3374 ($p < 0.05$)
sTNFRII				
β/glucan	–	–	−0.3227 ($p < 0.05$)	–
In Response to Candida Protein				
IL-1β/IL-10 ratio				
No stimulant	−0.2785 ($p < 0.05$)	–	–	–
zymosan	−0.3022 ($p < 0.02$)	–	–	–
IL-1β				
CL097	0.2382 ($p < 0.05$)	–	–	–

Table 7. Cont.

Correlation Coefficient	IL-1β/IL-10 Ratio Based ASD Subgroups			Non-ASD Controls (n = 41)
	High (n = 70) [1]	Normal (n = 74)	Low (n = 43)	
IL-10				
LPS	0.2709 ($p < 0.05$)	–	–	–
β-glucan	–	–	–	−0.323 ($p < 0.05$)
sTNFRII				
Zymosan	–	0.2433 ($p < 0.05$)	–	0.3507 ($p < 0.05$)
CL097	0.2969 ($p < 0.02$)	–	–	0.3165 ($p < 0.05$)
β-glucan	–	−0.2419 ($p < 0.05$)	–	0.3342 ($p < 0.05$)
IL-6				
CL097	0.3021 ($p < 0.05$)	–	–	–
β-glucan	0.261 ($p < 0.05$)	–	–	–
sTNFRII				
Zymosan	–	–	–	−0.3154 ($p < 0.05$)
CCL2				
No stimulant	–	–	0.3198 ($p < 0.05$)	–
Zymosan	–	–	–	−0.3658 ($p < 0.05$)
CL097	–	–	–	−0.3416 ($p < 0.05$)
β-glucan	–	–	–	−0.5169 ($p < 0.001$)

[1] Total sample numbers in each study group; [2] Correlation coefficient by Spearman test with p value shown in ( ) when p value is at least $p < 0.05$. [3] Culture conditions monocyte cytokines produced under.

We also observed significant correlations between IL-12 production by PBMCs and monocyte cytokine production, although IL-12 production did not differ between IL-1β/IL-10 based ASD subgroups (Table 8). Namely, the low ratio ASD subgroup revealed significant correlations between PBMC IL-12 production and PBMo cytokine production, while the other ASD subgroups and non-ASD controls revealed little correlations between these two parameters.

Table 8. Correlation between IL-12 production by PBMCs and monocyte cytokine production.

Correlation Coefficient	IL-1β/IL-10 Ratio Based ASD Subgroups			Non-ASD Controls (n = 41)
	High (n = 70) [1]	Normal (n = 74)	Low (n = 43)	
	In Response to β-Lactoglobulin			
IL-1β/IL-10 ratio				
No stimulant [3]	–	–	0.3867 ($p < 0.02$) [2]	–
IL-1β				
β-glucan	–	–	−0.3908 ($p < 0.02$)	–
IL-10				
Zymosan	−0.2832 ($p < 0.02$)	–	−0.4993 ($p < 0.005$)	0.338 ($p < 0.05$)
TNF-α				
β-glucan	–	–	−0.345 ($p < 0.05$)	–
IL-6				
LPS	0.2796 ($p < 0.05$)	–	–	–
Zymosan	–	–	−0.3165 ($p < 0.05$)	–
sTNFRII				
No stimulant	−0.3463 ($p < 0.01$)	–	–	–
LPS	–	–	−0.3762 ($p < 0.02$)	−0.342 ($p < 0.05$)
Zymosan	–	–	−0.4228 ($p < 0.01$)	−0.3346 ($p < 0.05$)
β-glucan	–	–	−0.4733 ($p < 0.005$)	–

Table 8. Cont.

Correlation Coefficient	IL-1β/IL-10 Ratio Based ASD Subgroups			Non-ASD Controls (n = 41)
	High (n = 70) [1]	Normal (n = 74)	Low (n = 43)	
TGF-β				
No stimulant	–	–	−0.4374 ($p < 0.01$)	–
LPS	–	–	−0.4476 ($p < 0.005$)	–
Zymosan	–	–	−0.4546 ($p < 0.005$)	–
CL097	–	–	−0.4602 ($p < 0.005$)	–
β-glucan	–	–	−0.4356 ($p < 0.01$)	–
In Response to Gliadin				
IL-1β/IL-10 ratio				
No stimulant	–	–	–	0.3964 ($p < 0.02$)
IL-1β				
β-glucan	–	0.2835 ($p < 0.02$)	–	–
IL-10				
Zymosan	−0.2667 ($p < 0.05$)	–	−0.3707 ($p < 0.02$)	–
TNF-α				
No stimulant	–	–	0.468 ($p < 0.005$)	–
LPS	–	0.255 ($p < 0.05$)	0.3284 ($p < 0.05$)	–
IL-6				
CL097	–	–	0.3248 ($p < 0.05$)	–
β-glucan	–	−0.2472 ($p < 0.05$)	–	–
sTNFRII				
No stimulant	−0.2898 ($p < 0.02$)	–	–	–
zymosan	−0.2466 ($p < 0.05$)	–	–	–
β-glucan	–	–	−0.4348 ($p < 0.005$)	–
TGF-β				
Zymosan	–	–	−0.3163 ($p < 0.05$)	–
β-glucan	–	–	−0.3341 ($p < 0.05$)	–
CCL2				
No stimulant	–	–	0.3084 ($p < 0.05$)	–
In Response to Candida Protein				
IL-1β/IL-10 ratio				
Zymosan	−0.3644 ($p < 0.005$)	–	–	–
CL097	–	–	–	−0.3143 ($p < 0.05$)
IL-10				
CL097	–	–	0.3205 ($p < 0.05$)	–
TNF-α				
CL097	–	–	0.3319 ($p < 0.05$)	–
TGF-β				
Zymosan	–	–	−0.3077 ($p < 0.05$)	–
CCL2				
No stimulant	−0.2456 ($p < 0.05$)	–	0.506 ($p < 0.0005$)	–
Zymosan	–	–	0.3125 ($p < 0.05$)	–
CL097	–	–	0.3431 ($p < 0.05$)	–

[1] Total sample numbers in each study group; [2] Correlation coefficient by Spearman test with p value shown in ( ) when p value is at least $p < 0.05$. [3] Culture conditions monocyte cytokines produced under.

3. Discussion

Changes in IL-1β/IL-10 ratios and monocyte cytokine profiles in the ASD subgroups, which we have reported before with the use of TLR agonists, were also found under the β-glucan stimulated cultures in this study. This finding indicates that the innate immune abnormalities observed in some ASD children involve both TLR and inflammasome mediated pathways. T cell cytokine profiles (IFN-γ, TNF-α, and IL-10) also differed among the IL-1β/IL-10 ratio based ASD subgroups under cultures stimulated with food proteins (β-LG and gliadin) and candida proteins. Moreover, T cell cytokine production revealed close correlations with monocyte cytokine production, specific to each ASD subgroup. These findings support our hypothesis of sustained effects of maladapted TI on adaptive immunity in some ASD children.

The immune system operates with two components, innate and adaptive immunity. Innate immunity exerts rapid Ag-non-specific immune responses to contain infection until Ag-specific adaptive immunity sets in to clear hazards from the human body [26–28]. As opposed to adaptive immunity, innate immunity has been thought to lack lasting effects, since innate immune responses are Ag non-specific. However, for the past few years, it became clear that innate immunity can generate lasting effects or IIM by inducing metabolic and epigenetic changes in innate immune cells [29,30]. The key difference of IIM from adaptive immune memory is that the 2nd stimuli to provoke IIM can be totally unrelated to the 1st stimuli.

The presence of IIM was first convincingly shown as non-specific effects of BCG. Namely, BCG vaccination led to a greater reduction of infant mortality than predicted for decrease in mortality caused by tuberculosis in epidemiological and then randomized prospective studies [31,32]. These findings were further confirmed in rodent IIM models: BCG vaccination reduced from *Candida albicans* in the absence of lymphocyte that generates adaptive immune responses [33]. TI is the term that was given to describe these non-specific effects of IMM. Further studies revealed that TI can be generated in various innate immune cells including monocyte-macrophage lineage cells, natural killer (NK) cells [34], and bone marrow progenitor cells of innate immunity [35,36].

Metabolic and epigenetic changes have been extensively studied in 'in vitro' models of TI with the use of β-glucan derived from *Candida albicans*. Others have shown that β-glucan stimulates inflammasome through dectin-1, resulting in activation of signaling pathways involving Akt/PTEN/mTOR/HIF-1α [37]. This will shift oxidative phosphorylation (ATP synthesis) to glycolysis, resulting in decreased basal cellular respiration, and increased consumption of glucose, thereby leading to increase in lactate production [37]. These metabolic changes also affect synthesis of cholesterol and phospholipids [13,38], leading the replenishment of the Krebs cycle through formation of glutamate and α-keto-glutamate, and finally accumulation of fumarate [13,38]. A high concentration of fumarate hinders enzymatic actions of H3K4 demethylase, eventually resulting in epigenetic reprogramming [38–40].

Pre-administration of proinflammatory innate cytokines (IL-1, TNF-α, and IL-6) provided protection against a variety of microbes [41]. Among the cytokines administered, IL-1 showed superior effects over TNF-α or IL-6 [41]. In humans, TI associated protection has been mainly implicated with IL-1β and other IL-1 families [22]. Given the role of IL-1β in TI, excessive, dysregulated production of IL-1β is likely to cause maladapted TI, and resultant pathogenic consequences. Patients with gene mutations that lead to the over-production of IL-1β are known to reveal inflammatory symptoms involving multiple organs including the brain [22,42]. Moreover, chronic inflammatory conditions, including neuropsychiatric conditions have been implicated with maladapted TI [29,43].

As opposed to TI, tolerance is another form of IIM, causing lasting hypo-responsiveness against stimuli of innate immunity which is bested studied in endotoxin tolerance [44]. Upon induction of endotoxin tolerance, innate immune cells were reported to produce less inflammatory cytokines (TNF-α, IL-12, IL-6), but generate more counter-regulatory cytokines (IL-10 and TGF-β) with the subsequent endotoxin challenge [45,46]. LPS, a representative endotoxin, exerts its actions through TLR4, that results in activation of downstream signaling pathways the myeloid differentiation factor 88 (MyD88) and the TIR-domain-containing adaptor-inducing interferon-β (TRIF) [17]. Under the state of endotoxin tolerance, suppression of activation of these pathways are shown to be accomplished through multiple stages; down-regulation of TLR4, suppressed recruitment of MyD88 and TRIF to TLR4, reduced activation of IL-1 receptor-associated kinase (IRAK)1 and IRAK4, diminished activity of nuclear factor κ chain of B cell (NFκB), and up-regulated expression of counter-regulatory molecules such as SHIP1 (SH2 domain-containing inositol phosphatase 1) [47]. Induction of innate immune tolerance appears crucial in maintaining brain homeostasis; impaired innate immune tolerance has been implicated with pathogenesis of chronic neurodegenerative disorders including Alzheimer's disease [29].

We have been analyzing monocyte functions in ASD subjects for the past 4–5 years, and we have reported variable differences in monocyte cytokine profiles in ASD subjects, which have been best reflected in IL-1β/IL-10 ratios [20]. This finding led us to subgroup ASD PBMo samples on the basis of IL-1β/IL-10 ratios generated by stimulating PBMo with a panel of TLR agonists [20]. The IL-1β/IL-10 ratio based subgrouping revealed notable changes in miRNA expression and mitochondrial respiration across the IL-1β/IL-10 based ASD subgroups [20]. In addition, we also found the IL-1β/IL-10 ratio based ASD subgroup specific associations between metabolic changes (mitochondrial respiration) and monocyte cytokine profiles [21]. This was also true when we examined correlations between serum miRNA levels and monocyte cytokine profiles in the IL-1β/IL-10 ratio based ASD subgroups (manuscript submitted for publication). In addition, it is our observation that the ASD subjects whose PBMo revealed low or high IL-1β/IL-10 ratios tend to reveal fluctuating behavioral symptoms following immune insults.

The above described findings indicate that the innate immune responses in the high and low IL-1β/IL-10 ratio ASD subgroups may be altered as a result of maladapted TI, leading to clinical pictures of chronic inflammation affecting multi-organs. To address this possibility, we assessed whether responses to β-glucan also differed in the IL-1β/IL-10 ratio based ASD subgroups. Our results revealed significant differences of IL-1β/IL-10 ratios and monocyte cytokine profiles across the IL-1β/IL-10 based ASD subgroups under β-glucan stimulated cultures (Table 5). If the previously observed changes of monocyte cytokine profile were only limited to TLR pathways, such changes would be more likely to be associated with defects specific to TLR mediated signaling pathways. β-glucan stimulates a connonical inflammasome pathway and amplifies signaling through the TLR pathway [25]. Thus, the fact that we observed similar changes under β-glucan stimulated cultures supports the role of maladapted TI in ASD subjects; TI has been reported in multiple signaling pathways associated with innate immunity [30].

This study also addressed how T cell cytokine profiles in response to recall Ags are associated with changes in innate immune responses in the IL-1β/IL-10 based ASD subgroups. TI induced excessive innate immune responses are likely to induce more exuberant adaptive responses, thereby increasing the risk of unwanted immune reactivity to benign environmental antigens such as food antigens. However, if chronic activation of adaptive immunity through maladapted TI is sustained, this may eventually lead to suppression of adaptive immunity, regaining immune homeostasis. Such secondary suppression of adaptive immunity could occur by clonal deletion or through actions exerted by regulatory T cells [48,49]. However, how dysregulated innate immune abnormalities (presumably maladapted TI) affect adaptive immune responses in ASD children is poorly understood. Since ASD subjects have a high frequency of GI symptoms and delayed type reactivity to common food proteins and candida proteins [50], we opted to check T cell cytokine profiles against representative food proteins and candida antigens, when assessing associations between T cell cytokine profiles and monocyte cytokine profiles.

With this analysis, we observed significant differences in the production of TNF-α and IL-10 in response to β-LG and gliadin between the IL-1β/IL-10 based ASD subgroups. Namely, the high ratio groups tended to reveal higher levels of these two cytokines than the other subgroups (Table 5). On the other hand, the normal and low ratio ASD subgroups revealed higher IFN-γ production in response to candida protein (Table 5). As for TNF-α in response to candida Ag, both the high and low IL-1β/IL-10 ratio subgroups revealed a higher TNF-α production (Table 5). In contrast, IL-10 production against candida Ag was lower in the ASD subgroups, with the normal ratio group being the lowest. These results indicate complex associations between adaptive immune responses and altered innate immune responses in the ASD subjects.

When correlations between T cell cytokine production against β-LG and gliadin and monocyte cytokine profiles were assessed, positive correlations between IFN-γ production and production of monocyte cytokines (IL-1β, IL-10, and IL-6) were predominantly observed in the normal ratio ASD subgroup (Table 6). In contrast, correlations between production of TNF-α, IL-10, and IL-12 by PBMCs in responses to these food proteins and monocyte cytokines were predominantly found in either the high ratio ASD subgroup (for TNF-α and IL-10), or the low ratio ASD subgroup (for IL-12) (Tables 7–9). Non-ASD controls revealed little correlations except for TNF-α production by PBMCs and TNF-α production by PBMo (Table 7). These results indicate that responses to benign environmental antigens, such as food proteins, appear to be differently affected by innate immune responses in the IL-1β/IL-10 based ASD subgroups, perhaps reflecting maladapted TI.

Table 9. Demographics of ASD subjects and non-ASD controls.

	ASD [1] Subjects (n = 152)	Non-ASD Controls (n = 41)
Age (years) [2] median, range average ± SD	10.0 (2.2–26.3) 11.2 ± 5.8	11.2 (1.9–29.6) 13.3 ± 8.0
Gender (M:F)	130:22 (85.5 %:14.5%)	24:17 (58.5%:41.5%)
Ethnicity	AA 11, Asian 34, Mixed 5, W 102	Asian 4, Mixed 6, W 31

[1] Abbreviations used; AA; African American, ASD; autism spectrum disorder, F; female, GI; gastrointestinal, M; male, NFA: non-IgE mediated food allergy, SD; standard deviation, W; Caucasian. [2] Age at the time of study enrollment is shown.

When correlations between T cell cytokine production against candida proteins and monocyte cytokine profiles were assessed, we observed similar results; predominant correlations with monocyte cytokines in the normal ratio group for IFN-γ production, with more predominant correlations in the high and/or low ratio ASD subgroups for TNF-α, IL-10, and IL-12 production by PBMCs (Tables 6–9). Non-ASD controls only revealed positive correlations between IL-10 production by PBMCs and monocyte cytokine productions (Table 8). Since we were testing cellular immune reactivity to benign environmental Ags (food proteins and candida which is a normal component of the gut microbiome), a lack of close associations of inflammatory T cell cytokine profiles against these benign Ags in the non-ASD controls, and monocyte cytokine profiles may indicate the establishment of immune tolerance in adaptive immunity. Negative correlations between IL-10 production against candida protein and monocyte cytokine production may also indicate the establishment of immune homeostasis in non-ASD controls (Table 8). While the presence of close associations between monocyte cytokine profiles and T cell cytokine profiles (especially inflammatory cytokines—IFN-γ, TNF-α, and IL-12) in the ASD subgroups may indicate on-going effects of innate immunity in the absence of oral tolerance; this may also reflect maladapted TI.

When we assessed the clinical features in the IL-1β/IL-10 based ASD subgroups, we observed a high frequency of GI symptoms and a history of NFA with favorable responses to dietary interventions (usually gluten-free, dairy-free diet), consistent with our previous reports [20,21]. The IL-1β/IL-10 low ratio subgroup tended to have a higher frequency of history of NFA. β-GL is thought to be a major milk protein component associated with delayed type cellular immune reactivity in predisposed individuals. Interestingly, in the low IL-1β/IL-10 ratio ASD subgroup, IL-12 production by PBMCs in response to β-GL, a component was negatively correlated with counter-regulatory monocyte cytokines (IL-10, sTNFRII, and TGF-β) (Table 9). In contrast, IL-10 production in response to the β-GL was mostly positively correlated with monocyte cytokines production in the low ratio ASD subgroup (Table 9). This may indicate that altered innate immune responses may be regulating T cell cytokine production in the direction of suppressing excessive responses to recall antigens. On the other hand, in the high ratio group, there are positive correlations between IFN-γ, TNF-α, and IL-10 production in response to β-GL and monocyte cytokines (both inflammatory and counter-regulatory cytokines). In the high ratio group, such negative regulations may not be properly in place. Alternatively, with immune stimuli, such negative regulations may be easily lost secondary to maladapted TI.

4. Materials and Methods

4.1. Study Subjects

This study protocol was approved as protocols 15:45 (approval on 28 April 2016) and 17:53 (approval on 26 April 2018) by the Institutional Review Board, Saint Peter's University Hospital, New Brunswick, NJ, USA. This study included both ASD and typically developing (TD), non-ASD control subjects. We obtained the signed consent forms prior to sample obtainment from parents or guardians when the study subjects were minor (<18 years of age) or were judged unable to give consent by him/herself due to intellectual disability. History of comorbidities including food allergy (FA), asthma, allergic rhinitis (AR), specific antibody deficiency (SAD), sleep disorder, and seizure disorders were assessed in ASD children by history taking and medical chart review. This study excluded subjects with chromosomal abnormalities, well defined gene mutations, or chronic diseases involving major organs, but did not exclude subjects with minor medical conditions highly prevalent in general population, such as seasonal allergy. In this study, both ASD and non-ASD, TD subjects were enrolled, and the signed consent forms were obtained prior to entering the study. Consent was obtained from parents/guardians if participant was a minor (<18 years old) or parents/guardians had custody. For ASD children, we also assessed whether they had a history of FA, asthma, AR, SAD, or seizure disorders. Subjects diagnosed with chromosomal abnormalities, other genetic diseases, or well characterized chronic medical conditions involving a major organ, were excluded from the study. Subjects with common minor medical conditions such as AR, mild to moderate asthma, eczema were not excluded from the study.

ASD subjects: ASD subjects ($n = 152$) were recruited from the Pediatric Allergy/Immunology Clinic. Diagnosis of ASD was made at various autism diagnostic centers, including ours. The ASD diagnosis was based on the Autism Diagnostic Observation Scale (ADOS) and/or Autism Diagnostic Interview-Revisited (ADI-R), and other standard measures. ASD subjects were also evaluated for their behavioral symptoms and sleep habits with the Aberrant Behavior Checklist (ABC) [51] and the Children's Sleep Habits Questionnaires (CSHQ) [52], respectively. Information regarding cognitive ability and adaptive skills were obtained from previous school evaluation records performed within 1 year of enrollment in the study; these results were based on standard measures such as the Woodcock-Johnson III test (for cognitive ability), and Vineland Adaptive Behavior Scale (VABS) (for adaptive skills) [53].

Non-ASD controls: A total of 41 non-ASD subjects served as controls. These subjects were recruited in the Pediatrics Subspecialty and General Pediatrics Clinics at our institution. These subjects were typically growing and satisfied our exclusion criteria.

Table 1 reveals demographics of study subjects. Gender difference did not reveal significant changes regarding monocyte cytokine profiles and IL-1β/IL-10 ratios in both ASD and non-ASD groups, as reported before [21].

Diagnosis of FA: IgE mediated FA was diagnosed with reactions to offending food, by affecting the skin, GI, and/or respiratory tract immediately (within 2 h) after intake with positive prick skin testing (PST) reactivity, and/or presence of food allergen-specific serum IgE. Non IgE mediated FA (NFA) was diagnosed if GI symptoms resolved, following implementation of a restricted diet (i.e., avoidance of offending food), and symptoms recurred with re-exposure to offending food [54]. NFA was also defined as being non-reactive to PFT and negative for serum IgE specific for food allergens [54].

Diagnosis of asthma and AR: AR and allergic conjunctivitis (AC) were diagnosed when subjects had corresponding clinical features along with positive PST reactivity and/or positive serum IgE specific to [55,56]. Asthma was diagnosed following the asthma guidelines from the Expert Panel Report 3 [57].

Antibody deficiency syndrome: When the subject revealed protective levels of antibodies in less than 11 of 14 serotypes of *Streptococcus pneumonia* after the booster dose of Pneumovax® or PCV13®, he/she was diagnosed with SAD [58]. Antibody (Ab) levels greater than 1.3 µg/mL were considered protective [58].

4.2. Sample Collection

Venous blood samples were obtained by physician in this study. We obtained one sample from each non-ASD control. As for ASD subjects, we obtained multiple blood samples from select ASD subjects ($n = 22$), in order to assess variability of T cell cytokine profiles. If parents or study subjects preferred, we applied a topical lidocaine/prilocaine cream (Emla cream®,IGI Laboratories, Buena, NJ, USA) to the site of venipuncture prior to blood sampling.

4.3. Cell Cultures

Ficoll–Hypaque density gradient centrifugation was used for separating PBMCs. From PBMCs, PBMo were further purified using magnetic beads labeled with anti-CD3, CD7, CD16, CD19, CD56, CD123, and glycophorin A (monocyte separation kit II—human, MILTENYI BIOTEC, Cambridge, MA, USA). Namely, this column depletes T, B, natural killer, and dendritic cells from PBMCs with combination of these antibodies.

Cytokine production by purified PBMo was induced by incubating cells overnight (2.5×10^5 cells/mL) with a panel of agonist of toll like receptors (TLRs). This assay system was designed to reflect the effects of microbial byproducts commonly encountered in real life. Lipopolysaccharide (LPS), a TLR4 agonist, represents a signaling pathway activated in response to a Gram negative (G (–)) bacteria. Zymosan, a TLR2/6 agonist, mimics an innate activation signal in response to G (+) bacteria and fungi. CL097, a TLR7/8 agonist, activates innate signaling pathways in response to ssRNA viruses that cause common respiratory infection. We adapted these stimuli in our assay system, since these innate immune stimuli have been widely used by others. In addition, candida heat extract as a source of β-glucan, dectin-1 agonist, was used as well as a representative C-lectin receptor agonist. PBMos were incubated overnight with LPS (0.1 µg/mL, GIBCO-BRL, Gaithersburg, MD, USA), zymosan (50 µg/mL, Sigma-Aldrich, St. Luis, Mo, USA), C097 (water-soluble derivative of imidazoquinoline, 20 µM, InvivoGen, San Diego, CA, USA), and candida heat extract (HCKA, heat killed candida albicans (10^7 cells/mL, InVivogen, San Diego, CA) as a source of β-glucan, a dectin 1 agonist, in RPMI 1640 with additives as previously described [59]. Overnight incubation (16–20 h) was adequate to induce the optimal responses in this setting. The culture supernatant was used for cytokine assays.

Production of T cell cytokines (IFN-γ, IL-5, TNF-α, IL-10, IL-12p40, IL-17, and TGF-β) was assessed by incubating PBMCs (10^6 cells/mL) with representative recall antigens including β-lactoglobulin (β-LG, 10 µg/mL, Sigma Aldrich), soy protein (5 µg/mL, Ross, Nutley, NJ, USA), gliadin (10 µg/mL, Sigma-Aldrich), milk protein (100 µg/mL, Ross), and candida protein (5 µg/mL, Greer, Lenoir, NC, USA) for 4 days in RPMI1540 with additives as reported previously [60]. As noted in our previous study, a 4 day incubation period resulted in the optimal production of these cytokines in this culture setting.

Levels of C-C chemokine ligand 2 (CCL2), CCL7, interferon-γ (IFN-γ), IL-1β, IL-5, IL-6, IL-10, IL-12p40, IL-17, transforming growth factor-β (TGF-β), tumor necrosis factor-α (TNF-α), and soluble TNF receptor II (sTNFRII) cytokines were measured by enzyme-linked immuno-sorbent assay (ELISA); 10–100 µL/well supernatants were used for ELISA. The OptEIA™ Reagent Sets (BD Biosciences, San Jose, CA, USA) were used for ELISA of IFN-γ, IL-1β, IL-6, IL-10, IL-12p40, and TNF-α. For CCL2, CCL7, IL-17 (IL-17A), sTNFRII, and TGF-β ELISA, reagents were obtained from BD Biosciences and R & D (Minneapolis, MN, USA). IL-23 ELISA kit was purchased from eBiosciences, San Diego, CA. Intra- and inter-variations of cytokine levels were less than 5%.

4.4. Categorizing ASD Samples on the Basis of IL-1β/IL-10 ratios

Previously, we reported that changes in the IL-1β/IL-10 ratios best reflect altered cytokine profiles and miRNA expression by PBMo [20]. We divided ASD samples into subgroups based on the IL-1β/IL-10 ratios produced by ASD PBMo, following the criteria used in our previous study [20], as outlined below. In this study, we used IL-1β/IL-10 ratios generated under cultures with medium only, LPS, zymosan, CL097, and candida heat extract as a source of β-glucan.

High IL-1β/IL-10 ratio subgroup: In this subgroup, ASD PBMo showed 2 standard deviation (SD) higher IL-1β/IL-10 ratios under at least one culture condition and/or 1 SD greater IL-1β/IL-10 ratios under more than two culture conditions, as compared to control PBMo.

Normal IL-1β/IL-10 ratio subgroup: ASD PBMo revealed IL-1β/IL-10 ratios less than +1 SD, and greater than −1 SD under all the culture conditions, or IL-1β/IL-10 ratios greater than 1 SD but less than 2 SD under only one culture condition, as compared to control PBMo.

Low IL-1β/IL-10 ratio subgroup: ASD PBMo revealed IL-1β/IL-10 ratios less than −1 SD under at least one culture condition, as compared to control PBMo.

Among 25 ASD subjects in whom we obtained blood samples at 2–4 time points, most subjects revealed that blood samples from these subjects were categorized in the same group except for six ASD subjects. PBMo from these six ASD subjects showed high ratios at 1–2 time points and normal/low ratios at one time point. Eleven ASD subjects revealed low ratios at 1–2 time points and normal ratios at one time point. When comparing their clinical characteristics, they were categorized as high and low IL-1β/IL-10 ratio groups, respectively.

4.5. Statistical Analysis

We used a two tailed Mann–Whitney test for comparison of two sets of numerical data. Comparison of multiple data sets was assessed by one-way ANOVA and/or Kruskal—Wallis test. Normality of the numerical data were assessed by skewness and kurtosis (Omnibus) with $\alpha = 0.2$. When assessing differences in frequency between two groups, we used the Fisher exact test. For assessing differences in frequency among multiple groups, we used the Chi-Square test and the Likelihood ratio. A linear association between two data sets was determined by Spearman test. A p value of less than 0.05 was considered nominally significant. Co-variance analysis was done with the use of general linear model for a fixed factor or for a variable factor. For assessing longitudinal changes, repeated measures of analysis of variance were used. NCSS19 (NCSS, LLC. Kaysville, UT, USA) was used for statistical analysis.

4.6. Availability of Data and Material

Clinical features of the ASD are available through NDAR data base (https://ndar.nih.gov/). The additional datasets used and/or analyzed during the current study are available from the corresponding author on reasonable request.

5. Conclusions

This study revealed similar changes in IL-1β/IL-10 ratios and monocyte cytokine profiles under β-glucan stimulated cultures as observed in the cultures stimulated with TLR agonist, indicating that changes in innate immune responses are not limited to TLR pathways. Correlations between the changes in monocyte cytokine profiles and T cell cytokine profiles in response to benign environmental Ags differed across the IL-1β/IL-10 based ASD subgroups. Such correlations were much less evident in non-ASD controls, supporting possible effects of maladapted TI in some ASD children. Further analysis of the status of innate immunity in association with TI or tolerance will be helpful in understanding the inflammatory subtype of ASD.

Author Contributions: H.J. was responsible for the study design, recruitment of the study subjects, collection of clinical information and blood samples, analysis of the overall data, and preparation of most of this manuscript. L.G. conducted cytokine production assays with the use of purified monocytes and conducted T cell cytokine production assay with the use of recall Ags.

Funding: This study was supported by funding from Autism Research Institute, San Diego, CA, Jonty Foundation, St. Paul, MN, and the Governor's Council for Medical Research and Treatment of Autism (CAUT16APL007), DHHS, Trenton, NJ.

Acknowledgments: We are thankful for L. Huguenin, Ph.D. for critically reviewing this manuscript.

Conflicts of Interest: There is no conflict of interest to declare. The funders had no role in the design of the study; in the collection, analyses, or interpretation of data; in the writing of the manuscript, or in the decision to publish the results.

Abbreviations

Ab	antibody
ABC	aberrant behavior checklist
AC	allergic conjunctivitis
ADHD	attention deficiency hyperactivity disorder
ADI-R	autism diagnostic inventory, revisited
ADOS	autism diagnostic observational scale
AED	anti-epileptic drugs
Ag	antigen
ANOVA	analysis of variance
AR	allergic rhinitis
ASD	autism spectrum disorder
BCG	Bacillus Calmette–Guérin
CCL2	CC-chemokine-ligand-2
CSHQ	Children's sleep habit questionnaire
ELISA	enzyme linked immune-sorbent assay
IL	interleukin
IIM	innate immune memory
LPS	lipopolysaccharide
MIA	maternal immune activation
miRNA	microRNA
mTOR	mammalian target of rapamycin
NFA	non-IgE mediated food allergy
PBMCs	peripheral blood mononuclear cells
PBMo	peripheral blood monocytes
PST	prick skin testing
SAD	specific antibody deficiency
SD	standard deviation
SSRI	selective serotonin receptor inhibitor
TGF	transforming growth factor
TI	trained immunity
TLR	toll like receptor
TNF	tumor necrosis factor
VABS	Vineland adaptive behavioral scale

References

1. Siniscalco, D.; Schultz, S.; Brigida, A.L.; Antonucci, N. Inflammation and Neuro-Immune Dysregulations in Autism Spectrum Disorders. *Pharmaceuticals* **2018**, *11*, 56. [CrossRef] [PubMed]
2. Cristiano, C.; Lama, A.; Lembo, F.; Mollica, M.P.; Calignano, A.; Mattace Raso, G. Interplay between Peripheral and Central Inflammation in Autism Spectrum Disorders: Possible Nutritional and Therapeutic Strategies. *Front. Physiol* **2018**, *9*, 184. [CrossRef] [PubMed]

3. Jiang, N.M.; Cowan, M.; Moonah, S.N.; Petri, W.A., Jr. The Impact of Systemic Inflammation on Neurodevelopment. *Trends Mol. Med.* **2018**, *24*, 794–804. [CrossRef] [PubMed]
4. Careaga, M.; Murai, T.; Bauman, M.D. Maternal Immune Activation and Autism Spectrum Disorder: From Rodents to Nonhuman and Human Primates. *Biol. Psychiatry* **2017**, *81*, 391–401. [CrossRef] [PubMed]
5. Pendyala, G.; Chou, S.; Jung, Y.; Coiro, P.; Spartz, E.; Padmashri, R.; Li, M.; Dunaevsky, A. Maternal Immune Activation Causes Behavioral Impairments and Altered Cerebellar Cytokine and Synaptic Protein Expression. *Neuropsychopharmacology* **2017**, *42*, 1435–1446. [CrossRef] [PubMed]
6. Rose, D.R.; Careaga, M.; Van de Water, J.; McAllister, K.; Bauman, M.D.; Ashwood, P. Long-term altered immune responses following fetal priming in a non-human primate model of maternal immune activation. *Brain Behav. Immun.* **2017**, *63*, 60–70. [CrossRef] [PubMed]
7. Guma, E.; Plitman, E.; Chakravarty, M.M. The role of maternal immune activation in altering the neurodevelopmental trajectories of offspring: A translational review of neuroimaging studies with implications for autism spectrum disorder and schizophrenia. *Neurosci. Biobehav. Rev.* **2019**, *104*, 141–157. [CrossRef] [PubMed]
8. Sarkar, T.; Patro, N.; Patro, I.K. Cumulative multiple early life hits-a potent threat leading to neurological disorders. *Brain Res. Bull.* **2019**, *147*, 58–68. [CrossRef] [PubMed]
9. Jyonouchi, H.; Geng, L.; Davidow, A.L. Cytokine profiles by peripheral blood monocytes are associated with changes in behavioral symptoms following immune insults in a subset of ASD subjects: An inflammatory subtype? *J. Neuroinflamm.* **2014**, *11*, 187. [CrossRef]
10. Jyonouchi, H.G.L.; Buyske, S. Interleukin-1β/Interleukin10 Ratio Produced by Monocytes as a Biomarker of Neuroinflammation in Autism. *J. Clin. Cell. Immunol.* **2017**, *8*, 1000503. [CrossRef]
11. Thom, R.P.; Keary, C.J.; Palumbo, M.L.; Ravichandran, C.T.; Mullett, J.E.; Hazen, E.P.; Neumeyer, A.M.; McDougle, C.J. Beyond the brain: A multi-system inflammatory subtype of autism spectrum disorder. *Psychopharmacology* **2019**. [CrossRef] [PubMed]
12. Netea, M.G.; Joosten, L.A.; Latz, E.; Mills, K.H.; Natoli, G.; Stunnenberg, H.G.; O'Neill, L.A.; Xavier, R.J. Trained immunity: A program of innate immune memory in health and disease. *Science* **2016**, *352*, aaf1098. [CrossRef] [PubMed]
13. Arts, R.J.; Novakovic, B.; Ter Horst, R.; Carvalho, A.; Bekkering, S.; Lachmandas, E.; Rodrigues, F.; Silvestre, R.; Cheng, S.C.; Wang, S.Y.; et al. Glutaminolysis and Fumarate Accumulation Integrate Immunometabolic and Epigenetic Programs in Trained Immunity. *Cell Metab.* **2016**, *24*, 807–819. [CrossRef] [PubMed]
14. Fok, E.T.; Davignon, L.; Fanucchi, S.; Mhlanga, M.M. The lncRNA Connection between Cellular Metabolism and Epigenetics in Trained Immunity. *Front. Immunol.* **2018**, *9*, 3184. [CrossRef] [PubMed]
15. Bekkering, S.; Arts, R.J.W.; Novakovic, B.; Kourtzelis, I.; van der Heijden, C.; Li, Y.; Popa, C.D.; Ter Horst, R.; van Tuijl, J.; Netea-Maier, R.T.; et al. Metabolic Induction of Trained Immunity through the Mevalonate Pathway. *Cell* **2018**, *172*, 135–146.e139. [CrossRef] [PubMed]
16. Sun, X.; Sun, J.; Shao, X.; Feng, J.; Yan, J.; Qin, Y. Inhibition of microRNA-155 modulates endotoxin tolerance by upregulating suppressor of cytokine signaling 1 in microglia. *Exp. Ther Med.* **2018**, *15*, 4709–4716. [CrossRef] [PubMed]
17. Vergadi, E.; Vaporidi, K.; Tsatsanis, C. Regulation of Endotoxin Tolerance and Compensatory Anti-inflammatory Response Syndrome by Non-coding RNAs. *Front. Immunol.* **2018**, *9*, 2705. [CrossRef] [PubMed]
18. Doxaki, C.; Kampranis, S.C.; Eliopoulos, A.G.; Spilianakis, C.; Tsatsanis, C. Coordinated Regulation of miR-155 and miR-146a Genes during Induction of Endotoxin Tolerance in Macrophages. *J. Immunol.* **2015**, *195*, 5750–5761. [CrossRef] [PubMed]
19. Ifrim, D.C.; Quintin, J.; Joosten, L.A.; Jacobs, C.; Jansen, T.; Jacobs, L.; Gow, N.A.; Williams, D.L.; van der Meer, J.W.; Netea, M.G. Trained immunity or tolerance: Opposing functional programs induced in human monocytes after engagement of various pattern recognition receptors. *Clin. Vaccine Immunol.* **2014**, *21*, 534–545. [CrossRef]
20. Jyonouchi, H.; Geng, L.; Streck, D.L.; Dermody, J.J.; Toruner, G.A. MicroRNA expression changes in association with changes in interleukin-1ss/interleukin10 ratios produced by monocytes in autism spectrum disorders: Their association with neuropsychiatric symptoms and comorbid conditions (observational study). *J. Neuroinflamm.* **2017**, *14*, 229. [CrossRef]

21. Jyonouchi, H.; Geng, L.; Rose, S.; Bennuri, S.C.; Frye, R.E. Variations in Mitochondrial Respiration Differ in IL-1ss/IL-10 Ratio Based Subgroups in Autism Spectrum Disorders. *Front. Psychiatry* **2019**, *10*, 71. [CrossRef] [PubMed]
22. Moorlag, S.; Roring, R.J.; Joosten, L.A.B.; Netea, M.G. The role of the interleukin-1 family in trained immunity. *Immunol. Rev.* **2018**, *281*, 28–39. [CrossRef] [PubMed]
23. Ifrim, D.C.; Quintin, J.; Meerstein-Kessel, L.; Plantinga, T.S.; Joosten, L.A.; van der Meer, J.W.; van de Veerdonk, F.L.; Netea, M.G. Defective trained immunity in patients with STAT-1-dependent chronic mucocutaneaous candidiasis. *Clin. Exp. Immunol.* **2015**, *181*, 434–440. [CrossRef] [PubMed]
24. Rodriguez, A.E.; Bogart, C.; Gilbert, C.M.; McCullers, J.A.; Smith, A.M.; Kanneganti, T.D.; Lupfer, C.R. Enhanced IL-1beta production is mediated by a TLR2-MYD88-NLRP3 signaling axis during coinfection with influenza A virus and Streptococcus pneumoniae. *PLoS ONE* **2019**, *14*, e0212236. [CrossRef] [PubMed]
25. Boxberger, N.; Hecker, M.; Zettl, U.K. Dysregulation of Inflammasome Priming and Activation by MicroRNAs in Human Immune-Mediated Diseases. *J. Immunol.* **2019**, *202*, 2177–2187. [CrossRef] [PubMed]
26. Krakauer, T. ; Inflammasomes, Autophagy, and Cell Death: The Trinity of Innate Host Defense against Intracellular Bacteria. *Mediat. Inflamm.* **2019**, *2019*, 2471215. [CrossRef] [PubMed]
27. McCoy, K.D.; Ronchi, F.; Geuking, M.B. Host-microbiota interactions and adaptive immunity. *Immunol. Rev.* **2017**, *279*, 63–69. [CrossRef] [PubMed]
28. Farber, D.L.; Netea, M.G.; Radbruch, A.; Rajewsky, K.; Zinkernagel, R.M. Immunological memory: Lessons from the past and a look to the future. *Nat. Rev. Immunol.* **2016**, *16*, 124–128. [CrossRef] [PubMed]
29. Sfera, A.; Gradini, R.; Cummings, M.; Diaz, E.; Price, A.I.; Osorio, C. Rusty Microglia: Trainers of Innate Immunity in Alzheimer's Disease. *Front. Neurol.* **2018**, *9*, 1062. [CrossRef] [PubMed]
30. Van der Heijden, C.; Noz, M.P.; Joosten, L.A.B.; Netea, M.G.; Riksen, N.P.; Keating, S.T. Epigenetics and Trained Immunity. *Antioxid Redox Signal.* **2018**, *29*, 1023–1040. [CrossRef]
31. Benn, C.S.; Netea, M.G.; Selin, L.K.; Aaby, P. A small jab—A big effect: Nonspecific immunomodulation by vaccines. *Trends Immunol.* **2013**, *34*, 431–439. [CrossRef] [PubMed]
32. Aaby, P.; Roth, A.; Ravn, H.; Napirna, B.M.; Rodrigues, A.; Lisse, I.M.; Stensballe, L.; Diness, B.R.; Lausch, K.R.; Lund, N.; et al. Randomized trial of BCG vaccination at birth to low-birth-weight children: Beneficial nonspecific effects in the neonatal period? *J. Infect. Dis.* **2011**, *204*, 245–252. [CrossRef] [PubMed]
33. Kleinnijenhuis, J.; Quintin, J.; Preijers, F.; Joosten, L.A.; Ifrim, D.C.; Saeed, S.; Jacobs, C.; van Loenhout, J.; de Jong, D.; Stunnenberg, H.G.; et al. Bacille Calmette-Guerin induces NOD2-dependent nonspecific protection from reinfection via epigenetic reprogramming of monocytes. *Proc. Natl. Acad. Sci. USA* **2012**, *109*, 17537–17542. [CrossRef] [PubMed]
34. Sun, J.C.; Beilke, J.N.; Lanier, L.L. Adaptive immune features of natural killer cells. *Nature* **2009**, *457*, 557–561. [CrossRef] [PubMed]
35. Mitroulis, I.; Ruppova, K.; Wang, B.; Chen, L.S.; Grzybek, M.; Grinenko, T.; Eugster, A.; Troullinaki, M.; Palladini, A.; Kourtzelis, I.; et al. Modulation of Myelopoiesis Progenitors Is an Integral Component of Trained Immunity. *Cell* **2018**, *172*, 147–161.e112. [CrossRef] [PubMed]
36. Kaufmann, E.; Sanz, J.; Dunn, J.L.; Khan, N.; Mendonca, L.E.; Pacis, A.; Tzelepis, F.; Pernet, E.; Dumaine, A.; Grenier, J.C.; et al. BCG Educates Hematopoietic Stem Cells to Generate Protective Innate Immunity against Tuberculosis. *Cell* **2018**, *172*, 176–190.e119. [CrossRef]
37. Cheng, S.C.; Quintin, J.; Cramer, R.A.; Shepardson, K.M.; Saeed, S.; Kumar, V.; Giamarellos-Bourboulis, E.J.; Martens, J.H.; Rao, N.A.; Aghajanirefah, A.; et al. mTOR-and HIF-1alpha-mediated aerobic glycolysis as metabolic basis for trained immunity. *Science* **2014**, *345*, 1250684. [CrossRef]
38. Arts, R.J.; Joosten, L.A.; Netea, M.G. Immunometabolic circuits in trained immunity. *Semin. Immunol.* **2016**, *28*, 425–430. [CrossRef]
39. Saeed, S.; Quintin, J.; Kerstens, H.H.; Rao, N.A.; Aghajanirefah, A.; Matarese, F.; Cheng, S.C.; Ratter, J.; Berentsen, K.; van der Ent, M.A.; et al. Epigenetic programming of monocyte-to-macrophage differentiation and trained innate immunity. *Science* **2014**, *345*, 1251086. [CrossRef]
40. Novakovic, B.; Habibi, E.; Wang, S.Y.; Arts, R.J.W.; Davar, R.; Megchelenbrink, W.; Kim, B.; Kuznetsova, T.; Kox, M.; Zwaag, J.; et al. Beta-Glucan Reverses the Epigenetic State of LPS-Induced Immunological Tolerance. *Cell* **2016**, *167*, 1354–1368.e1314. [CrossRef]
41. Netea, M.; van der Meer, J.W. Trained Immunity: An Ancient Way of Remembering. *Cell Host Microbe* **2017**, *21*, 297–300. [CrossRef] [PubMed]

42. Keddie, S.; Parker, T.; Lachmann, H.J.; Ginsberg, L. Cryopyearin-Associated Periodic Fever Syndrome and the Nervous System. *Curr. Treat. Options Neurol.* **2018**, *20*, 43. [CrossRef] [PubMed]
43. Salam, A.P.; Borsini, A.; Zunszain, P.A. Trained innate immunity: A salient factor in the pathogenesis of neuroimmune psychiatric disorders. *Mol. Psychiatry* **2018**, *23*, 170–176. [CrossRef] [PubMed]
44. Seeley, J.J.; Baker, R.G.; Mohamed, G.; Bruns, T.; Hayden, M.S.; Deshmukh, S.D.; Freedberg, D.E.; Ghosh, S. Induction of innate immune memory via microRNA targeting of chromatin remodelling factors. *Nature* **2018**, *559*, 114–119. [CrossRef] [PubMed]
45. Del Fresno, C.; Garcia-Rio, F.; Gomez-Pinam, V.; Soares-Schanoski, A.; Fernandez-Ruiz, I.; Jurado, T.; Kajiji, T.; Shu, C.; Marin, E.; Gutierrez del Arroyo, A.; et al. Potent phagocytic activity with impaired antigen presentation identifying lipopolysaccharide-tolerant human monocytes: Demonstration in isolated monocytes from cystic fibrosis patients. *J. Immunol.* **2009**, *182*, 6494–6507. [CrossRef]
46. Nahid, M.A.; Satoh, M.; Chan, E.K. MicroRNA in TLR signaling and endotoxin tolerance. *Cell Mol. Immunol.* **2011**, *8*, 388–403. [CrossRef]
47. Biswas, S.K.; Lopez-Collazo, E. Endotoxin tolerance: New mechanisms, molecules and clinical significance. *Trends Immunol.* **2009**, *30*, 475–487. [CrossRef]
48. Attias, M.; Al-Aubodah, T.; Piccirillo, C.A. Mechanisms of human FoxP3(+) Treg cell development and function in health and disease. *Clin. Exp. Immunol.* **2019**, *197*, 36–51.
49. Okeke, E.B.; Uzonna, J.E. The Pivotal Role of Regulatory T Cells in the Regulation of Innate Immune Cells. *Front. Immunol.* **2019**, *10*, 680. [CrossRef]
50. Jyonouchi, H.; Geng, L.; Ruby, A.; Reddy, C.; Zimmerman-Bier, B. Evaluation of an association between gastrointestinal symptoms and cytokine production against common dietary proteins in children with autism spectrum disorders. *J. Pediatr.* **2005**, *146*, 605–610. [CrossRef]
51. Aman, M.G.; Singh, N.N.; Stewart, A.W.; Field, C.J. The aberrant behavior checklist: A behavior rating scale for the assessment of treatment effects. *Am. J. Ment. Defic.* **1985**, *89*, 485–491. [PubMed]
52. Owens, J.A.; Spirito, A.; McGuinn, M. The Children's Sleep Habits Questionnaire (CSHQ): Psychometric properties of a survey instrument for school-aged children. *Sleep* **2000**, *23*, 1043–1051. [CrossRef] [PubMed]
53. Sparrow, S.B.C.D.; Vineland, D.V. *Adaptive Behavior Scales Survey Form Manual*; American Guidance Service: Cirde Pines, MN, USA, 1985.
54. Boyce, J.A.; Assa'ad, A.; Burks, A.W.; Jones, S.M.; Sampson, H.A.; Wood, R.A.; Plaut, M.; Cooper, S.F.; Fenton, M.J.; Arshad, S.H.; et al. Guidelines for the diagnosis and management of food allergy in the United States: Report of the NIAID-sponsored expert panel. *J. Allergy Clin. Immunol.* **2010**, *126*, S1–S58. [CrossRef] [PubMed]
55. Butrus, S.; Portela, R. Ocular allergy: Diagnosis and treatment. *Ophthalmol. Clin. N. Am.* **2005**, *18*, 485–492.
56. Nassef, M.; Shapiro, G.; Casale, T.B. Identifying and managing rhinitis and its subtypes: Allergic and nonallergic components—A consensus report and materials from the Respiratory and Allergic Disease Foundation. *Curr. Med. Res. Opin* **2006**, *22*, 2541–2548. [CrossRef] [PubMed]
57. Expert Panel Report 3 (EPR-3). Guidelines for the Diagnosis and Management of Asthma-Summary Report 2007. *J. Allergy Clin. Immunol.* **2007**, *120*, S94–S138. [CrossRef]
58. Orange, J.S.; Ballow, M.; Stiehm, E.R.; Ballas, Z.K.; Chinen, J.; De La Morena, M.; Kumararatne, D.; Harville, T.O.; Hesterberg, P.; Koleilat, M.; et al. Use and interpretation of diagnostic vaccination in primary immunodeficiency: A working group report of the Basic and Clinical Immunology Interest Section of the American Academy of Allergy, Asthma & Immunology. *J. Allergy Clin. Immunol.* **2012**, *130*, S1–S24.
59. Jyonouchi, H.; Geng, L.; Ruby, A.; Zimmerman-Bier, B. Dysregulated innate immune responses in young children with autism spectrum disorders: Their relationship to gastrointestinal symptoms and dietary intervention. *Neuropsychobiology* **2005**, *51*, 77–85. [CrossRef]
60. Jyonouchi, H.; Geng, L.; Cushing-Ruby, A.; Quraishi, H. Impact of innate immunity in a subset of children with autism spectrum disorders: A case control study. *J. Neuroinflamm.* **2008**, *5*, 52. [CrossRef]

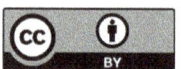

© 2019 by the authors. Licensee MDPI, Basel, Switzerland. This article is an open access article distributed under the terms and conditions of the Creative Commons Attribution (CC BY) license (http://creativecommons.org/licenses/by/4.0/).

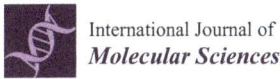

Article

Gender Related Changes in Gene Expression Induced by Valproic Acid in A Mouse Model of Autism and the Correction by S-adenosyl Methionine. Does It Explain the Gender Differences in Autistic Like Behavior?

Liza Weinstein-Fudim [1], Zivanit Ergaz [1], Gadi Turgeman [2], Joseph Yanai [1], Moshe Szyf [3] and Asher Ornoy [1,*]

[1] Department of Medical Neurobiology, Hebrew University Hadassah Medical School, Jerusalem 91120, Israel; liza.weinstein-f@mail.huji.ac.il (L.W.-F.); Zivanit@hadassah.org.il (Z.E.); josephy@ekmd.huji.ac.il (J.Y.)
[2] Department of Molecular Biology and Pre-Medical Studies, Ariel University, Ariel 40700, Israel; gadit@ariel.ac.il
[3] Department of Pharmacology and Therapeutics, McGill University Medical School, Montreal, QC H4A3J1, Canada; moshe.szyf@gmail.com
* Correspondence: ornoy@cc.huji.ac.il; Tel.: +972-2-6758-329

Received: 27 September 2019; Accepted: 22 October 2019; Published: 24 October 2019

Abstract: In previous studies we produced autism like behavioral changes in mice by Valproic acid (VPA) with significant differences between genders. S-adenosine methionine (SAM) prevented the autism like behavior in both genders. The expression of 770 genes of pathways involved in neurophysiology and neuropathology was studied in the prefrontal cortex of 60 days old male and female mice using the NanoString nCounter. In females, VPA induced statistically significant changes in the expression of 146 genes; 71 genes were upregulated and 75 downregulated. In males, VPA changed the expression of only 19 genes, 16 were upregulated and 3 downregulated. Eight genes were similarly changed in both genders. When considering only the genes that were changed by at least 50%, VPA changed the expression of 15 genes in females and 3 in males. Only Nts was similarly downregulated in both genders. SAM normalized the expression of most changed genes in both genders. We presume that genes that are involved in autism like behavior in our model were similarly changed in both genders and corrected by SAM. The behavioral and other differences between genders may be related to genes that were differently affected by VPA in males and females and/or differently affected by SAM.

Keywords: ASD; epigenetics; mice; postnatal VPA injection; SAM; gene expression; nanostring

---

1. Introduction

Autism spectrum disorder (ASD) is a complex neurodevelopmental disorder characterized by impaired social communication and social interactions and restrictive stereotyped behaviors and interests. ASD core symptoms are frequently accompanied by developmental delay, anxiety and cognitive deficits [1–3]. Currently, the prevalence of ASD is 1 in 59 children, at an earlier onset of children prior to 3 years of age [4]. ASD is more prevalent in males, with the average male to female ratio 4:1 [4]. This male bias that can be partially explained by specific genetic differences between males and females had various impacts on both research and clinical practice [5]. Furthermore, autistic male and female demonstrate different phenotypes; females were usually reported to have lower social and communicative problems and fewer restricted and repetitive behaviors than males [6–8]. The age of diagnosis is also on average later in autistic females than males, and females may often be missed by current diagnostic procedures [9].

Although ASD is a highly heritable disorder, prenatal and early postnatal exposures to environmental toxicants (i.e., pollutants, insecticides and pesticides) or maternal infections as well as epigenetic alterations are hypothesized to contribute to the development of ASD. Nevertheless, the underlying cause is still unclear [1–3,10]. Moreover, currently there are no biochemical or molecular markers for the diagnosis of ASD.

Animal models enable the use of preclinical tools to understand the role of genetic mutations and environmental factors in the etiology of ASD. Hence, there are several rodent models in which ASD-like symptoms were produced by exposure of the pregnant dams to a teratogenic agent, especially valproic acid (VPA), during different stages of gestation, and a few following early postnatal insults [2,10,11].

VPA is an antiepileptic drug that has also been used for bipolar disorder, migraine headaches and as a mood stabilizer [12,13]. VPA exposure during pregnancy, especially during the organogenesis period, is associated with various teratogenic effects including high risk of major anomalies, mainly spina bifida. VPA during pregnancy also leads to 5–10 fold increased rate of ASD in the offspring [3,14]. Similarly, rodents exposed to VPA during different stages of pregnancy exhibit behavioral deficits including delayed developmental milestones, stereotypic and self-injurious behavior and impaired social behavior similar to those observed in autistic patients [11,15–19]. Therefore, VPA rodent model became a robust, widely used, environmental preclinical model of ASD with face construct and predictive validity [20].

Interestingly, while the male to female ratio observed in human ASD is 4:1, the male to female ratio in ASD children exposed to VPA during pregnancy is nearly 1:1 [21] or 2:1 [22].

As in human, there are behavioral differences between male and female rodents exposed to VPA. Male mice exposed to VPA exhibited social impairment and reduced social interaction, manifested by lack of preference for a stranger mouse in the three-chamber test [23–25]. On the other hand, increased repetitive behavior and anxiety-like behaviors was reported in both males and females [23,26].

It is important to remember that most cases of ASD in human are genetic in origin and not related to the use of specific drugs or chemicals during pregnancy. There are also distinct neurobehavioral differences in human with ASD when compared to animal models. For example, there is a wide range of cognitive abilities in human from normal to severe retardation (1,2), while learning is often impaired in the VPA animal model.

The mechanism(s) by which VPA exposure during pregnancy causes autistic-like behaviors in both human and rodent offspring are still far to be clear. Among the proposed mechanisms are: Folic acid deficiency, effects on Wnt signaling, increased oxidative stress [11], alternations in serotonin homeostasis [27] and in the activity of gamma amino butyrate (GABA) neurotransmitter, and neuronal spine density changes. Other suggested pathways are derangement of the serotonergic, dopaminergic and/or oxytocinergic systems. In addition, VPA is an epigenetic modulator and a potent histone deacetylase (HDAC) class l and ll inhibitor [9,11–13]. Histone deacetylases removes acetyl groups from the tail of core histones, and regulates chromatin condensation and gene expression. Mice exposed prenatally to VPA demonstrate transient increase in acetylated histone levels [28].

Recently, more and more studies suggest that multifactorial conditions of ASD result from epigenetic changes, i.e., heritable changes in gene expression via a number of mechanisms including DNA methylation, histone modifications and ATP-dependent chromatin remodeling, without changing the underlying DNA sequence.

Choi et al. [29] demonstrated that the effect of prenatal VPA exposure in offspring could be paternally transmitted from the first up to the third generation. They detected autistic-like behaviors and increased postsynaptic markers of excitatory neurons in VPA-exposed F2 and F3 generations similar to those impairments detected in F1 VPA prenatally exposed mice. Furthermore, because the transmission experiments were performed with non- exposed female mice, the transmission is paternal and it is not influenced by any in utero exposures. They also reported congenital malformations only in

F1 generation of VPA exposed mice, suggesting that VPA-induced congenital defects are mediated by a mechanism other than transmissible epigenetic changes. Their findings support the transgenerational epigenetic inheritance in the etiology of ASD.

So far, genetic studies identified more than 1000 genes that contribute to ASD risk [30]. Nevertheless, specific cellular abnormalities that link genes with behavior remain obscure. Most studies exploring gene alternation in VPA exposed rodents focused on specific set of genes or genes involved in the process of interest [31–33]. Only a few studies demonstrated comprehensive genetic analysis. Zhang et al. [34] performed transcriptome analysis in the prefrontal cortex of male rats prenatally exposed to VPA. They reported 3228 differently expressed genes and 637 genes differently spliced in the VPA group compared to controls, including genes involved in neurological diseases such as Huntington's disease, Alzheimer's disease and Parkinson's disease. VPA also changed the expression of genes associated with neurogenesis, generation of neurons, neuron projection development, neuron differentiation and synaptic development.

Kotajima-Murakami et al. [35] treated prenatally VPA exposed pups with intraperitoneal injection of rapamycin for 2 consecutive days. The mammalian target of rapamycin (mTOR) signaling pathway plays a crucial role in cell growth, proliferation and metabolism. Mice prenatally exposed to VPA exhibited the aberrant expression of genes associated with the mTOR signaling pathway, and rapamycin treatment recovered changes in the expression of some genes.

Hill et al. [36] explored changes in methylation of CpG islands in the frontal cortex of mice prenatally exposed to VPA as well as mice exposed to other toxicants including lead and manganese. They reported lower regulation and overexpression of Chd7 gene essential for neural crest cell migration and patterning in all treatment groups.

Several brain structures and functions have been suggested to underlie behavioral abnormalities of ASD including the prefrontal cerebral cortex [37], the cerebellum, the hippocampus and the basolateral amygdala [38]. The prefrontal cerebral cortex is affected in ASD at the neuronal development and synaptic functionality levels. Studies found alternations such as Hyper-Connectivity and Hyper-Plasticity in the pyramidal network in the medial prefrontal cortex [39]. Thus, we decided to focus on this part of the brain in our study.

S Adenosyl methionine (SAM) is the principal biological methyl donor involved in multiple biochemical reactions and critical for regulation of cell growth, differentiation, and function and biosynthesis of hormones and neurotransmitters [40]. SAM has also been shown to be involved in reduction of oxidative stress [41–44]. Villalobos et al. [41] showed that SAM modulates cellular oxidative status, mainly by inhibiting lipid peroxidation and enhancing glutathione system in the brain of rat model of brain ischemia-reperfusion.

Reduction in SAM levels has been found in neurological conditions such as Alzheimer disease [45]. Numerous studies have therefore explored the efficiency of treatment of depression and other neuropsychiatric conditions by SAM administration [46–49]. A few studies indicated that gender might impact the antidepressant efficacy of SAM, with greater therapeutic effect found in males [50].

In our recent study [23] we injected four-day-old mice with a single dose of 300 mg/kg of VPA and tested them on a variety of neurobehavioral tests during postnatal days 50 to 59. The mice exhibited typical ASD-like behavior, with differences between males and females in some of the tests. Lower preference for social novelty and stereotyped repetitive behaviors were more prominent in males, while impaired re-learning ability were more prominent in females. In addition we evaluated oxidative stress parameters in the prefrontal cortex and liver on day 60. Enhanced oxidative stress was observed in the prefrontal cortex, demonstrated by changes in the activity of Superoxide dismutase (SOD) and Catalase (CAT) enzymes and increased lipid peroxidation in VPA treated mice. In general oxidative stress parameters were more prominent in females. There were no changes in the redox potential of the liver, implying that the oxidative stress was induced only in the brain as a result of the epigenetic changes induced by the VPA. The co-administration of VPA and SAM alleviated most ASD like neurobehavioral symptoms and normalized the redox potential in the prefrontal cortex [23].

Our current research focuses on the gene expression changes in the VPA treated mice. In this study, we aimed to evaluate the effects of early postnatal VPA administration on ASD like behavior and the therapeutic effect of SAM on the VPA exposed mice by measuring the changes in the expression of genes involved in various neurobiological pathways. In addition we aimed to evaluate the differences in the gene expression between males and females in order to understand the cause of the ASD like behavioral variance between genders.

2. Results

As there were significant gender differences in the expression of genes, the data is described separately for males and for females. In females, VPA injection induced statistically significant changes in the expression of 146 genes, 71 genes were upregulated and 75 genes were downregulated. In males, VPA changed the expression of 19 genes, 16 were upregulated and 3 genes were downregulated. Nine of these genes were similarly changed in both genders (See Figures 1 and 2).

Gene ontology functional enrichment analysis for the genes significantly changed by VPA in females revealed several pathways associated with Huntington disease, Alzheimer's disease, Prostate cancer, focal adhesion, calcium and PIK3-signaling (Table 1). Of special importance for our study are pathways of associated diseases involving cognitive impairment, namely Alzheimer's disease and Huntington's disease (supplementary Figure S1). In both pathways, key genes were upregulated in VPA exposed females (i.e., APP & Htt). Furthermore, Huntington's disease pathway share mechanisms with epigenetic modulation of DNA and gene repression, including HDAC - a putative target for VPA (supplementary Figure S1A). However, in males, no statistical significant pathway was detected. We therefore, continued to explore the data by focusing on specific genes with a cut-off of 50% de-regulation of expression, and their possible role as key genes.

Figure 1A,B represent heat map of mRNA levels of genes involved in neuropathological pathways at the prefrontal cortex. For each gene the expression was normalized to the geometrical mean of 7 housekeeping genes and the negative and positive technical controls. Each vertical column represents one animal belonging to the treatment group indicated in the upper panel while each horizontal lane represents the normalized mRNA counts for one gene. The colors represent the expression of each gene among the different treated animals (red and blue represent strong and weak expression, respectively). As observed, there were many genes whose expression was significantly changed by VPA. More of these genes were up or downregulated in females compared to males.

For strict selection we decided to focus on genes with at least 50% change by VPA. With the restriction of 50% change in comparison to controls, there were 15 genes in females and 3 genes in males whose expression was changed by VPA. Only one of these genes, Nts, was similarly downregulated in both genders, as described in Tables 2 and 3.

Table 2 shows the percent of change by VPA compared to controls for each gene in females, whether the change is corrected by SAM administration or not. Six genes were upregulated and 9 were downregulated. The affected genes are involved in various pathways; 6 are involved in neurotransmission, 5 in neuroplasticity and 6 in neuroinflammation. Note that 4 of the genes also appear in Sfari database for genes reported in human ASD. These genes are involved in neurotransmission and neuroinflammation (Table 2).

Table 3 shows the percent of change by VPA compared to controls for each gene in males, whether the change was corrected by SAM administration or not. VPA changed the expression of 3 genes, 2 were upregulated and one was downregulated. The biological pathway of these genes varies, as seen in the table. None of these genes was reported in SFARI database for genes reported in human ASD.

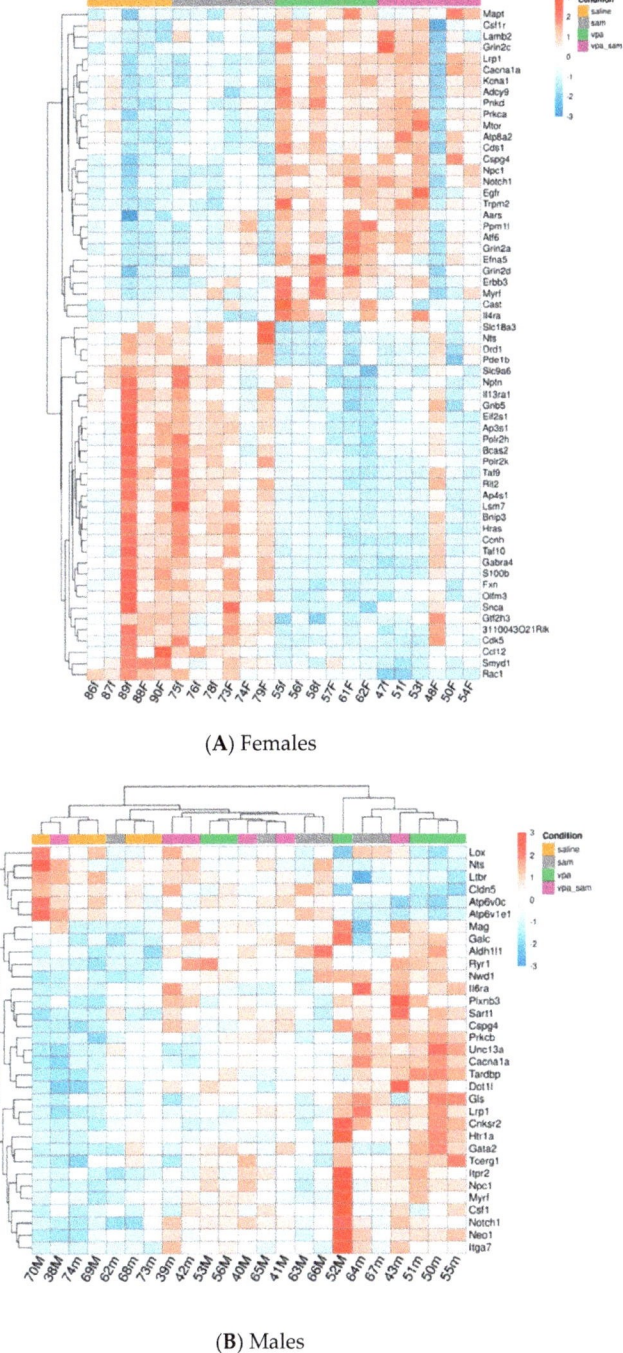

Figure 1. Effect of VPA and SAM administration on the gene expression in the prefrontal cortex. Heat map of the genes significantly changed by VPA in the different groups: **A**. females, **B**. males. Each heat map consists of two NanoString panels (12 samples).

Table 1. Functional enrichment analysis of the genes significantly changed by VPA in females and males.

	Category	Term	Count	%	p Value	Genes	Fold Enrichment
	KEGG_PATHWAY	mmu04510: Focal adhesion	22	6%	0.011	PRKCA, EGFR, COL4A2, HRAS, COL4A1, FLT1, MAP2K1, PIK3CB, IGF1, PRKCG, BAD, CTNNB1, IGF1R, MAPK1, LAMB2, TNR, ITGA7, RAC1, PDGFRB, PIK3CA, PAK1, FN1	1.630
	KEGG_PATHWAY	mmu03022: Basal transcription factors	9	3%	0.025	TAF10, MNAT1, CCNH, GTF2H3, TAF9, CDK7, TAF6L, GTF2B, TBPL1	2.222
	KEGG_PATHWAY	mmu05016: Huntington's disease	18	5%	0.025	POLR2H, HTT, CREBBP, DNAH1, SOD1, PPARGC1A, TFAM, AP2B1, EP300, PLCB4, HDAC2, GNAQ, CASP9, SP1, GRIN2B, BAX, TBPL1, HAP1	1.626
Females	KEGG_PATHWAY	mmu05215: Prostate cancer	17	5%	0.026	EGFR, HRAS, MAP2K1, PIK3CB, CREBBP, IGF1, BAD, CTNNB1, IGF1R, MAPK1, CDKN1A, ATF4, EP300, CASP9, PDGFRB, PIK3CA, MTOR	1.657
	KEGG_PATHWAY	mmu04151: PI3K-Akt signaling pathway	31	9%	0.029	HRAS, IL4RA, PPP2R5C, IGF1R, LAMB2, CASP9, TNR, RAC1, PIK3CA, PRKAA2, INSR, CSF1R, FN1, PRKCA, EGFR, COL4A2, FLT1, COL4A1, MAP2K1, PIK3CB, IGF1, BAD, MAPK1, CDKN1A, ATF4, ITGA7, PDGFRB, GNB5, EFNA5, PPP2R5E, MTOR	1.383
	KEGG_PATHWAY	mmu05010: Alzheimer's disease	21	6%	0.038	CDK5R1, ADAM10, SNCA, GRIN2A, BAD, CDK5, ATF6, MAPK1, APP, PLCB4, LRP1, GNAQ, CASP9, GRIN2B, GRIN2C, MAPT, RYR3, GRIN2D, BACE1, PPP3CC, CACNA1C	1.496
	KEGG_PATHWAY	mmu04020: Calcium signaling pathway	22	6%	0.044	PRKCA, EGFR, SLC8A1, DRD1, ADORA2A, ERBB3, GRIN2A, PRKCG, ATP2B3, PLCB4, GNAQ, ADCY9, PDE1B, GRIN2C, RYR3, GRIN2D, PDGFRB, PPP3CC, RYR2, CACNA1C, CACNA1A, CACNA1B	1.455

Table 2. Genes changed by VPA at least by 50% in females and the normalization by SAM *.

Gene.	Official Full Name	Up (+)/down(−) Regulated by VPA	% Change	Adjusted p Value	Neuroinflammation	Neuroplasticity, Development & Aging	Metabolism	Compartmentalization and Structural Integrity	Neurotransmission		Normalized by SAM Administration
Smyd1	SET and MYND domain containing 1	(−)	−63%	0.001951	−	+	−	−	−		−
Cspg4	chondroitin sulfate proteoglycan 4	(+)	51%	0.01074	+	+	−	−	−		−
Nts	neurotensin	(−)	−71%	0.01074	−	−	−	+	−		+
Il4ra	interleukin 4 receptor, alpha	(+)	63%	0.01097	+	−	−	−	−		−
Ccl12	chemokine (C-C motif) ligand 12	(−)	−58%	0.01461	+	+	+	+	+		−
Drd1	dopamine receptor D1	(−)	−57%	0.01567	−	−	−	+	+	Reported in human and animal SFARI data base.	+
Slc18a3	solute carrier family 18 (vesicular monoamine), member 3	(−)	−58%	0.02247	−	−	−	+	+		+
Notch1	notch 1	(+)	51%	0.02426	−	+	−	−	−		−
Ppm1l	protein phosphatase 1 (formerly 2C)-like	(+)	60%	0.02426	+	−	−	−	−		+
Grin2a	glutamate receptor, ionotropic, NMDA2A (epsilon 1)	(+)	61%	0.02478	−	−	−	+	+	Reported in human SFARI data base.	+
Chat	choline acetyltransferase	(−)	−56%	0.03445	−	−	+	+	+		+
Cd40	CD40 antigen	(−)	−55%	0.04037	+	−	−	+	−		−
Cd4	CD4 antigen	(−)	−55%	0.0411	−	−	−	+	−		−
Adora2a	adenosine A2a receptor	(−)	−59%	0.05169	−	−	−	−	+	Reported in human and animal SFARI data base.	+
Flt1	FMS-like tyrosine kinase 1	(+)	83%	0.05169	+	+	−	−	−	Reported in human SFARI data base.	+

* The genes are ordered by the significance of the adjusted p value.

Table 3. Genes changed by VPA at least by 50% in males and the normalization by SAM *.

Gene.	Official Full Name	Up(+)/down(−) Regulated by VPA	% Change	Adjusted p Value	Neuroinflammation	Compartmentalization and Structural Integrity	Neurotransmission	Normalized by SAM Administration
Ryr1	ryanodine receptor 1, skeletal muscle	(+)	61%	0.007544	−	−	+	+
Nts **	neurotensin	(−)	−76%	0.03878	−	+	−	+
Itga7	integrin alpha 7	(+)	53%	0.04183	−	+	−	+

* The genes were ordered by the significance of the adjusted p value. ** Nts was also similarly downregulated in females.

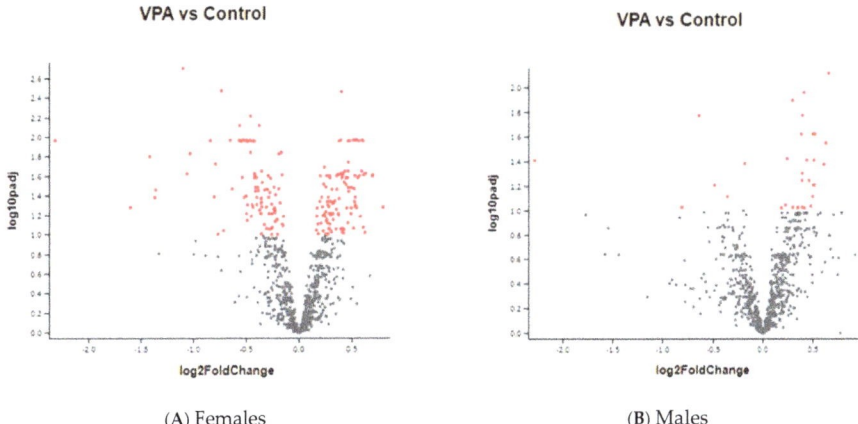

(A) Females   (B) Males

Figure 2. (**A,B**) are a volcano plot of log 2 fold-change (x-axis) versus −log 10 adjusted *p*-value (y-axis, representing the probability that the gene is differentially expressed). Every dot represents one gene. Red dots: genes with statistically significant change compared to controls. Grey dots: no statistical change. More genes were up or down regulated in females compared to males. In males, most of the genes whose expression was changed by VPA were upregulated.

SAM Administration to Controls

SAM alone did not affect gene expression in males. In females, only one gene, Lsr (lipolysis stimulated lipoprotein receptor) was significantly downregulated by SAM administration (adjusted *p* value 0.008764).

SAM administration to VPA exposed mice: Co-administration of SAM with VPA normalized in females the expression of 8 of 15 genes that were significantly affected (for at least 50%) by VPA and their expression was similar to their expression in controls (Table 2). Three of these genes were upregulated by VPA and 5 were downregulated. All 4 genes that were reported in the Sfari database of human and animal genes involved in ASD were normalized by SAM.

In males, SAM corrected the expression of all three genes that were changed by VPA at least 50% (Table 3). Note that the gene Nts was similarly downregulated by VPA and corrected by SAM in both genders.

Table 4 shows 8 genes that were significantly changed in the same direction by VPA in both genders and the percent of change was similar. Of these genes, only Nts gene changed by more than 50% (Table 4). Two of these 8 genes were reported in the Sfari database of human and animal genes involved in ASD: Unc13a and Cacna1a. These two genes were normalized by SAM administration only in males.

Table 4. Genes whose expression was significantly changed in the same direction by VPA in males and females and their correction by SAM *.

Gene.	Official Full Name	% Change Males	Adjusted p Value-Males	% Change Females	Adjusted p Value-Females	Neuroplasticity, Development & Aging	Metabolism	Compartmentalization and Structural Integrity	Neuron-Glia interaction	Neurotransmission	Normalized by SAM Males	Normalized by SAM Females	
Npc1	Niemann-Pick type C1	31%	0.01089	26%	0.003442	−	+	−	−	−	+	−	
Plxnb3	plexin B3	34%	0.02376	40%	0.0259	+	−	−	−	−	−	+	Reported in human SFARI database
Unc13a	unc-13 homolog A (C. elegans)	0.24	0.02376	0.23	0.04218	−	−	+	−	+	+	−	
Myrf	myelin regulatory factor	48%	0.0281	30%	0.02347	−	−	−	+	−	+	+	
Notch1	notch 1	0.43	0.03878	0.51	0.02426	+	−	+	−	−	−	+	
Nts	neurotensin	−76%	0.03878	−71%	0.01074	−	−	+	−	−	+	−	
Itga7	integrin alpha 7	0.53	0.04183	0.3	0.04599	−	−	+	−	−	+	−	
Cacna1a	voltage-dependent, P/Q type, alpha 1A subunit	25%	0.0497	36%	0.02478	+	−	+	−	+	+	−	Reported in human SFARI database

* The genes were ordered by the significance of the adjusted p value.

3. Discussion

In this study we explored the regulation of gene expression in the prefrontal cortex of adult male and female mice by VPA and the possible correction of these changes by SAM. We found that early postnatal injection of VPA induced statistically significant differences ($p < 0.05$) in the expression of many genes. In females, the expression of 146 genes was changed, 15 of them being changed by more than 50%. In males, the expression of 19 genes was significantly changed by VPA, 3 of them being changed more than 50%.

VPA is a broad-spectrum antiepileptic drug with a wide range of clinical effects. While normally VPA is considered to be a safe drug with only few side effects, during pregnancy it may cause severe teratogenic effects in the embryo and fetus [11]. VPA is a strong HDAC inhibitor, playing an important role in transcriptional regulation; thus it is reasonable to assume that gene expression changes detected in the prefrontal cortex of 60 day old adult mice results from VPA induced epigenetic modifications accumulating during early postnatal developmental stages in the brain. Indeed VPA –induced changes in gene expression were reported by several investigators [31–33].

S-adenosyl methionine (SAM) is an important biological methyl donor which provides the methyl groups for histone or nucleic acid modification and phosphatidylcholine production, tuning regulation of gene expression [51].

In the current study we treated VPA injected pups with SAM. In males, 75% of VPA induced differently expressed genes were "repaired" by SAM administration; in females more genes were affected by VPA and only 52% of VPA- affected genes normalized by SAM. These results correlate with our previously reported behavioral findings that demonstrated greater beneficial effect of SAM in males in most of the behavioral tests compared to females [23]. In the behavioral analysis of our study, a composite ASD score combined of the social novelty preference, T-maze test and self-grooming assay was calculated for each mouse. An elevated score in the VPA group with correction in the SAM treatment group was noted both in females and males. However, differences were higher in males compared to females.

Male-to-female prevalence ratio of ASD is estimated to be about 4.5 [52]. This strong male predominance suggests the existence of different genetic involvement in the pathogenesis of ASD. In our study, the VPA –induced changes in gene expression were indeed different between the genders.

Most studies using the VPA model have predominantly explored the male sex and gender differences in autistic like behavioral phenotypes were reported only in few studies. Autistic male mice and rats were reported to display less social interest and had impairment in social novelty preference [28,53], decreased ability of nest-building [54] increased anxiety like behaviors, increased repetitive/stereotypic-like activity and lower sensitivity to pain [24]. Only few studies reported impaired social behavior in females as that was generally less pronounced than in males [55].

In our previous study, both genders exhibited autistic-like behaviors with differences in several neurological functions. Females were more prone to present anxiety-related traits as observed in the open field (center duration) and Elevated plus maze (head dipping); males displayed greater impairment in social novelty preference, grooming frequency and cognitive rigidity (T-maze) implying that the autistic-like behavior was stronger in males in spite of fewer VPA-affected genes. The differences were also reflected in the higher autism composite score induced by VPA in males [23].

We will therefore discuss the role of the genes whose expression was significantly changed by VPA and corrected by SAM and are already known to be related to ASD and/or to several common psychiatric and neurodegenerative diseases of the brain.

Only one gene, Nts, was similarly downregulated by more than 50% in males and females and its expression was normalized by SAM administration. Hence, this gene deserves special consideration.

Neurotensin (NTS) is a 13-amino-acid peptide which acts as a principal neuromodulator in the central nervous system. NTS was reported to be involved in mediating visceral analgesia [56], vocal communication and social behaviors [57], maternal aggression during offspring defense [58], sleep-wake regulation, anxiety, depressive-like behaviors [59] and locomotor activity [60]. The Nts system has been implicated in the pathophysiology of several psychiatric and neurological disorders, such as schizophrenia [61], anxiety [62] and depression [63]. Nts-expressing neurons modulate and interact with major neurotransmitter systems, including the dopaminergic [64,65], glutamatergic [66–68], gabaergic [69] and cholinergic [70] systems. NTS has strong interactions with dopamine and in the rat prefrontal cortex Nts is exclusively localized in dopamine axons [71].

In mammals, the Nts biological effects are mediated through two G-protein coupled receptors, Nts1 and Nts2, and one single-transmembrane receptor, Ntsr3 /sortilin [61,72,73]. Activation of Nts1 receptor by the selective agonist PD149163 reduced locomotor activity in mice with dose dependent effects [74]. This agonist also improved memory performance in male Norway rats [75]. Two studies reported elevated NTS levels in the serum of autistic children [76,77] that may occur as a result of inflammatory processes [78,79].

Although Nts seems to be involved in pathways and brain areas critical for social behavior, it received very little research attention regarding its possible role in the etiology of ASD. Kirsten et al. established a mouse model for ASD by prenatal Lipopolysaccharide exposure and reported autistic like behavior and reduced NTS (protein) plasma levels in male offspring. Postnatal treatment with the anti-diabetic drug Pioglitazone corrected social and communication deficits and abolished the reduction in the NTS levels [80,81]. We found reduced Nts mRNA levels in VPA exposed male and female mice that were corrected by SAM administration. In our previous behavioral analysis we detected increased anxiety-like behaviors, manifested by reduced frequency of head dipping in the VPA exposed male and female mice in the elevated plus maze test. A possible connection between reduced NTS protein activity and lower performance in the same behavioral test was described also by Normandeau et al. [82] in a mouse model of chronic stress.

In our previous study [23] we also detected significantly decreased time spent in the center of the arena in the open field, especially in females. These anxiety-related behaviors normalized by co-administration of SAM. Similar anxiety-related phenotype in the open field activity test was described by Fitzpatrick et al. [59] in Nts Receptor1 knockout male mice, with less distance traveled in the open field, less time spent in the center and more time spent in the corners than the wild-type controls.

Since Nts was the single gene similarly downregulated by VPA more than 50% and corrected by SAM in both genders, it is tempting to presume that downregulation of Nts may induce autistic like behavior. As Nts was not yet reported in Sfari data base as possibly related to ASD in animals or man, this issue needs further studies.

In addition to Nts, we have detected 8 genes that changed in both genders, with significant statistical difference from control (but less than 50% change). The similarity in the VPA-induced changes and the fact that both genders had ASD like behavior, may imply that several of these genes are indeed related to the autistic like behavior of the VPA treated animals. Two of these genes: Unc13a and Cacna1a also appear in Sfari database for genes reported in human/animal ASD. Since SAM improved the autistic –like behavior in both genders, we may decrease the number of candidate genes only to those that were corrected by SAM.

The expression of Unc13a and Cacna1a was upregulated in both genders, but normalized by SAM only in males. Unc13a, a neurotransmitter release regulator at nerve cell synapses, single-nucleotide exchange in the Unc13a gene, was reported in a number of disorders including delayed cognitive development, speech impairment, ASD, and ADHD [83].

Cacna1a encodes for the alpha-1A subunit of a neuronal ion calcium channel, which is predominantly expressed in neuronal tissue. CACNA1A loss-of-function mutations are associated with cognitive impairment including intellectual disability, ADHD and ASD [84]. Both genes are involved in glutamatergic synaptic neurotransmission and significantly associated with major depressive disorder [85]. Glutamate is considered to be a central excitatory neurotransmitter in CNS synaptic transmission and is involved in learning, memory and synaptic plasticity. Hence, the gender differences in the gene expression involved in glutamatergic pathways may explain the sex differences in the pathology of ASD.

Adults with ASD have regional abnormalities in subcortical glutamatergic neurotransmission that are associated with variations in social development [86]. Reduction in glutamate metabolism in ASD was reported in the basal ganglia [86], anterior cingulate cortex and the thalamus [87], while increased glutamate metabolism was found in the amygdala-hippocampal region of ASD individuals [88].

In a Shank2-mutant mouse model of ASD, Won et al. reported marked decrease in NMDA (*N*-methyl-*D*-aspartate) glutamate receptor (NMDAR) function which was accompanied by ASD-like behaviors including impaired social interaction, reduced social communication by ultrasonic vocalizations, and repetitive behavior, increased anxiety-like behavior and impaired spatial learning and memory. Furthermore, treatment of mice with a positive allosteric modulator of metabotropic glutamate receptor 5 (mGluR5) which normalized NMDAR function were found to have enhances social interaction.

A recently published review by Wickens et al. [89] described sex differences in the glutamatergic system contribution to psychiatric diseases with male predominance in schizophrenia, ASD and ADHD, and female predominance in Alzheimer's disease and major depressive disorder. Furthermore, they described overall increase in glutamatergic transmission in females in most of these diseases that may play a protective role and lead to differences in symptomatology. Our findings support the involvement of sex specific alternations in the glutamatergic system in ASD pathophysiology. More studies are needed to estimate how glutamate dysfunction differentially affects males and females in context to ASD phenotype.

3.1. Genes Whose Expression Was Significantly Changed in Females

We will focus on genes previously reported in ASD: Drd1, Adora2a, Grin2a and Flt1. The expression of Drd1 and Adora2a was decreased and the expression of Flt1 and Grin2a was increased after VPA injection. All these genes were normalized by SAM administration. In addition, we will also focus on Nlrp3 gene that has been upregulated by almost 250% from controls and on Chat gene- of importance in acetyl choline metabolism that was downregulated by 55% and normalized by SAM.

The dopamine D1 receptor (Drd1) is among the most important postsynaptic effectors of dopamine function in the central nervous system. Drd1 regulates neuronal growth and development, mediates behavioral responses, and is involved in modulation of Drd2 mediated events. Drd1 was reported to be involved in social cognition [90]. Mutant Drd1 male rats have significantly reduced sociability and decreased interest in social novelty accompanied by decreased ultrasonic vocalization [91].

Adora2a: Adenosine A2A receptors are closely intertwined with the dopamine neurotransmitter system, are co-localized and have functional interactions with dopamine D2 receptors [92,93].

Adora2a is located on 22q11.23 chromosome, while deletions and duplications of chromosome 22q11.2 are associated with higher rates of ASD and psychotic symptoms [94]. Polymorphisms in Adora2a have been associated with schizophrenia, psychosis and anxiety [95–97]. Furthermore, Freitag et al. [98] found an association between single variant of Adora2a gene and increased autistic symptoms in human. Squillace et al. [99] revealed dramatically blunted Drd2 and Adora2a neurotransmission in BTBR strain of autistic mice, a finding that could play a role in the social deficits exhibited by these animals.

The Grin2a gene encodes the glutamate-binding GluN2A subunit of the N-methyl-D-aspartate receptors (NMDARs)- a glutamate gated cation channels that mediates the slow component of excitatory synaptic transmission [100]. NMDARs play essential roles in normal brain function, including learning, memory, synaptic plasticity, motor and sensory processes, and nervous system development. Grin2a mutations were identified in children with specific language impairment, speech disorders and epilepsy [101,102]. In our study VPA induced upregulation of Grin2a gene. Up regulation of GRIN2A receptor was also found in the prefrontal cortex of patients with major depression [103,104].

Flt1 (VegfR1) - Vascular endothelial growth factor receptor- 1 is a Tyrosine-protein kinase that acts as a cell-surface receptor for VEGF, a well-known major angiogenesis stimulating factor. Flt1 was reported to be involved in the regulation of angiogenesis, cell survival and cell migration, and acts as a negative regulator of embryonic angiogenesis [105,106]. In our study, the expression of Flt1 gene was upregulated by 83% after VPA exposure, and normalized by SAM. Higher prefrontal cortex expression of Flt1 was associated with worse cognitive trajectories in Alzheimer disease patients [107].

Upregulation of the Flt1 gene was also described by Hu et al. [108] in a study that examined the gene expression profiling on DNA microarrays of lymphoblastoid cell lines derived from five monozygotic twin pairs discordant in severity for ASD and language impairment. There was a positive association between the severity of the autistic phenotype exhibited by the twins (higher or lower expression in the more severely affected twin relative to the other twin) and the expression level of several genes involved in neurological function, including Flt1.

The expression of Chat was reduced by 56% in females but not in males. However, we decided to focus on this gene because of its importance in neuronal pathways.

Choline acetyltransferase (Chat) encodes CHAT enzyme which catalyzes the biosynthesis of the neurotransmitter acetylcholine. Acetylcholine is one of the most important neurotransmitters controlling the parasympathetic and the sympathetic autonomic nervous system as well as the somatic motor system. Furthermore, Acetylcholine is a major neurotransmitter in the CNS, involved in many functions, including control of locomotor activity, emotional behavior, and higher cognitive processes such as attention, learning and memory processes [109–111]. Changes in cholinergic neurotransmission are associated with a variety of important neurological disorders including Alzheimer's disease, schizophrenia, Parkinson's disease, epilepsy, attention-deficit hyperactivity disorder, mild cognitive impairment and also ASD [110,112]. Cholinergic agents such as Donepezil have been proposed for treatment of ASD symptoms [113].

Wang et al. [114] examined the role of the nicotinic cholinergic system on social and repetitive behavior in BTBR mouse model of ASD. They treated autistic mice for 4 weeks with different doses of nicotine (50, 100, 200 and 400 µg/mL), an agonist of nicotinic acetylcholine receptor subtypes that is also known to upregulate the expression of various nAChR (acetylcholine receptor) subtypes. They reported that high doses of nicotine (200 and 400 µg/mL) significantly decreased repetitive self-grooming behavior in BTBR mice compared to baseline, while lower doses of nicotine (100 µg/mL) increased social interactions in BTBR mice in the three chambers social interaction test. The authors combined male and female data because they did not find any gender differences. In our previous study males, but not females, exposed to VPA showed significantly increased grooming frequency and lower preference for social novelty and preference to familiar social stimuli in the Social interaction test, which was normalized by the co-administration of SAM [23].

Although, dysfunction of the cholinergic system may underlie autism-related behavioral symptoms, we did not find any evidence from the literature connecting between the involvements of Chat to ASD etiology, especially not in VPA-induced ASD. Furthermore, studies analyzing tissue samples from deceased autistic adults reported no alteration of CHAT biochemical activity in the cerebellum [115] and in the frontal and parietal cerebral cortex [116]. Despite these reports, studies of other neurological disorders suggested significant involvement of CHAT enzyme alternations and described its possible connection to behavioral changes. Hence, further studies should be carried out to elucidate the possible role of Chat in the etiology of ASD

Down-regulation of Chat as well as other cholinergic signaling genes was demonstrated in a chronic restraint stress rat model of depression, in which rats display depression-like behaviors such as anhedonia and mood despair [117]. In Alzheimer patients Chat activity is significantly decreased in the cerebral cortex and hippocampus and it seems to correlate with the severity of the dementia [118].

In our previous study [23], in the water T maze assessing reversal learning, cognitive rigidity and repetitive behavior, the learning curve for detecting the new location of a hidden platform was significantly less effective and there were greater latencies in trials only in the VPA-exposed females compared to controls. This higher latency was normalized by the co-addition of SAM. In males we did not find any differences in the water T maze test, in parallel to normal expression of Chat gene.

3.2. Genes Whose Expression Was Significantly Changed Only in Males

In addition to Nts 3, Ryr1 and Itga7 were all upregulated by VPA. The expression of all these genes was normalized by SAM administration. None of these genes was reported to be related to ASD.

Ryr1- ryanodine receptor 1 plays a central role in the regulation of intracellular calcium (Ca^{2+}) homeostasis, which is crucial for neuron survival and function. Ryrs exist in three isoforms (Ryr 1–3). Ryr2–3 is predominantly expressed in Purkinje cells of the cerebellum and cerebral cortex and in the hippocampus [119] and is involved in modulation of learning and memory functions [120]. Ryr1 also plays a critical role in calcium release and muscle contraction in skeletal muscle [121].

Gene ontology functional enrichment analysis for the genes significantly changed by VPA in females, demonstrated potential shared mechanism with neurodegenerative diseases such as Alzheimer's disease and Huntington's disease, as our Nlrp3 analysis suggest. Thus, GO term analysis suggests that common pathways underlay common symptoms in different pathologies. Studying such common pathways may have implication to several diseases including ASD. Nevertheless, we could not find shared pathways between females and males. However, it is still possible that individual genes whose expression was similarly changed by VPA and corrected by SAM play a role in the autistic like behavior of both genders. Such a candidate gene is Nts. The differences in the behavioral pattern between VPA treated males and females may be related to the change in the expression of genes that are differently affected between genders or not corrected by SAM. However, from our data it is impossible to point out to the genes that are specifically responsible for the ASD like behavioral changes.

4. Materials and Methods

4.1. Animals

Male and female (four days old) outbred ICR albino pups were injected subcutaneously on postnatal day 4, either with 300 mg/Kg body weight of VPA dissolved in normal saline or normal saline (NS). The dose chosen was the minimal dose that was reported to produce ASD in mice offspring. This time is developmentally equivalent to months 7–8 of human pregnancy. Each of these two groups (VPA and NS treated) were further subdivided into two groups- one receiving daily by intraoral gavage, from day 5 for 3 days, 30 mg/Kg body weight of SAM dissolved in NS, and the other receiving NS. Each treatment or control group consisted of 12–16 males and a similar number of female mice.

Twenty four hours after VPA injection pups were given daily for 3 consecutive days 30 mg/kg SAM by intragastric lavage. On day 60, the animals were euthanized; brains (prefrontal cerebral cortex) were removed for molecular studies. All pups were handled similarly in the animal quarters under optimal temperature and light. The University of Ariel Ethics committee for experiments on animals received approval for the study (IL-109-06-16, 6th July 2016). The more complete data on the experimental design and the results of the neurobehavioral tests were published elsewhere [23].

4.2. RNA Extraction and Gene Expression Analysis

Total RNA was extracted from the right prefrontal cortex of the mice using the RNA/DNA/protein purification plus kit (47700; Norgen, Thorold, ON, Canada) according to the manufacturer's protocol. RNA was quantified at absorbance of 260nm. An OD260/280 ratio between 1.8 and 2.2 was considered for further processing.

Gene expression analysis was performed for 24 samples of each gender, 6 in each group, using the NanoString nCounter system (NanoString Technologies, Seattle, WA, USA) that provides a simple way to profile specific nucleic acid molecules in a complex mixture. The system is based on direct digital detection of mRNA molecules utilizing target-specific, color-coded probe pairs that can hybridize directly to target molecules. The expression level of mRNA molecules is measured by counting the number of times the barcode for that molecule is detected by a digital analyzer. It does not require the conversion of mRNA to cDNA by reverse transcription or the amplification of the resulting cDNA by PCR. The system does not need amplification and is sensitive enough to detect low abundance molecules.

The data is expressed by the number of mRNA molecules In 100 ng/uL of RNA. It can simultaneously quantify up to 800 different interesting targets in a single reaction, making it ideal for miRNA profiling and targeted mRNA expression analysis [122]. We used the Mouse Neuropathology Panel that includes 770 genes covering pathways involved in neurophysiology, neurodegeneration and other nervous system diseases, and 10 internal reference genes for data normalization.

4.3. Gene Functional Enrichment

Gene Ontology for Functional enrichment of pathways (KEGG) was performed for genes which were found to be significantly altered by VPA using DAVID bioinformatics resources 6.8 [123]. The total list of 770 genes related for neuropathology that were tested in the array was used as background. Significantly enriched pathways were selected by p value (<0.05) and fold enrichment (>1.3) [124,125].

4.4. Statistical Analysis

NanoString analysis was performed on 6 samples from each group and each gender. This large sample size allows detecting and referring also to small but statistically significant changes in gene expression.

Gene expression data were analyzed by two-way ANOVA, in the first time with control as the reference group, and the second time with VPA as the reference group.

NanoString analysis was performed on 6 samples from each group and each gender. This large sample size allows detecting and referring also to small but statistically significant changes in gene expression.

Gene expression data were analyzed by the R package DESeq2, v1.22.1 [126]. Since samples were measured in two batches, the statistical model included both the treatment and the batch. After normalization by the internal reference genes, Wald test was used to compare the different conditions, using default parameters, including the significance threshold of Benjamini-Hochberg FDR (p adj) less than 0.05. Further filtering of significant genes required a change in expression of at least 50% relative to the control group.

NanoString assay is reported to be reliable, high-throughput assay used to simultaneously screen for gene expression changes in clinical practice [127,128]. Studies that used the NanoString n-counter system usually did not use rtPCR analysis for validation [129–132].

5. Conclusions

Most of the genes whose expression were changed by VPA and corrected by SAM seem to be involved in ASD and/or several other diseases of the nervous system, or in cognition and memory. These include genes involved in neuronal function and in inflammation. Genes of these two groups were also described as being associated with human ASD. The fact that SAM normalized their function may also explain the reversal of the autistic like behavior and reduction of brain oxidative stress observed in our previous studies. The changes induced by VPA in several pathways (Alzheimer's disease and Huntington's disease) were observed only in females. Since these changes are gender specific, they might not be related to the ASD like behavioral changes manifested in females and males. This emphasizes that only changes in the expression of individual genes may be related to the autistic like behavior. Unfortunately, our data do not enable us to correctly point to the gene/s that may be responsible for the autistic like behavior induced by VPA, but point to a number of genes possibly involved, especially those similarly changed by VPA in both genders and "corrected" by SAM such as Nts or Myrf. Early postnatal administration of SAM alone had very little effect on gene expression. Methylation of DNA occurs via the methyl donor SAM, and maintenance of adequate SAM circulating concentrations are, in part, dependent on folic acid and vitamin B12 [133]. Because most of the epigenetic programming accrue during prenatal development, it is reasonable that SAM effects as a methyl donor on the methylation pattern will be lower after birth. Indeed, in a different study we found that SAM administration during mid-pregnancy to ICR mice caused many significant changes in gene expression in the prefrontal cortex of the neonates (to be published).

Supplementary Materials: The following is available online at http://www.mdpi.com/1422-0067/20/21/5278/s1, Figure S1: KEGG pathway analysis in females exposed to VPA. The distribution of differentially expressed genes in prefrontal cortex of females exposed to VPA compared with controls in (A) Huntington's disease pathway and (B) Alzheimer's disease pathway. Significantly, deregulated genes are marked with red star, detected using DAVID/KEGG enrichment analysis of the Nanostring array.

Author Contributions: This study is part of the PhD thesis of L.W.-F. All other researchers on the list: Z.E.; G.T.; J.Y.; M.S. and A.O. are part of the team of the investigators who conceptualized and planned these studies and evaluated the results. A.O. is the head of the laboratory of Teratology where much of the study was performed and L.W.-F's instructor. All authors read the manuscript and added their comments, bringing the manuscript to its current final form.

Funding: This research was partially supported by the Harris Foundation Grant, Chicago, USA.

Acknowledgments: We thank the bioinformatics unit of the Hebrew University Hadassah Medical School who helped in the evaluation of the molecular data. Liza Weinstein-Fudim served for partial fulfilment of the requirements for a PhD of the Hebrew University

Conflicts of Interest: The authors declare no conflict of interest.

Abbreviations

ASD	Autism Spectrum disorder
VPA	Valproic Acid
SAM	S- Adenosyl Methionine
SFARI	Simons Foundation Autism Research Initiative
ADHD	Attention Deficit Hyperactivity Disorder
CAT	Catalase
SOD	Superoxide Dismutase
HDAC	Histone deacetylase
NMDA	N-methyl-D-aspartate
VEGF	Vascular endothelial growth factor
CHAT	Choline acetyltransferase

References

1. American Psychiatric Association. *Diagnostic and Statistical Manual of Mental Disorders*, 5th ed.; Association, A.P., Ed.; American Psychiatric Association: Washington DC, USA, 2013; pp. 50–59.
2. Ornoy, A.; Weinstein-Fudim, L.; Ergaz, Z. Prenatal factors associated with autism spectrum disorder (ASD). *Reprod. Toxicol.* **2015**, *56*, 155–169. [CrossRef] [PubMed]
3. Developmental Disabilities Monitoring Network Surveillance Year Principal Investigators, Centers for Disease, and Prevention. Prevalence of autism spectrum disorder among children aged 8 years-autism and developmental disabilities monitoring network, 11 sites, United States, 2010. *MMWR Surveill. Summ.* **2014**, *63*, 1–21.
4. Baio, J.; Wiggins, L.; Christensen, D.L.; Maenner, M.J.; Daniels, J.; Warren, Z.; Kurzius-Spencer, M.; Zahorodny, W.; Robinson, C.; Rosenberg, C.R.; et al. Prevalence of Autism Spectrum Disorder Among Children Aged 8 Years—Autism and Developmental Disabilities Monitoring Network, 11 Sites, United States, 2014. *MMWR Surveill. Summ.* **2018**, *67*, 1–23. [CrossRef] [PubMed]
5. Lai, M.C.; Lombardo, M.V.; Auyeung, B.; Chakrabarti, B.; Baron-Cohen, S. Sex/gender differences and autism: Setting the scene for future research. *J. Am. Acad. Child Adolesc. Psychiatry* **2015**, *54*, 11–24. [CrossRef] [PubMed]
6. Beggiato, A.; Peyre, H.; Maruani, A.; Scheid, I.; Rastam, M.; Amsellem, F.; Gillberg, C.I.; Leboyer, M.; Bourgeron, T.; Gillberg, C.; et al. Gender differences in autism spectrum disorders: Divergence among specific core symptoms. *Autism Res.* **2017**, *10*, 680–689. [CrossRef] [PubMed]
7. Szatmari, P.; Liu, X.Q.; Goldberg, J.; Zwaigenbaum, L.; Paterson, A.D.; Woodbury-Smith, M.; Georgiades, S.; Duku, E.; Thompson, A. Sex differences in repetitive stereotyped behaviors in autism: Implications for genetic liability. *Am. J. Med. Genet. B Neuropsychiatr. Genet.* **2012**, *159*, 5–12. [CrossRef] [PubMed]

8. Van Wijngaarden-Cremers, P.J.; van Eeten, E.; Groen, W.B.; Van Deurzen, P.A.; Oosterling, I.J.; Van der Gaag, R.J. Gender and age differences in the core triad of impairments in autism spectrum disorders: A systematic review and meta-analysis. *J. Autism Dev. Disord.* **2014**, *44*, 627–635. [CrossRef]
9. Loomes, R.; Hull, L.; Mandy, W.P.L. What Is the Male-to-Female Ratio in Autism Spectrum Disorder? A Systematic Review and Meta-Analysis. *J. Am. Acad. Child Adolesc. Psychiatry* **2017**, *56*, 466–474. [CrossRef]
10. Rodier, P.M.; Ingram, J.L.; Tisdale, B.; Nelson, S.; Romano, J. Embryological origin for autism: Developmental anomalies of the cranial nerve motor nuclei. *J. Comp. Neurol.* **1996**, *370*, 247–261. [CrossRef]
11. Ornoy, A. Valproic acid in pregnancy: How much are we endangering the embryo and fetus? *Reprod. Toxicol.* **2009**, *28*, 1–10. [CrossRef]
12. Silberstein, S.D. Preventive migraine treatment. *Neurol. Clin.* **2009**, *27*, 429–443. [CrossRef] [PubMed]
13. Post, M.R.; Weiss, S.R. Tolerance to the prophylactic effects of carbamazepine and related mood stabilizers in the treatment of bipolar disorders. *CNS Neurosci.* **2011**, *17*, 649–660. [CrossRef] [PubMed]
14. Williams, G.; King, J.; Cunningham, M.; Stephan, M.; Kerr, B.; Hersh, J.H. Fetal valproate syndrome and autism: Additional evidence of an association. *Dev. Med. Child Neurol.* **2001**, *43*, 202–206. [CrossRef] [PubMed]
15. Wagner, G.C.; Reuhl, K.R.; Cheh, M.; McRae, P.; Halladay, A.K. A New Neurobehavioral Model of Autism in Mice: Pre- and Postnatal Exposure to Sodium Valproate. *J. Autism Dev. Disord.* **2006**, *36*, 779–793. [CrossRef]
16. Bambini-Junior, V.; Rodrigues, L.; Behr, G.A.; Moreira, J.C.F.; Riesgo, R.; Gottfried, C. Animal model of autism induced by prenatal exposure to valproate: Behavioral changes and liver parameters. *Brain Res.* **2011**, *1408*, 8–16. [CrossRef]
17. Kolozsi, E.; MacKenzie, R.; Roullet, F.; Decatanzaro, D.; Foster, J. Prenatal exposure to valproic acid leads to reduced expression of synaptic adhesion molecule neuroligin 3 in mice. *Neuroscience* **2009**, *163*, 1201–1210. [CrossRef]
18. Rodier, P.M.; Ingram, J.L.; Tisdale, B.; Croog, V.J. Linking etiologies in humans and animal models: Studies of autism. *Reprod. Toxicol.* **1997**, *11*, 417–422. [CrossRef]
19. Ingram, J.L.; Peckham, S.M.; Tisdale, B.; Rodier, P.M. Prenatal exposure of rats to valproic acid reproduces the cerebellar anomalies associated with autism. *Neurotoxicol. Teratol.* **2000**, *22*, 319–324. [CrossRef]
20. Nicolini, C.; Fahnestock, M. The valproic acid-induced rodent model of autism. *Exp. Neurol.* **2018**, *299*, 217–227. [CrossRef]
21. Rasalam, A.; Hailey, H.; Williams, J.; Moore, S.; Turnpenny, P.; Lloyd, D.; Dean, J. Characteristics of fetal anticonvulsant syndrome associated autistic disorder. *Dev. Med. Child Neurol.* **2005**, *47*, 551–555. [CrossRef]
22. Jeon, S.J.; Gonzales, E.L.; Mabunga, D.F.N.; Valencia, S.T.; Kim, D.G.; Kim, Y.; Adil, K.J.L.; Shin, D.; Park, D.; Shin, C.Y. Sex-specific Behavioral Features of Rodent Models of Autism Spectrum Disorder. *Exp. Neurobiol.* **2018**, *27*, 321–343. [CrossRef] [PubMed]
23. Ornoy, A.; Weinstein-Fudim, L.; Tfilin, M.; Ergaz, Z.; Yanai, J.; Szyf, M.; Turgeman, G. S-adenosyl methionine prevents ASD like behaviors triggered by early postnatal valproic acid exposure in very young mice. *Neurotoxicol. Teratol.* **2019**, *71*, 64–74. [CrossRef] [PubMed]
24. Schneider, T.; Roman, A.; Basta-Kaim, A.; Kubera, M.; Budziszewska, B.; Schneider, K.; Przewłocki, R. Gender-specific behavioral and immunological alterations in an animal model of autism induced by prenatal exposure to valproic acid. *Psychoneuroendocrinology* **2008**, *33*, 728–740. [CrossRef] [PubMed]
25. Kazlauskas, N.; Seiffe, A.; Campolongo, M.; Zappala, C.; Depino, A.M. Sex-specific effects of prenatal valproic acid exposure on sociability and neuroinflammation: Relevance for susceptibility and resilience in autism. *Psychoneuroendocrinology* **2019**, *110*, 104441. [CrossRef]
26. Sailer, L.; Duclot, F.; Wang, Z.; Kabbaj, M. Consequences of prenatal exposure to valproic acid in the socially monogamous prairie voles. *Sci. Rep.* **2019**, *9*, 2453. [CrossRef]
27. Mabunga, D.F.N.; Gonzales, E.L.T.; Kim, J.-W.; Kim, K.C.; Shin, C.Y. Exploring the Validity of Valproic Acid Animal Model of Autism. *Exp. Neurobiol.* **2015**, *24*, 285–300. [CrossRef]
28. Kataoka, S.; Takuma, K.; Hara, Y.; Maeda, Y.; Ago, Y.; Matsuda, T. Autism-like behaviours with transient histone hyperacetylation in mice treated prenatally with valproic acid. *Int. J. Neuropsychopharmacol.* **2013**, *16*, 91–103. [CrossRef]
29. Choi, C.S.; Gonzales, E.L.; Kim, K.C.; Yang, S.M.; Kim, J.-W.; Mabunga, D.F.; Cheong, J.H.; Han, S.-H.; Bahn, G.H.; Shin, C.Y. The transgenerational inheritance of autism-like phenotypes in mice exposed to valproic acid during pregnancy. *Sci. Rep.* **2016**, *6*, 36250. [CrossRef]

30. Wiśniowiecka-Kowalnik, B.; Nowakowska, B.A. Genetics and epigenetics of autism spectrum disorder-current evidence in the field. *J. Appl. Genet.* **2019**, *60*, 37–47. [CrossRef]
31. Lauber, E.; Filice, F.; Schwaller, B. Prenatal Valproate Exposure Differentially Affects Parvalbumin-Expressing Neurons and Related Circuits in the Cortex and Striatum of Mice. *Front. Mol. Neurosci.* **2016**, *9*, 150. [CrossRef]
32. Hou, Q.; Wang, Y.; Li, Y.; Chen, D.; Yang, F.; Wang, S. A Developmental Study of Abnormal Behaviors and Altered GABAergic Signaling in the VPA-Treated Rat Model of Autism. *Front. Behav. Neurosci.* **2018**, *12*, 182. [CrossRef] [PubMed]
33. Qin, L.; Dai, X.; Yin, Y.; Yin, Y. Valproic acid exposure sequentially activates Wnt and mTOR pathways in rats. *Mol. Cell. Neurosci.* **2016**, *75*, 27–35. [CrossRef] [PubMed]
34. Zhang, R.; Zhou, J.; Ren, J.; Sun, S.; Di, Y.; Wang, H.; An, X.; Zhang, K.; Zhang, J.; Qian, Z.; et al. Transcriptional and splicing dysregulation in the prefrontal cortex in valproic acid rat model of autism. *Reprod. Toxicol.* **2018**, *77*, 53–61. [CrossRef] [PubMed]
35. Kotajima-Murakami, H.; Kobayashi, T.; Kashii, H.; Sato, A.; Hagino, Y.; Tanaka, M.; Nishito, Y.; Takamatsu, Y.; Uchino, S.; Ikeda, K. Effects of rapamycin on social interaction deficits and gene expression in mice exposed to valproic acid in utero. *Mol. Brain* **2019**, *12*, 3. [CrossRef] [PubMed]
36. Hill, D.S.; Cabrera, R.; Schultz, D.W.; Zhu, H.; Lu, W.; Finnell, R.H.; Wlodarczyk, B.J. Autism-Like Behavior and Epigenetic Changes Associated with Autism as Consequences of in UteroExposure to Environmental Pollutants in a Mouse Model. *Behav. Neurol.* **2015**, *2015*, 426263. [CrossRef]
37. Bezgin, G.; Lewis, J.D.; Evans, A.C. Developmental changes of cortical white-gray contrast as predictors of autism diagnosis and severity. *Transl. Psychiatry* **2018**, *8*, 249. [CrossRef]
38. Wang, X.; Guo, J.; Song, Y.; Wang, Q.; Hu, S.; Gou, L.; Gao, Y. Decreased Number and Expression of nNOS-Positive Interneurons in Basolateral Amygdala in Two Mouse Models of Autism. *Front. Cell. Neurosci.* **2018**, *12*, 251. [CrossRef]
39. Rinaldi, T.; Perrodin, C.; Markram, H. Hyper-Connectivity and Hyper-Plasticity in the Medial Prefrontal Cortex in the Valproic Acid Animal Model of Autism. *Front. Neural Circuits* **2008**, *2*, 4. [CrossRef]
40. Otero-Losada, M.E.; Rubio, M.C. Acute changes in 5-HT metabolism after S-adenosyl-L-methionine administration. *Gen. Pharmacol. Vasc. Syst.* **1989**, *20*, 403–406. [CrossRef]
41. Villalobos, M.; De La Cruz, J.P.; Cuerda, M.; Ortiz, P.; Smith-Agreda, J.; De La Cuesta, F.S. Effect of S-adenosyl-l-methionine on rat brain oxidative stress damage in a combined model of permanent focal ischemia and global ischemia-reperfusion. *Brain Res.* **2000**, *883*, 31–40. [CrossRef]
42. Gonzalez-Correa, J.A.; De La Cruz, J.P.; Martin-Aurioles, E.; Lopez-Egea, M.A.; Ortiz, P.; De La Cuesta, F.S.; Gonzalez-Correa, J.A.; Martin-Aurioles, E.; Lopez-Egea, M.A. Effects ofS-adenosyl-L-methionine on hepatic and renal oxidative stress in an experimental model of acute biliary obstruction in rats. *Hepatology* **1997**, *26*, 121–127. [CrossRef] [PubMed]
43. Li, Q.; Cui, J.; Fang, C.; Liu, M.; Min, G.; Li, L. S-Adenosylmethionine Attenuates Oxidative Stress and Neuroinflammation Induced by Amyloid-beta Through Modulation of Glutathione Metabolism. *J. Alzheimers Dis.* **2017**, *58*, 549–558. [CrossRef] [PubMed]
44. Yoon, S.-Y.; Hong, G.H.; Kwon, H.-S.; Park, S.; Park, S.Y.; Shin, B.; Kim, T.-B.; Moon, H.-B.; Cho, Y.S. S-adenosylmethionine reduces airway inflammation and fibrosis in a murine model of chronic severe asthma via suppression of oxidative stress. *Exp. Mol. Med.* **2016**, *48*, e236. [CrossRef] [PubMed]
45. Morrison, L.D.; Smith, D.D.; Kish, S.J. Brain S-adenosylmethionine levels are severely decreased in Alzheimer's disease. *J. Neurochem.* **1996**, *67*, 1328–1331. [CrossRef]
46. Mischoulon, D.; Price, L.H.; Carpenter, L.L.; Tyrka, A.R.; Papakostas, G.I.; Baer, L.; Dording, C.M.; Clain, A.J.; Durham, K.; Walker, R.; et al. A double-blind, randomized, placebo-controlled clinical trial of S-adenosyl-L-methionine (SAMe) versus escitalopram in major depressive disorder. *J. Clin. Psychiatry* **2014**, *75*, 370–376. [CrossRef] [PubMed]
47. Sarris, J.; Murphy, J.; Mischoulon, D.; Papakostas, G.I.; Fava, M.; Berk, M.; Ng, C.H. Adjunctive Nutraceuticals for Depression: A Systematic Review and Meta-Analyses. *Am. J. Psychiatry* **2016**, *173*, 575–587. [CrossRef]
48. Williams, A.-L.; Girard, C.; Jui, D.; Sabina, A.; Katz, D.L. S-adenosylmethionine (SAMe) as treatment for depression: A systematic review. *Clin. Investig. Med.* **2005**, *28*, 132–139.

49. Sharma, A.; Gerbarg, P.; Bottiglieri, T.; Massoumi, L.; Carpenter, L.L.; Lavretsky, H.; Muskin, P.R.; Brown, R.P.; Mischoulon, D. S-Adenosylmethionine (SAMe) for Neuropsychiatric Disorders: A Clinician-Oriented Review of Research. *J. Clin. Psychiatry* **2017**, *78*, e656–e667. [CrossRef]
50. Sarris, J.; Price, L.H.; Carpenter, L.L.; Tyrka, A.R.; Ng, C.H.; Papakostas, G.I.; Jaeger, A.; Fava, M.; Mischoulon, D. Is S-Adenosyl Methionine (SAMe) for Depression Only Effective in Males? A Re-Analysis of Data from a Randomized Clinical Trial. *Pharmacopsychiatry* **2015**, *48*, 141–144. [CrossRef]
51. Ding, W.; Higgins, D.P.; Yadav, D.K.; Godbole, A.A.; Pukkila-Worley, R.; Walker, A.K. Stress-responsive and metabolic gene regulation are altered in low S-adenosylmethionine. *PLoS Genet.* **2018**, *14*, e1007812. [CrossRef]
52. Christensen, D.L.; Baio, J.; Van Naarden Braun, K.; Bilder, D.; Charles, J.; Constantino, J.N.; Daniels, J.; Durkin, M.S.; Fitzgerald, R.T.; Kurzius-Spencer, M.; et al. Prevalence and Characteristics of Autism Spectrum Disorder Among Children Aged 8 Years-Autism and Developmental Disabilities Monitoring Network, 11 Sites, United States, 2012. *MMWR Surveill. Summ.* **2016**, *65*, 1–23. [CrossRef] [PubMed]
53. Cho, H.; Kim, C.H.; Knight, E.Q.; Oh, H.W.; Park, B.; Kim, D.G.; Park, H.-J. Changes in brain metabolic connectivity underlie autistic-like social deficits in a rat model of autism spectrum disorder. *Sci. Rep.* **2017**, *7*, 13213. [CrossRef] [PubMed]
54. Kim, K.C.; Cho, K.S.; Yang, S.M.; Gonzales, E.L.; Valencia, S.; Eun, P.H.; Choi, C.S.; Mabunga, D.F.; Kim, J.-W.; Noh, J.K.; et al. Sex Differences in Autism-Like Behavioral Phenotypes and Postsynaptic Receptors Expression in the Prefrontal Cortex of TERT Transgenic Mice. *Biomol. Ther.* **2017**, *25*, 374–382. [CrossRef] [PubMed]
55. Win-Shwe, T.-T.; Nway, N.C.; Imai, M.; Lwin, T.-T.; Mar, O.; Watanabe, H. Social behavior, neuroimmune markers and glutamic acid decarboxylase levels in a rat model of valproic acid-induced autism. *J. Toxicol. Sci.* **2018**, *43*, 631–643. [CrossRef] [PubMed]
56. Smith, K.E.; Boules, M.; Williams, K.; Richelson, E. NTS1 and NTS2 mediate analgesia following neurotensin analog treatment in a mouse model for visceral pain. *Behav. Brain Res.* **2012**, *232*, 93–97. [CrossRef] [PubMed]
57. Merullo, D.P.; Cordes, M.A.; Devries, M.S.; Stevenson, S.A.; Riters, L.V. Neurotensin neural mRNA expression correlates with vocal communication and other highly-motivated social behaviors in male European starlings. *Physiol. Behav.* **2015**, *151*, 155–161. [CrossRef]
58. Gammie, S.C.; D'Anna, K.L.; Gerstein, H.; Stevenson, S.A. Neurotensin inversely modulates maternal aggression. *Neuroscience* **2009**, *158*, 1215–1223. [CrossRef]
59. Fitzpatrick, K.; Winrow, C.J.; Gotter, A.L.; Millstein, J.; Arbuzova, J.; Brunner, J.; Kasarskis, A.; Vitaterna, M.H.; Renger, J.J.; Turek, F.W. Altered Sleep and Affect in the Neurotensin Receptor 1 Knockout Mouse. *Sleep* **2012**, *35*, 949–956. [CrossRef]
60. Levitas-Djerbi, T.; Sagi, D.; Lebenthal-Loinger, I.; Lerer-Goldshtein, T.; Appelbaum, L. Neurotensin Enhances Locomotor Activity and Arousal, and Inhibits Melanin-Concentrating Hormone Signalings. *Neuroendocrinology* **2019**, in press. [CrossRef]
61. Cáceda, R.; Kinkead, B.; Nemeroff, C.B. Neurotensin: Role in psychiatric and neurological diseases. *Peptides* **2006**, *27*, 2385–2404. [CrossRef]
62. Shilling, P.D.; Feifel, D. The neurotensin-1 receptor agonist PD149163 blocks fear-potentiated startle. *Pharmacol. Biochem. Behav.* **2008**, *90*, 748–752. [CrossRef] [PubMed]
63. Cervo, L.; Rossi, C.; Tatarczyńska, E.; Samanin, R. Antidepressant-like effect of neurotensin administered in the ventral tegmental area in the forced swimming test. *Psychopharmacology* **1992**, *109*, 369–372. [CrossRef] [PubMed]
64. Binder, E.B.; Kinkead, B.; Owens, M.J.; Nemeroff, C.B. Neurotensin and dopamine interactions. *Pharmacol. Rev.* **2001**, *53*, 453–486. [PubMed]
65. Dobner, P.R. Multitasking with neurotensin in the central nervous system. *Cell. Mol. Life Sci.* **2005**, *62*, 1946–1963. [CrossRef] [PubMed]
66. Yin, H.H.; Adermark, L.; Lovinger, D.M. Neurotensin reduces glutamatergic transmission in the dorsolateral striatum via retrograde endocannabinoid signaling. *Neuropharmacology* **2008**, *54*, 79–86. [CrossRef]
67. Kadiri, N.; Rodeau, J.L.; Schlichter, R.; Hugel, S. Neurotensin inhibits background K+ channels and facilitates glutamatergic transmission in rat spinal cord dorsal horn. *Eur. J. Neurosci.* **2011**, *34*, 1230–1240. [CrossRef]
68. Ferraro, L.; Tomasini, M.C.; Mazza, R.; Fuxe, K.; Fournier, J.; Tanganelli, S.; Antonelli, T. Neurotensin receptors as modulators of glutamatergic transmission. *Brain Res. Rev.* **2008**, *58*, 365–373. [CrossRef]

69. Rakovska, A.; Giovannini, M.; Corte, L.; Kalfin, R.; Bianchi, L.; Pepeu, G. Neurotensin modulation of acetylcholine and gaba release from the rat hippocampus: An in vivo microdialysis study. *Neurochem. Int.* **1998**, *33*, 335–340. [CrossRef]
70. Petkova-Kirova, P.; Rakovska, A.; Della Corte, L.; Zaekova, G.; Radomirov, R.; Mayer, A. Neurotensin modulation of acetylcholine, GABA, and aspartate release from rat prefrontal cortex studied in vivo with microdialysis. *Brain Res. Bull.* **2008**, *77*, 129–135. [CrossRef]
71. Petrie, K.A.; Schmidt, D.; Bubser, M.; Fadel, J.; Carraway, R.E.; Deutch, A.Y. Neurotensin Activates GABAergic Interneurons in the Prefrontal Cortex. *J. Neurosci.* **2005**, *25*, 1629–1636. [CrossRef]
72. Vincent, J.-P.; Mazella, J.; Kitabgi, P. Neurotensin and neurotensin receptors. *Trends Pharmacol. Sci.* **1999**, *20*, 302–309. [CrossRef]
73. Martin, S.; Vincent, J.-P.; Mazella, J. Involvement of the Neurotensin Receptor-3 in the Neurotensin-Induced Migration of Human Microglia. *J. Neurosci.* **2003**, *23*, 1198–1205. [CrossRef] [PubMed]
74. Vadnie, C.A.; Hinton, D.J.; Choi, S.; Choi, Y.; Ruby, C.L.; Oliveros, A.; Prieto, M.L.; Park, J.H.; Choi, D.-S. Activation of neurotensin receptor type 1 attenuates locomotor activity. *Neuropharmacology* **2014**, *85*, 482–492. [CrossRef] [PubMed]
75. Keiser, A.A.; Matazel, K.S.; Esser, M.K.; Feifel, D.; Prus, A.J. Systemic administration of the neurotensin NTS-receptor agonist PD149163 improves performance on a memory task in naturally deficient male brown Norway rats. *Exp. Clin. Psychopharmacol.* **2014**, *22*, 541–547. [CrossRef] [PubMed]
76. Angelidou, A.; Francis, K.; Vasiadi, M.; Alysandratos, K.-D.; Zhang, B.; Theoharides, A.; Lykouras, L.; Sideri, K.; Kalogeromitros, D.; Theoharides, T.C. Neurotensin is increased in serum of young children with autistic disorder. *J. Neuroinflamm.* **2010**, *7*, 48. [CrossRef]
77. Tsilioni, I.; Dodman, N.; Petra, A.I.; Taliou, A.; Francis, K.; Moon-Fanelli, A.; Shuster, L.; Theoharides, T.C. Elevated serum neurotensin and CRH levels in children with autistic spectrum disorders and tail-chasing Bull Terriers with a phenotype similar to autism. *Transl. Psychiatry* **2014**, *4*, e466. [CrossRef]
78. Patel, A.B.; Tsilioni, I.; Leeman, S.E.; Theoharides, T.C. Neurotensin stimulates sortilin and mTOR in human microglia inhibitable by methoxyluteolin, a potential therapeutic target for autism. *Proc. Natl. Acad. Sci. USA* **2016**, *113*, E7049–E7058. [CrossRef]
79. Ghanizadeh, A. Targeting neurotensin as a potential novel approach for the treatment of autism. *J. Neuroinflamm.* **2010**, *7*, 58. [CrossRef]
80. Kirsten, T.B.; Casarin, R.C.; Bernardi, M.M.; Felicio, L.F. Pioglitazone abolishes autistic-like behaviors via the IL-6 pathway. *PLoS ONE* **2018**, *13*, e0197060. [CrossRef]
81. Kirsten, T.B.; Casarin, R.C.; Bernardi, M.M.; Felicio, L.F. Pioglitazone abolishes cognition impairments as well as BDNF and neurotensin disturbances in a rat model of autism. *Biol. Open* **2019**, *8*, bio041327. [CrossRef]
82. Normandeau, C.P.; Ventura-Silva, A.P.; Hawken, E.R.; Angelis, S.; Sjaarda, C.; Liu, X.; Pego, J.M.; Dumont, E.C. A Key Role for Neurotensin in Chronic-Stress-Induced Anxiety-Like Behavior in Rats. *Neuropsychopharmacology* **2018**, *43*, 285–293. [CrossRef] [PubMed]
83. Lipstein, N.; Verhoeven-Duif, N.M.; Michelassi, F.E.; Calloway, N.; Van Hasselt, P.M.; Pienkowska, K.; Van Haaften, G.; Van Haelst, M.M.; Van Empelen, R.; Cuppen, I.; et al. Synaptic UNC13A protein variant causes increased neurotransmission and dyskinetic movement disorder. *J. Clin. Investig.* **2017**, *127*, 1005–1018. [CrossRef] [PubMed]
84. Damaj, L.; Lupien-Meilleur, A.; Lortie, A.; Riou, E.; Ospina, L.H.; Gagnon, L.; Vanasse, C.; Rossignol, E. CACNA1A haploinsufficiency causes cognitive impairment, autism and epileptic encephalopathy with mild cerebellar symptoms. *Eur. J. Hum. Genet.* **2015**, *23*, 1505–1512. [CrossRef] [PubMed]
85. Lee, P.H.; Perlis, R.H.; Jung, J.-Y.; Byrne, E.M.; Rueckert, E.; Siburian, R.; Haddad, S.; Mayerfeld, C.E.; Heath, A.C.; Pergadia, M.L.; et al. Multi-locus genome-wide association analysis supports the role of glutamatergic synaptic transmission in the etiology of major depressive disorder. *Transl. Psychiatry* **2012**, *2*, e184. [CrossRef] [PubMed]
86. Horder, J.; Lavender, T.; Mendez, M.A.; O'Gorman, R.; Daly, E.; Craig, M.C.; Lythgoe, D.J.; Barker, G.J.; Murphy, D.G. Reduced subcortical glutamate/glutamine in adults with autism spectrum disorders: A [H] MRS study. *Transl. Psychiatry* **2013**, *3*, e279. [CrossRef]
87. Bernardi, S.; Anagnostou, E.; Shen, J.; Kolevzon, A.; Buxbaum, J.D.; Hollander, E.; Hof, P.R.; Fan, J. In vivo 1H-magnetic resonance spectroscopy study of the attentional networks in autism. *Brain Res.* **2011**, *1380*, 198–205. [CrossRef]

88. Page, L.A.; Daly, E.; Schmitz, N.; Simmons, A.; Toal, F.; Deeley, Q.; Ambery, F.; McAlonan, G.M.; Murphy, K.C.; Murphy, D.G.M. In Vivo 1 H-Magnetic Resonance Spectroscopy Study of Amygdala-Hippocampal and Parietal Regions in Autism. *Am. J. Psychiatry* **2006**, *163*, 2189–2192. [CrossRef]
89. Wickens, M.M.; Bangasser, D.A.; Briand, L.A. Sex Differences in Psychiatric Disease: A Focus on the Glutamate System. *Front. Mol. Neurosci.* **2018**, *11*, 197. [CrossRef]
90. Plavén-Sigray, P.; Gustavsson, P.; Farde, L.; Borg, J.; Stenkrona, P.; Nyberg, L.; Bäckman, L.; Červenka, S. Dopamine D1 receptor availability is related to social behavior: A positron emission tomography study. *NeuroImage* **2014**, *102*, 590–595. [CrossRef]
91. Homberg, J.R.; Olivier, J.D.A.; VandenBroeke, M.; Youn, J.; Ellenbroek, A.K.; Karel, P.; Shan, L.; Van Boxtel, R.; Ooms, S.; Balemans, M.; et al. The role of the dopamine D1 receptor in social cognition: Studies using a novel genetic rat model. *Dis. Model. Mech.* **2016**, *9*, 1147–1158. [CrossRef]
92. Canals, M.; Marcellino, D.; Fanelli, F.; Ciruela, F.; de Benedetti, P.; Goldberg, S.R.; Neve, K.; Fuxe, K.; Agnati, L.F.; Woods, A.S.; et al. Adenosine A2A-dopamine D2 receptor-receptor heteromerization: Qualitative and quantitative assessment by fluorescence and bioluminescence energy transfer. *J. Biol. Chem.* **2003**, *278*, 46741–46749. [CrossRef] [PubMed]
93. Collins, A.G.E.; Frank, M.J. Opponent actor learning (OpAL): Modeling interactive effects of striatal dopamine on reinforcement learning and choice incentive. *Psychol. Rev.* **2014**, *121*, 337–366. [CrossRef] [PubMed]
94. Vorstman, J.A.; Morcus, M.E.; Duijff, S.N.; Klaassen, P.W.; Heineman-de Boer, J.A.; Beemer, F.A.; Swaab, H.; Kahn, R.S.; van Engeland, H. The 22q11.2 deletion in children: High rate of autistic disorders and early onset of psychotic symptoms. *J. Am. Acad. Child Adolesc. Psychiatry* **2006**, *45*, 1104–1113. [CrossRef] [PubMed]
95. Deckert, J.; Rietschel, M.; Wildenauer, D.; Bondy, B.; Ertl, M.A.; Knapp, M.; Schofield, P.R.; Albus, M.; Maier, W.; Propping, P. Human adenosine A2a receptor (A2aAR) gene: Systematic mutation screening in patients with schizophrenia. *J. Neural Transm.* **1996**, *103*, 1447–1455. [CrossRef] [PubMed]
96. Hong, C.-J.; Liu, H.-C.; Liu, T.-Y.; Liao, D.-L.; Tsai, S.-J. Association studies of the adenosine A2a receptor (1976T > C) genetic polymorphism in Parkinson's disease and schizophrenia. *J. Neural Transm.* **2005**, *112*, 1503–1510. [CrossRef] [PubMed]
97. Hohoff, C.; Mullings, E.L.; Heatherley, S.V.; Freitag, C.M.; Neumann, L.C.; Domschke, K.; Krakowitzky, P.; Rothermundt, M.; Keck, M.E.; Erhardt, A.; et al. Adenosine A2A receptor gene: Evidence for association of risk variants with panic disorder and anxious personality. *J. Psychiatr. Res.* **2010**, *44*, 930–937. [CrossRef]
98. Freitag, C.M.; Agelopoulos, K.; Huy, E.; Rothermundt, M.; Krakowitzky, P.; Meyer, J.; Deckert, J.; von Gontard, A.; Hohoff, C. Adenosine A (2A) receptor gene (ADORA2A) variants may increase autistic symptoms and anxiety in autism spectrum disorder. *Eur. Child Adolesc. Psychiatry* **2010**, *19*, 67–74. [CrossRef]
99. Squillace, M.; Dodero, L.; Federici, M.; Migliarini, S.; Errico, F.; Napolitano, F.; Krashia, P.; Di Maio, A.; Galbusera, A.; Bifone, A.; et al. Dysfunctional dopaminergic neurotransmission in asocial BTBR mice. *Transl. Psychiatry* **2014**, *4*, e427. [CrossRef]
100. Traynelis, S.F.; Wollmuth, L.P.; McBain, C.J.; Menniti, F.S.; Vance, K.M.; Ogden, K.K.; Hansen, K.B.; Yuan, H.; Myers, S.J.; Dingledine, R. Glutamate receptor ion channels: Structure, regulation, and function. *Pharmacol. Rev.* **2010**, *62*, 405–496. [CrossRef]
101. Chen, X.S.; Reader, R.H.; Hoischen, A.; Veltman, J.A.; Simpson, N.H.; Francks, C.; Newbury, D.F.; Fisher, S.E. Next-generation DNA sequencing identifies novel gene variants and pathways involved in specific language impairment. *Sci. Rep.* **2017**, *7*, 46105. [CrossRef]
102. Gao, K.; Tankovic, A.; Zhang, Y.; Kusumoto, H.; Zhang, J.; Chen, W.; Xiangwei, W.; Shaulsky, G.H.; Hu, C.; Traynelis, S.F.; et al. A de novo loss-of-function GRIN2A mutation associated with childhood focal epilepsy and acquired epileptic aphasia. *PLoS ONE* **2017**, *12*, e0170818. [CrossRef] [PubMed]
103. Goswami, D.B.; Jernigan, C.S.; Chandran, A.; Iyo, A.H.; May, W.L.; Austin, M.C.; Stockmeier, C.A.; Karolewicz, B. Gene expression analysis of novel genes in the prefrontal cortex of major depressive disorder subjects. *Prog. Neuropsychopharmacol. Biol. Psychiatry* **2013**, *43*, 126–133. [CrossRef]
104. Kaut, O.; Schmitt, I.; Hofmann, A.; Hoffmann, P.; Schlaepfer, T.E.; Wüllner, U.; Hurlemann, R. Aberrant NMDA receptor DNA methylation detected by epigenome-wide analysis of hippocampus and prefrontal cortex in major depression. *Eur. Arch. Psychiatry Clin. Neurosci.* **2015**, *265*, 331–341. [CrossRef] [PubMed]
105. Lee, H.K.; Chauhan, S.K.; Kay, E.; Dana, R. Flt-1 regulates vascular endothelial cell migration via a protein tyrosine kinase-7–dependent pathway. *Blood* **2011**, *117*, 5762–5771. [CrossRef] [PubMed]

106. Shibuya, M. Differential roles of vascular endothelial growth factor receptor-1 and receptor-2 in angiogenesis. *J. Biochem. Mol. Biol.* **2006**, *39*, 469–478. [CrossRef]
107. Mahoney, E.R.; Dumitrescu, L.; Moore, A.M.; Cambronero, F.E.; De Jager, P.L.; Koran, M.E.I.; Petyuk, V.A.; Robinson, R.A.S.; Goyal, S.; Schneider, J.A.; et al. Brain expression of the vascular endothelial growth factor gene family in cognitive aging and alzheimer's disease. *Mol. Psychiatry* **2019**, in press. [CrossRef]
108. Hu, V.W.; Frank, B.C.; Heine, S.; Lee, N.H.; Quackenbush, J. Gene expression profiling of lymphoblastoid cell lines from monozygotic twins discordant in severity of autism reveals differential regulation of neurologically relevant genes. *BMC Genom.* **2006**, *7*, 118.
109. Maurer, S.V.; Williams, C.L. The Cholinergic System Modulates Memory and Hippocampal Plasticity via Its Interactions with Non-Neuronal Cells. *Front. Immunol.* **2017**, *8*, 1489. [CrossRef]
110. Ballinger, E.C.; Ananth, M.; Talmage, D.A.; Role, L.W. Basal Forebrain Cholinergic Circuits and Signaling in Cognition and Cognitive Decline. *Neuron* **2016**, *91*, 1199–1218. [CrossRef]
111. Drenan, R.M.; Grady, S.R.; Steele, A.D.; McKinney, S.; Patzlaff, N.E.; McIntosh, J.M.; Marks, M.J.; Miwa, J.M.; Lester, H.A. Cholinergic modulation of locomotion and striatal dopamine release is mediated by alpha6alpha4* nicotinic acetylcholine receptors. *J. Neurosci.* **2010**, *30*, 9877–9889. [CrossRef]
112. Sarter, M.; Lustig, C.; Taylor, S.F. Cholinergic contributions to the cognitive symptoms of schizophrenia and the viability of cholinergic treatments. *Neuropharmacology* **2012**, *62*, 1544–1553. [CrossRef] [PubMed]
113. Hardan, A.Y.; Handen, B.L. A Retrospective Open Trial of Adjunctive Donepezil in Children and Adolescents with Autistic Disorder. *J. Child Adolesc. Psychopharmacol.* **2002**, *12*, 237–241. [CrossRef] [PubMed]
114. Wang, L.; Almeida, L.E.F.; Spornick, N.A.; Kenyon, N.; Kamimura, S.; Khaibullina, A.; Nouraie, M.; Quezado, Z.M.N. Modulation of social deficits and repetitive behaviors in a mouse model of autism: The role of the nicotinic cholinergic system. *Psychopharmacology* **2015**, *232*, 4303–4316. [CrossRef] [PubMed]
115. Lee, M.; Martin-Ruiz, C.; Graham, A.; Court, J.; Jaros, E.; Perry, R.; Iversen, P.; Bauman, M.; Perry, E. Nicotinic receptor abnormalities in the cerebellar cortex in autism. *Brain* **2002**, *125*, 1483–1495. [CrossRef]
116. Perry, E.K.; Lee, M.L.; Martin-Ruiz, C.M.; Court, J.A.; Volsen, S.G.; Merrit, J.; Folly, E.; Iversen, P.E.; Bauman, M.L.; Perry, R.H.; et al. Cholinergic Activity in Autism: Abnormalities in the Cerebral Cortex and Basal Forebrain. *Am. J. Psychiatry* **2001**, *158*, 1058–1066. [CrossRef]
117. Han, S.; Yang, S.H.; Kim, J.Y.; Mo, S.; Yang, E.; Song, K.M.; Ham, B.-J.; Mechawar, N.; Turecki, G.; Lee, H.W.; et al. Author Correction: Down-regulation of cholinergic signaling in the habenula induces anhedonia-like behavior. *Sci. Rep.* **2017**, *7*, 17090. [CrossRef]
118. Bierer, L.M.; Haroutunian, V.; Gabriel, S.; Knott, P.J.; Carlin, L.S.; Purohit, D.P.; Perl, D.P.; Schmeidler, J.; Kanof, P.; Davis, K.L. Neurochemical correlates of dementia severity in Alzheimer's disease: Relative importance of the cholinergic deficits. *J. Neurochem.* **1995**, *64*, 749–760. [CrossRef]
119. Giannini, G.; Conti, A.; Mammarella, S.; Scrobogna, M.; Sorrentino, V. The ryanodine receptor/calcium channel genes are widely and differentially expressed in murine brain and peripheral tissues. *J. Cell Boil.* **1995**, *128*, 893–904. [CrossRef]
120. Galeotti, N.; Quattrone, A.; Vivoli, E.; Norcini, M.; Bartolini, A.; Ghelardini, C. Different involvement of type 1, 2, and 3 ryanodine receptors in memory processes. *Learn. Mem.* **2008**, *15*, 315–323. [CrossRef]
121. Hernandez-Ochoa, E.O.; Pratt, S.J.P.; Lovering, R.M.; Schneider, M.F. Critical Role of Intracellular RyR1 Calcium Release Channels in Skeletal Muscle Function and Disease. *Front. Physiol.* **2015**, *6*, 420. [CrossRef]
122. Kulkarni, M.M. Digital multiplexed gene expression analysis using the NanoString nCounter system. *Curr. Protoc. Mol. Biol.* **2011**. [CrossRef]
123. da Huang, W.; Sherman, B.T.; Lempicki, R.A. Bioinformatics enrichment tools: Paths toward the comprehensive functional analysis of large gene lists. *Nucleic Acids Res.* **2009**, *37*, 1–13. [CrossRef] [PubMed]
124. Salman, M.M.; Sheilabi, M.A.; Bhattacharyya, D.; Kitchen, P.; Conner, A.C.; Bill, R.M.; Woodroofe, M.N.; Conner, M.T.; Princivalle, A.P. Transcriptome analysis suggests a role for the differential expression of cerebral aquaporins and the MAPK signalling pathway in human temporal lobe epilepsy. *Eur. J. Neurosci.* **2017**, *46*, 2121–2132. [CrossRef] [PubMed]
125. Salman, M.M.; Kitchen, P.; Woodroofe, M.N.; Bill, R.M.; Conner, A.C.; Heath, P.R.; Conner, M.T. Transcriptome Analysis of Gene Expression Provides New Insights into the Effect of Mild Therapeutic Hypothermia on Primary Human Cortical Astrocytes Cultured under Hypoxia. *Front. Cell. Neurosci.* **2017**, *11*, 386. [CrossRef]
126. Love, M.I.; Huber, W.; Anders, S. Moderated estimation of fold change and dispersion for RNA-seq data with DESeq2. *Genome Boil.* **2014**, *15*, 550. [CrossRef]

127. Kim, S.T.; Do, I.G.; Lee, J.; Sohn, I.; Kim, K.M.; Kang, W.K. The NanoString-based multigene assay as a novel platform to screen EGFR, HER2, and MET in patients with advanced gastric cancer. *Clin. Transl. Oncol.* **2015**, *17*, 462–468. [CrossRef]
128. Leal, L.F.; Evangelista, A.F.; De Paula, F.E.; Almeida, G.C.; Carloni, A.C.; Saggioro, F.; Stavale, J.N.; Malheiros, S.M.; Mançano, B.; De Oliveira, M.A.; et al. Reproducibility of the NanoString 22-gene molecular subgroup assay for improved prognostic prediction of medulloblastoma. *Neuropathology* **2018**, *38*, 475–483. [CrossRef]
129. Łastowska, M.; Trubicka, J.; Niemira, M.; Paczkowska-Abdulsalam, M.; Karkucińska-Więckowska, A.; Kaleta, M.; Drogosiewicz, M.; Perek-Polnik, M.; Kretowski, A.; Cukrowska, B.; et al. Medulloblastoma with transitional features between Group 3 and Group 4 is associated with good prognosis. *J. Neuro-Oncol.* **2018**, *138*, 231–240. [CrossRef]
130. Zapka, P.; Dorner, E.; Dreschmann, V.; Sakamato, N.; Kristiansen, G.; Calaminus, G.; Vokuhl, C.; Leuschner, I.; Pietsch, T. Type, Frequency, and Spatial Distribution of Immune Cell Infiltrates in CNS Germinomas: Evidence for Inflammatory and Immunosuppressive Mechanisms. *J. Neuropathol. Exp. Neurol.* **2018**, *77*, 119–127. [CrossRef]
131. Solomon, I.H.; De Girolami, U.; Chettimada, S.; Misra, V.; Singer, E.J.; Gabuzda, D. Brain and liver pathology, amyloid deposition, and interferon responses among older HIV-positive patients in the late HAART era. *BMC Infect. Dis.* **2017**, *17*, 151. [CrossRef]
132. Prokopec, S.D.; Watson, J.D.; Waggott, D.M.; Smith, A.B.; Wu, A.H.; Okey, A.B.; Pohjanvirta, R.; Boutros, P.C. Systematic evaluation of medium-throughput mRNA abundance platforms. *RNA* **2013**, *19*, 51–62. [CrossRef] [PubMed]
133. Oldridge, N.B.; Streiner, D.L. The health belief model: Predicting compliance and dropout in cardiac rehabilitation. *Med. Sci. Sports Exerc.* **1990**, *22*, 678–683. [CrossRef] [PubMed]

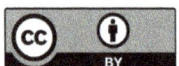

© 2019 by the authors. Licensee MDPI, Basel, Switzerland. This article is an open access article distributed under the terms and conditions of the Creative Commons Attribution (CC BY) license (http://creativecommons.org/licenses/by/4.0/).

MDPI
St. Alban-Anlage 66
4052 Basel
Switzerland
Tel. +41 61 683 77 34
Fax +41 61 302 89 18
www.mdpi.com

International Journal of Molecular Sciences Editorial Office
E-mail: ijms@mdpi.com
www.mdpi.com/journal/ijms